Cambridge History of Medicine

EDITORS: CHARLES WEBSTER AND CHARLES ROSENBERG

Hospital life in Enlightenment Scotland

Hospital life
in Enlightenment Scotland

CARE AND TEACHING AT THE
ROYAL INFIRMARY OF EDINBURGH

GUENTER B. RISSE
University of Wisconsin

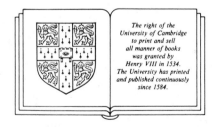

The right of the
University of Cambridge
to print and sell
all manner of books
was granted by
Henry VIII in 1534.
The University has printed
and published continuously
since 1584.

CAMBRIDGE UNIVERSITY PRESS

CAMBRIDGE

LONDON   NEW YORK   NEW ROCHELLE

MELBOURNE   SYDNEY

Published by the Press Syndicate of the University of Cambridge
The Pitt Building, Trumpington Street, Cambridge CB2 1RP
32 East 57th Street, New York, NY 10022, USA
10 Stamford Road, Oakleigh, Melbourne 3166, Australia

First published 1986

Printed in the United States of America

Library of Congress Cataloging in Publication Data
Risse, Guenter B., 1932–
Hospital life in enlightenment Scotland.
(Cambridge history of medicine)
Bibliography: p.
Includes index.
1. Royal Infirmary of Edinburgh – History.
2. Hospitals – Scotland – Edinburgh (Lothian) – History –
18th century.   3. Poor – Hospital care – Scotland –
Edinburgh (Lothian) – History – 18th century.
4. Scotland – History – 18th century.   I. Title.
II. Series.   [DNLM: 1. Royal Infirmary of Edinburgh.
2. Health Services – history – Scotland.   3. Hospitals –
history – Scotland.   4. Hospitals, Teaching – history –
Scotland. WX 28 FS2 R5h]
RA988.E4R67   1986   362.1′1′094134   85-16614

British Library Cataloguing in Publication Data
Risse, Guenter, B.
Hospial life in Enlightenment Scotland : care
and teaching at the Royal Infirmary of Edinburgh
– (Cambridge history of medicine)
1. Royal Infirmary of Edinburgh – History
I. Title
362.1′1′094134   RA988.E4R6
ISBN 0 521 30518 7

To my parents

Contents

List of tables and figures

FIGURES

Acknowledgments

Most of the research for this book was carried out in Edinburgh, Scotland. For their help and gracious hospitality I would first like to thank Joan P. S. Ferguson, Librarian, Royal College of Physicians, Edinburgh. Miss Ferguson not only guided me through the college's rich manuscript collection but ordered microfilms of the student notebooks and lecture notes and patiently answered subsequent queries. My gratitude also extends to Dr. J. T. Hall, Sub-librarian, Special Collections, Edinburgh University Library, and his assistant, Marjorie Robertson, as well as to Dorothy H. Wardle, Librarian, Royal College of Surgeons, Edinburgh, and Walter H. Mackey, City Archivist, Department of Administration, City of Edinburgh District Council. I am likewise indebted to Pat Strong, Permanent Secretary, the Royal Medical Society of Edinburgh, and the staffs at the Scottish Record Office, National Library of Scotland, and Edinburgh Room, Edinburgh City Library. A special note of thanks must go to Rosemary M. Gibson, successor to the late P. M. Eaves Walton as Archivist in the Medical Archive Center of the University of Edinburgh. She generously shared her expertise and allowed the microfilming of folios belonging to the infirmary's General Register of Patients. To the staff of the Wellcome History of Medicine and Science Unit, Department of History, University of Edinburgh, my appreciation for all the courtesies extended to me during my last research trip of 1982.

On the other side of the Atlantic I would like to thank Dorothy T. Hanks, Reference Librarian, History of Medicine Division, National Library of Medicine, Bethesda, MD, and Richard J. Wolfe, Curator of Rare Books and Manuscripts, Boston Medical Library, for their help in locating further student casebooks. I am grateful to Blanche L. Singer, interlibrary loan librarian at the W. S. Middleton Health Sciences Library, University of Wisconsin, for getting much of this material to me. A number of graduate students working for the University of Wisconsin Department of the History of Medicine helped to sift the numerous entries of the General Register of Patients, especially Roy J. DeCarvalho, Rennie Schoepflin, and Kathryn Holtgraver. To William J. Raynor from the Computer Sciences Department at the University of Wisconsin goes my appreciation for introducing me to the world of codes and computers.

Several colleagues took particular interest in my project and deserve special thanks. Foremost among them is Stephanie Blackden, then a postdoctoral research fellow at the History of Medicine and Science Unit in Edinburgh, who repeatedly checked patients' lists, microfilmed documents, and generously shared her expertise in Scottish history. Useful suggestions came from David Hamilton, Helen Brock, William B. Howie, and Haldane P. Tait. Nearer to home I am indebted to Glenn Sonnedecker, John Parascandola, and J. Worth Estes for their valuable advice regarding eighteenth-century pharmacy and prescription routines. My thanks also to Toby Gelfand, who read the chapter on medical education, and Ann G. Carmichael, who viewed early drafts of the chapters concerned with diseases and medical practice. Particular thanks go to the Program Committee of the American Association for the History of Medicine responsible for organizing the fifty-third annual meeting in Boston and selecting my paper on Edinburgh hospital practice. Favorable responses to my presentation provided the necessary impetus to pursue further research and conceive of an entire book devoted to the subject. I would also like to thank Charles Rosenberg, who not only encouraged me to complete the project but also promptly read my first draft and made valuable suggestions to improve the manuscript.

I would like to acknowledge the assistance of both the University of Wisconsin Medical School and the American Philosophical Society for granting me two research awards that made travel to Edinburgh possible in 1977 and again in 1982. To Lloyd G. Stevenson, Lester S. King, Rosemary Stevens, and William Coleman I extend my appreciation for supporting the project and recommending me for the latter awards. Carolyn F. Hackler flawlessly typed the entire manuscript, successfully deciphering my handwritten notes and instructions. Her devotion to the project and numberless hours in front of the word processor were key ingredients in rendering the text into its final form.

Last but not least I want to express deep gratitude to my family for putting up with my absences during long hours of research, computations, and writing. Without their encouragement this book would probably never have been completed.

Madison, Wisconsin

Introduction

In contemporary society university-affiliated hospitals play a central role in the progress of medicine. They are often vast bureaucratic enterprises attempting to balance the needs of patient care with those of professional education, all within the context and resources of the society that they have pledged to serve. At the same time, modern university hospitals are poised at the cutting edge of advances in the medical sciences, decisively contributing to the design and performance of clinical research. Thus, as convergent points of science, education, and practice, these establishments usually confer distinction on the institutions of higher learning to which they are linked and high professional status on their teachers, while attracting hopeful patients to the wards from near and far. Because of their importance, university hospitals are not only local architectural landmarks noted on maps or depicted on postcards but also sources of convenient employment and civic pride.[1]

Quite similar characteristics can be noted for the hospital that constitutes the focal point of this study: the Royal Infirmary of Edinburgh. As will be seen, its inception in 1729 and its subsequent development were the culmination of years of fund-raising by several groups with differing interests and agendas. British infirmaries were part of a comprehensive program to institutionalize the poor under the banner of a vigorous philanthropic movement fueled by religious and humanistic concerns. Whatever the expense involved, erecting such hospitals also seemed to make economic sense to eighteenth-century leaders, who believed that medical efforts could restore sizable numbers of workers to their previous health and productivity, thereby decreasing welfare costs and even expanding the population. Leading physicians and surgeons, in turn, recognized the usefulness of such hospitals for the clinical instruction of future health professionals.[2]

The development of both the Royal Infirmary and the Edinburgh Medical School owes a great deal to the scientific and educational ideas adopted by the Scottish Enlightenment. In less than a century after the Union of 1707 with England, Scotland underwent a dramatic transformation from a poor, backward country into a prosperous British province. At the same time, Edinburgh, no longer the seat of royalty, became known as the "Athens of the North," the hub of a remarkable social and cultural development. With broad participation of aristocrats, literati, philosophers, lawyers, and medical men, Edinburgh played a leading role in the formulation of a new Scottish ideology of self-improvement.[3]

Medicine played an important role within the framework of ideas guiding the Scottish Enlightenment. Medical men actively participated in the educational program launched in the 1720s that was designed to provide useful knowledge to Scottish citizens. In fact, after 1750 the University of Edinburgh became a prominent international center of medical learning, a mecca not only for industrious Scots but also for English students, especially those barred from Oxford and Cambridge for religious reasons. In addition, foreigners eagerly flocked to Edinburgh for the purpose of attending medical lectures, arriving from other European countries and America with their letters of introduction.[4]

From its inception, the Edinburgh infirmary became meshed into this educational program. Its wards provided not only opportunities for the observation of individuals afflicted with diseases common to Scotland but occasions to watch and learn from those entrusted with the care of the sick. Beginning in 1732, discussion, analysis, and publication of individual clinical cases seen in the hospital contributed to the practical training of the medical profession.[5] Thus, from the very beginning, the infirmary took its place among Edinburgh's institutions devoted to educational pursuits, a group that also included the university and several learned societies.[6]

In spite of its modest size, the hospital in time became an important factor in the success of medical education at Edinburgh. As the medical faculty expanded after mid-century and the number of matriculating students rose dramatically, the infirmary furnished the locus for an organized clinical teaching program that combined bedside instruction with systematic lectures and that had few peers in Europe. In 1748 the hospital began to sponsor a course of clinical lectures under university auspices, devoted to the formal discussion of important infirmary cases and given by the most prestigious Edinburgh professors.[7]

Besides participating in the training of future medical professionals, the Edinburgh infirmary also responded to the economic improvement plans of the Scottish Enlightenment. One of the ostensible reasons given for its creation was the idea that providing hospital care for the working poor would be financially advantageous both to them and to society at large. Helping patients recover in an institutional setting such as the infirmary would decrease the impact of sickness on their lives and those of their dependents. If cures could be achieved, the poor would presumably return to productive jobs and thus avoid becoming public burdens. Such purely economic considerations, widely held in Britain and elsewhere as part of the mercantilist doctrine, were closely linked to questions of public welfare.

Edinburgh's governing class also strongly adhered to the humanitarian precepts of the Enlightenment; they demonstrated through their sponsorship of the infirmary their sense of responsibility for protecting the lower ranks of society.[8]

Another consideration with strong economic implications was the flow of Scottish students and their money to England and other European countries for the completion of medical studies. Copying the Dutch model of a hospital-based clinical instruction, the founders of the Edinburgh infirmary made such studies available locally, eventually setting up (in 1750) an independent teaching ward to be directed by a university professor during the academic year. As more foreign students came to study in Edinburgh during the 1770s and 1780s, this unit was increased in size, and hospital revenues obtained from the sale of admission tickets to the students helped pay a substantial portion of the infirmary's operating expenses.

During the second half of the eighteenth century, the Edinburgh infirmary therefore became part of the city's network of influence, patronage, and power. Appointments to its governing board and medical staff conferred prestige and furthered social and professional status. Among the managers and subscribers were key figures of Edinburgh's governmental and intellectual circles. Its roster of volunteer and salaried physicians and surgeons contained the names of the most prominent individuals then practicing in the capital. The same criteria were applied in the selection of ordinary physicians, medical and surgical clerks, and student dressers. Financial arrangements with both the Royal Army and Navy during wartime and before brought substantial revenues to the hospital, as well as the goodwill of powerful commissioners, many of them Edinburgh graduates. At one point, the infirmary even turned lender for the municipal government, giving to the city fathers funds originally earmarked by the king for invalid soldiers.

Lastly, one must see the Edinburgh infirmary as an important factor in the conscious drive toward modernity and national achievement fueled by the Scottish Enlightenment. Its establishment in 1729 as the first such institution in Britain outside London was meant to indicate that Edinburgh could provide its sick poor with the type of charitable assistance that was available in the English capital. Decades later, as is demonstrated by the large flow of foreign students through its wards, the infirmary became well known beyond the borders of Scotland, and its organization, architecture, and staff were taken as models for similar institutions in Britain and abroad.[9] Contemporaries were impressed by its cleanliness, low mortality, and valuable in-house pharmacopoeia.[10] In that sense, the Royal Infirmary of Edinburgh fulfilled the most ambitious goals of the Enlightenment reformers who sought to promote the good of the old kingdom and make Scotland look respectable in the eyes of the world.

Eighteenth-century hospitals have not fared well in the historical literature. With few exceptions, one simply finds single narratives of particular institutions written in commemoration of special anniversaries. These accounts are mostly repositories of information about prominent persons and events shaping the hospital or tales of scientific progress depicting technological innovations. Building plans, staff rosters, and extant regulations sprinkle the overall story, which usually unfolds outside the social and political context of the times.[11]

Unfortunately, such purely descriptive and anecdotal histories of hospitals have hitherto failed to probe the actual nature and mechanisms of hospital confinement during the eighteenth century. Patients and diseases are usually relegated to a few statistical charts without analysis. Comments about medical treatment appear seldom and then are summarily dismissed as "crude compilations of a blundering empiricism."[12] The tendency has been to stress the great progress made in medicine since that time of wanton bleeding and purging.

Based on a number of historical accounts, the standard contemporary judgment is that eighteenth-century hospitals were "hot-beds of infection" and "gateways to death." This impression, articulated by widely read authors such as Thomas McKeown[13] and Michel Foucault,[14] now unfortunately permeates much of the general literature on hospitals, casting a dark shadow on all eighteenth-century efforts to care for the sick.[15] At that time the value of hospital confinement had already prompted lively discussions, but before blanket indictments are made the problem needs further analysis and definition.

In his comprehensive study of British infirmaries, Brian Abel-Smith remarked that "little is known about what hospitals actually did for particular patients and diseases." At the same time, however, he expressed the hope that "detailed analysis of the case records of individual hospitals" would eventually furnish information about those who were admitted, their ailments, and their treatment.[16] Given the often fragmentary evidence still available, Abel-Smith's recommendations have hitherto been difficult to implement. Many eighteenth-century British hospitals kept admissions and financial records as part of their accountability to charitable subscribers, but the practice of writing down periodic notes about the institutional progress of patients was still in its preliminary stages and never implemented on a wide scale. Whatever survived the vagaries of time in the form of registers, minutes, and reports often fell victim to more recent paper-recycling efforts undertaken during wartime shortages.

In the case of the Edinburgh infirmary, however, scholars can find a virtual bonanza of documentation, at least for the period 1770–1800, which constitutes the focus of this work. Given the hospital's prominence in Edinburgh society and medical education, its authorities were forced to develop a detailed accounting system, including a register of patients, individual ward journals, and yearly statistics concerning admissions, discharges, and deaths. Moreover, the hospital managers kept extensive minutes of their monthly meetings, issued yearly financial reports, published updated rules to regulate the flow of patients through the institution, and determined duties of the medical and ancillary staff. Since the hospital was affiliated with the University of Edinburgh, additional information can be obtained from official academic regulations and student matriculation records.

Most important of all, the present attempt to reconstruct the activities taking place in the Royal Infirmary of Edinburgh relies on records left by medical students who enrolled in the course of clinical lectures given in the hospital. These students were periodically allowed to copy from official records complete cases of patients admitted to the teaching ward. Each case history contained the name of the individual, symptomatology, diagnosis, treatment, and daily progress notes describing the entire clinical evolution, together with adjustments in therapy. The copying was usually executed prior to presentation and discussion of these patients by professors in charge of the teaching ward and the clinical course. Moreover, several students took down verbatim all the remarks made in class by these academics, thereby providing another unique and invaluable document for the study of eighteenth-century diagnostics and therapeutics (see Figure I.1 and Appendixes A and B).

Fourteen student casebooks copied between 1771 and 1799 and containing 808 individual clinical histories constitute the core of the data utilized for the present analysis. They were supplemented by the 3,047 entries randomly extracted from the surviving folios of the infirmary's General Register of Patients for the same years. Together they furnish a great deal of information about the kind of patients admitted to the hospital, including age, sex, and occupation. Admission and discharge dates allow for estimates of length of hospitalization, types of discharge, and mortality rates. Effects of the medical regimen and clinical complications can be gathered from the patient histories. Finally, from remarks made by the Edinburgh professors during their clinical lectures, we can gain a good understanding of the reasons given for therapeutic intervention and choice of specific modes of treatment.

All of these materials permit an in-depth examination of hospital life at the Royal Infirmary of Edinburgh during the last decades of the eighteenth century. Diseases seen in the wards have here retained their original designations and medical meanings, merely being brought together into categories arranged by bodily systems. This approach should provide readers with a general overview of the disease ecology encountered in the institution. Many historians succumb to the temptation of retrospective medical diagnoses, using specific modern criteria and terminology to recast older and ambiguous disease entities. The resulting distortion of historical data often proves misleading, creating additional problems of interpretation.

Lastly, attention has been given to both the content and methods of the

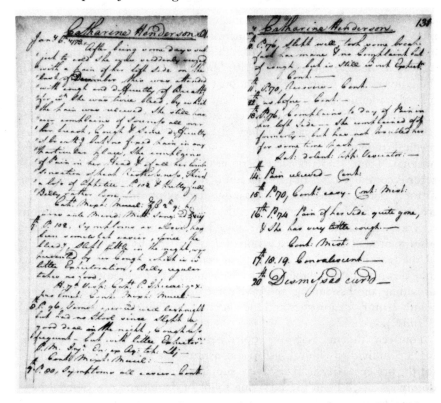

Figure I.1. Case of Catherine Henderson, in James Gregory, Clinical lectures and cases, 1789–1796, MSS B51, National Library of Medicine, Bethesda, MD

teaching made available to medical students and surgical apprentices, since clinical instruction was one of the important institutional functions. In the final analysis, this work tries to recreate the "state of the medical art" as reflected in the care of hospital patients admitted between 1770 and 1800 to one of the leading establishments of its kind in Europe.

1

The sick poor and voluntary hospitals

"DESIROUS OF ACCOMMODATION IN THE HOUSE": THE ROAD TO HOSPITAL ADMISSION

The persons to be received into the hospital . . . want that which makes poverty tolerable. They would want no more but to be re-established in their former health, to return to their labor and industry, and be no further burdensome to the public. Are these real objects of charity?[1]

On Wednesday, January 9, 1780, Margaret ("Peggy") Carmichael was brought into the Royal Infirmary of Edinburgh in a "stupid, comatose state," unable to give "any distinct account of herself." Her face was flushed, the skin very warm and "marbled at the arms," the breathing laborious. Barely twenty years old, Peggy suffered from one of the most commonly perceived ailments of the eighteenth century: a fever. Her complaints had begun nine days earlier, in a household already ravaged by disease. Her mother had died three weeks earlier, also the victim of a fever, and her father, Andrew, who had taken care of his wife, was now a patient in the teaching ward of the hospital, fortunately convalescing from a similar ailment.[2]

Before the week was out, Peggy's eight-year-old sister Mary and brother Pat, barely three, were also sent to the infirmary with fevers. They were joined on January 18 by their grandmother, Margaret Clunie, a seventy-nine-year-old woman who, alone and exhausted from the ordeal of caring for the children, had been confined to her bed for days, tormented by a persistent cough.[3]

The Carmichael family lived in Edinburgh, "in Grass Market opposite Paxton," on the western edge of an expanding provincial city boasting at this time a population of about seventy-five thousand. Peggy's father was by occupation a carter, one of those "deserving" or "industrious" poor willing to work and fend for their families as long as health allowed. Like most members of the "lower ranks" of society, the Carmichaels were periodically exposed to sickness, which "seized" the laboring population and "chained" the afflicted to their cots or worn-out blankets strewn on hard and dirty floors.[4]

Time and again the fragile self-sufficiency of these families was undermined by illness. When it affected the breadwinner, sickness caused direct economic hardship to the entire family, but even when the wife fell ill, "so much of her husband's time is employed in attending to her and supplying her place in the care of the children" that the effects were similar.[5] Economic hardship was the rule, beginning with the sale of all belongings to buy food, and followed by expulsion from the dwellings the family occupied because of their inability to pay rent or the neighbors' fear of contagion. Many people, their savings exhausted and debts mounting because of illness in their families, found themselves thrown into prison by impatient creditors.

Poor families such as the Carmichaels lived in low, damp cellars or the upper floors of Edinburgh's high-rise houses, densely packed together into narrow, single rooms. Fever supposedly originated from poisonous vapors arising within the stale or putrid air, heavy with the "exhalations" emitted by the many dirty bodies crowded into small, windowless chambers.[6]

The poor held a variety of notions about the causes of their ailments. Respiratory ills were often blamed on excessive exposure to cold air, especially during frosty nights, whereas "fevers" were thought to ensue after drinks of cold water when people were in a state of "heat" or perspiration, especially after dancing throughout the night.[7] One woman suffering from a "catarrh" went so far as to attribute her complaints "to carrying a great weight pressing against her chest."[8] Another was convinced that a "disagreeable smell," probably all too frequent in Edinburgh, "had made her very faintish," precipitating an episode of cough and fever.[9]

During winters, respiratory ailments, including "consumption" – probably pulmonary tuberculosis – were attributed to "much hardship and poor living" in miserable hovels scattered throughout the city. They were frequent "especially among the vulgar who from the state of their houses and employments are exposed to repeated attacks of cold."[10] Under the circumstances, hospitalization created an attractive alternative. "He is a poor indigent man without house of family," read one 1795 clinical history, referring to a forty-two-year-old porter, "and to him accommodations of an hospital are luxuries . . . what he seemed most to want was shelter and protection during the severe wintry months."[11]

Breathing difficulties associated with respiratory and circulatory problems were exacerbated by Edinburgh's most common and unavoidable activity: climbing stairs. The city was built on the top of a high ridge, and the sides of its houses, many of them ten to twelve stories high, clung on the rocks. Each floor in the buildings could be reached only through endless and crowded stairways, most of them too narrow to permit passage of a casket on the way to its burial. Thus reaching quarters reserved for the poor on the upper floors of such tenements severely strained the already weakened constitutions of many would-be patients.

Rheumatic complaints, quite common among Edinburgh dwellers, were blamed on dampness or "violent fits of anger," repeated exposure to cold when sweating, or "stoppage of menstrual flow."[12] The latter phenomenon was widely believed to be responsible for a great number of ailments, and emotions were held to play key roles in occurrences ranging from dyspepsia and ascites to miscarriages and cancer. In one instance jaundice was said to have "appeared a day after she experienced a violent emotion: terror."[13] Another woman connected her daily febrile fits to "excessive grief at having lost her husband and three sons in the last months and [being] thus left friendless with a small family."[14]

Other people succumbed to illness after long and exhausting walks, the only reliable and inexpensive transportation method employed by the poor. A stroll from the nearby port of Leith during the winter months caused one woman to experience severe chills and fever; another, still weak from her delivery and presently nursing and carrying a six-month-old infant, "returned walking from Glasgow and is very much fatigued."[15] An extreme case was an eighty-two-year-old man who complained of an affection on his foot resembling gout after completing a six-hundred-mile walk.[16]

Given the frequency of infectious diseases affecting the population, "exposure to the contagion of fever" was frequently listed as the reason for seeking hospital admission. Sometimes a mother and her small child, both suffering from the same sickness, hoped to be accepted, and even entire families, such as the Carmichaels, presented themselves at the gates, no one left to care for them at home. In one instance a recently married barber and his wife were brought in together with identical febrile complaints. On other occasions the terse clinical notes merely mention the fact that "several people in the neighborhood are ill." In the case of a soldier called "Littlefear," a guard at the Edinburgh Castle, exposure to contagion "occurred in a room at the castle in which a person labored under a fever."[17] Entire families comprising up to six members were all brought in for treatment at the same time.[18]

There were many examples of accidents requiring surgical attention. The considerable height of Edinburgh's buildings could prove fatal for those who fell down stairs or out of windows, often in a state of alcoholic stupor produced by "congenial dissipations." Others slipped from rooftops or trees, sustaining skull and leg fractures. Being struck by falling stones or bricks from crumbling buildings was another hazard. Dodging such lethal missiles was a common Edinburgh exercise.[19] One servant lost consciousness after being forced under a large mass of snow sliding from the roof of a tall building.

Other injuries were associated with the usual means of transportation winding their way through the narrow streets and alleys of the city. A coach driver negotiating a difficult passage fell from his seat, and one wheel of the vehicle ran over his left leg, shattering it. A man driving a chaise fell to the pavement, bruising not only the side of his body but also his head, with sudden visual impairment. Another, more fortunate laborer only broke his ribs.[20] Farm-related incidents were not uncommon. Euphemia Ross, a servant, "received a stroke from the front of a cow upon the pit of her stomach" and vomited clotted blood for several weeks; a ploughman "thrown on his back by the falling of a heap of earth" suffered from paralysis of both legs.[21]

Fights and brawls took their toll. A drunken bitmaker, for example, was knocked down on New Year's Eve during a scuffle with other merrymakers, the victim of a blow over his forehead. A musician was kicked in the back and kept coughing up bright red blood for weeks. A caskmaker was hit in the eye, "having been ill-treated and left exposed all night by companions with whom he had been drinking."[22] In several instances people said to have been suffering from epileptic fits or partial paralysis of the legs fell on the pavement. One was a young boy with two considerable skull depressions presumed to have occurred at birth.[23] Other clinical histories recorded some unusual mishaps. One man walking on the street was suddenly struck by a cask rolling down a hill, and a woman injured her chest when she was blown against the door of a building by a strong gust of wind.[24]

Among those seeking medical assistance were a number of leadworkers, a silver refiner, and a painter, all exposed to lead or mercury fumes that they blamed for severe abdominal cramps. Apparently one of the leadworks was located in Leith near Edinburgh, but it is not clear whether all affected individuals worked there.[25] A mason suffered a corneal injury from a stone fragment that had struck his eye as he was chiseling, a nurse became acutely ill while attending a smallpox patient, and a glassmaker suddenly exposed to hot and cold air blamed the temperature changes for his respiratory ailment. Finally, the member of a band who kept playing his French horn for several hours each night found blowing the instrument painful; he continued spitting up fresh blood as well as finding it in his horn after the performances.[26]

Whether suddenly struck or chronically invalided, few Scotsmen were deserted at the time of sickness. Indeed, one contemporary observer condemned the traditional practice of having "idle visitors crowding around the sickbed," since these persons ran the risk of becoming infected in fever cases or, worse yet, carrying communicable diseases "from house to house, from village to village." Reassurance provided by such "innocent marks of attention" could be nullified if the sick person concluded that such displays of social solidarity meant the disease would have a fatal outcome.[27]

In Edinburgh the sick poor showed a considerable willingness to seek hospital admission and medical advice. Almost half of all persons (40%) "desirous of accommodation" at the Royal Infirmary of Edinburgh had been ill for fewer than ten days and could thus be characterized as suffering from acute disease. These people were on the average younger than any other group of prospective patients (26 years old) and to a greater extent female. An additional 13% reported longer-lasting, subacute complaints (ten to thirty days' duration). The rest, mostly males, had chronic conditions lasting for at least a month.[28] The hospital was by no means a last resort.

When sickness struck, the poor not only consoled each other, they took therapeutic matters into their own hands and prescribed for each other. Almost half of all patients coming to the hospital admitted that they had received some form of prior treatment.[29] The remedies ranged from common practices such as gargling with alum whey for sore throat or drinking seawater for skin troubles to more serious treatments usually prescribed by physicians, surgeons, and apothecaries. One woman admitted being cured of ague in England by a Roman Catholic priest who administered to her a large dose of nutmeg and alum; a man stopped his diarrhea with French brandy and cinnamon.[30] Bloodletting was also frequently employed by laypersons.[31]

A considerable number of sick people admitted previous visits to hospitals. Most of them had already been several times in the Royal Infirmary of Edinburgh, but a few acknowledged stays in similar English institutions.[32] For example, one man with fluid in his chest spent six months at the Newcastle Infirmary, then traveled up to Edinburgh for another opinion.[33] Clearly, then, in time of illness, the Carmichael family and other lower-class inhabitants of Edinburgh and its vicinity had recourse to one type of establishment belonging to the crusade of charity developed in Britain: the voluntary hospital. To understand better both the context and the methods of medical care employed at the Royal Infirmary of Edinburgh, it is essential first to examine the origins, philosophy, and organization of the British hospital movement.

THE ORIGINS OF THE BRITISH HOSPITAL MOVEMENT

From admiration to this parent God,
Some gen'rous souls, with pious energy
Presum's to imitate the SOVEREIGN GOOD,
By heaping blessings on their fellow creatures.
T'was then the reign of charity began;
And Hospitals were rear'd to heal the sick,
And raise the poor man who had none to help him.[34]

Contemporaries praised the eighteenth-century hospital movement as the most noteworthy philanthropic achievement of the century. Unlike other European countries, especially France and Germany, Britain in 1700 possessed only five hospitals for care of the sick poor, all of them located in the city of London.[35] The man responsible for this situation was Henry VIII, who after two centuries of gradual decay and administrative corruption had in 1545 abolished the city's medieval hospices for care and shelter, together with other religious institutions. Faced with a growing number of inhabitants later in the sixteenth century, the secular authorities of London were allowed to reopen and establish a few hospitals in the city under royal auspices and financed by private donations. Bequests came mainly from the wealthy merchant class, which insisted on efficient institutional management and integration with the city's official medical establishment. In the late sixteenth and the seventeenth centuries private contributions became an acceptable practice and indeed an honored charitable tradition. Sick, old, and infirm people from the lower classes of society living in London composed the population housed in these institutions.[36]

By the early eighteenth century available hospital facilities in London proved totally inadequate in the face of growing urbanization. Although the population was no longer periodically visited by the plague, contemporary conditions fostered the spread of smallpox, consumption, and numerous fevers that especially affected newcomers and children.[37] As one contemporary author remarked: "Cities are now the graves of young infants. They are drains of the human species . . . Close streets, alleys, lanes and habitations of the poor inhibit free ventilation and circulation of air."[38]

Although the Poor Laws had already established mechanisms for dealing with paupers at local parish levels, no comparable welfare program addressed the needs of the working poor. Since they were willing to work, a fact that implied acceptance of the Puritan work ethic, these British men and women and their children were considered to be "deserving" of assistance, including charitable support and free medical care in hospitals and dispensaries. The proposition "it is as much the duty of the poor to labour when they are able as it is for the rich to help them when they are sick" summarized the unwritten contract established between the social classes.[39]

Medicalization of society

To a considerable extent interest in the work force was dictated by the mercantilist ideology that prevailed in most eighteenth-century European countries. Among newly perceived requirements of national power was the need for a growing and healthy population capable of furnishing enough manpower for the production of crops and goods, maintenance of significant standing armies, and payment of taxes and rents. If national ascendancy and economical well-being were linked to an expanding society, it seemed clear that geopolitical objectives could be implemented only with a population whose material welfare was significantly improved. To be successful, this policy had to include steps designed to better the health of workers. As a result, the new strategies of European mercantilism radically changed the limited focus of earlier medical activities, thus propelling questions of health and disease to the forefront of social policy.[40]

Consequently, medicine in the eighteenth century dramatically expanded the scope of its activities under the impact of powerful social and political forces. The so-called medicalization of society allowed physicians not only to reach new sectors of the burgeoning middle class but for the first time in history to make contact with significant sectors of the populace. The range of health-related activities widened to include greater emphasis on environmental health, infant and maternal welfare, and military and naval medicine, as well as mass treatment of the population in newly erected hospitals and dispensaries. The underlying premise was that sickness could be controlled, removed, and perhaps even prevented by conscious and deliberate application of enlightened views about health and disease.[41]

In many European countries, notably France and Germany, such health-related activities were quickly supported by effective and centralized bureaucratic organizations that came into being during the seventeenth and eighteenth centuries.[42] Mercantilist efforts to improve health and size of the British population were forced to rely largely on private initiatives, rather than on governmental action. One tradition originating in the seventeenth century actually sought to achieve social and medical reforms through the use of vital statistics. This information was gathered and repeatedly published to impress upon the prosperous upper and especially middle classes the need for reforms and thereby perhaps to mobilize them into action. Although some roots for this statistical direction can also be traced to Henry VIII, particularly the inception of parish registers and London bills of mortality, employment of numbers as tools for administrative reform occurred only after 1650. Beginning with John Graunt's *Natural and Political Observations upon the Bills of Mortality* published in 1662, and William Petty's *Essays in Political Arithmetik* of 1687, Britons gathered demographic data to convince potential reformers of the deplorable health conditions that existed among working people.[43]

Concepts of health and sickness

In the eighteenth century, calls for the improvement of the populace were clearly based on an optimistic outlook regarding the role and benefits of medicine. Elaborated by a number of prominent Enlightenment thinkers, these ideas implied confidence that diseases could eventually be eradicated, since health was a natural bodily condition: Health could in fact be maintained and illness averted. In time, such notions began to permeate all health-related activities, including hospital care. Thus Enlightenment views profoundly shaped contemporary conceptions of wellness and illness, encouraged the search for factors responsible for sickness, and contributed to new strategies of medical intervention.[44]

An important program of health conservation based on the classical model of the so-called non-naturals and designed for the upper and middle classes of society was already in place.[45] The non-naturals comprised a number of environmental agents such as air, food, and drink; natural bodily functions like motion and rest, wakefulness and sleep, and retention and evacuation of nutritive substances; and finally mental activities, including the passions. Together, these factors were considered responsible for human health, and their skillful manipulation became a convenient platform for launching a comprehensive plan of disease prevention.[46]

Among those who subscribed to Enlightenment values, health was a key ideal to strive for, a state of bodily and psychological wellness conducive to a more enjoyable and longer life. Measures to preserve a healthy balance of all bodily functions were a responsibility that individuals had to assume on their own, with or without medical assistance. To be successful, each person had to acquire sufficient knowledge of the effects wrought by the non-naturals on his or her own nature and bodily constitution. "There does not exist a definition of health applicable to everyone," asserted Arnulfe d'Aumont, a French physician who wrote the article on this subject for Diderot's *Encyclopédie;* "each person had his own state of well-being."[47]

Sickness was therefore regarded as an avoidable problem, even though it constantly threatened both individuals and communities at large. The effects of disease resulted in much personal suffering coupled with financial losses for the afflicted, their families, and ultimately the state. In consonance with the doctrine of non-naturals, measures needed to be taken to prevent the appearance of disease or to check its dissemination. "Hygiene," proclaimed d'Aumont, who also wrote on this theme for the *Encyclopédie,* "is a term that serves to designate the first of two medical procedures, namely the one concerning the conduct necessary to follow for maintaining the state of existing health."[48] Fresh air, enough food, personal cleanliness, and sufficient exercise and rest, as well as control of the passions, were recommended. Hygiene was not a strictly medical policy, and lay reluctance to seek advice from healers was often matched by professional unwillingness to deal with nontherapeutic issues. To fill the resulting information gap, a number of popular manuals were written during the eighteenth century to serve in part as self-help guides regarding hygienic matters.[49]

Of course, the more traditional role of medicine was to restore lost health by fighting the "contra-naturals," meaning diseases and their causes and effects. As in preceding centuries, the aim of eighteenth-century medical treatment was to aid and supplement the healing power of nature inherent in the human constitution. While taking different positions about the rationale underlying specific measures and the degree of therapeutic activism, both lay and medical authors expressed considerable optimism about future developments. It was widely believed that medicine would prosper if physicians could improve their understanding of the diseases afflicting humankind. Systematic observations such as those that could be conducted in hospitals were expected to provide more precise and therefore useful information.

Not surprisingly, the lower classes of European society did not always share such cheerful views of wellness, sickness prevention, and medical treatment. Their own concepts of health and illness were not necessarily linked to the biological models and rational causalities adopted by professional medicine. To the deeply religious, human imperfection since the Fall in the Garden of Eden was reflected in a permanent vulnerability to sickness and thus periodic visitations by dreadful diseases. For many, illness ultimately remained a mysterious event, unpredictable yet inevitable and governed by divine forces or blind fate. Observed one British physician: "The general notion of all illiterate persons is a kind of irresistible fatality, and they are too apt, in diseases, to commit all to God . . . Possibly many years must yet elapse before the whole kingdome will be awakened to a just sense of its interest and safety, before custom and prejudice are done away and ignorance enlightened."[50]

Referring to his hospitalized roommates at the Devon and Exeter Hospital around 1800, one patient remarked that "most delight in supernatural things, death tokens and departed spirits, and awful voices heard and judgments dire sent down from heaven." Claiming as an artist to be one "whom Providence has blessed with juster notions and sublimer views of the divine economy," this man tried to generate pity instead of scorn for the sick poor with "uninstructed minds" housed in the institution. In his opinion their deeply grafted grotesque "ideas" about illness arose from a "sense of divine wrath."[51]

Despite religious views that prompted prayers and visits to the priest, popular healing favored an interventionist approach, using homemade remedies to palliate bothersome complaints. Many of the treatments employed herbal concoctions prepared from traditional recipes. If circumstances allowed, self-proclaimed folk healers or traveling drug peddlers were consulted in addition to family members and friends. These various measures reveal a universal and pragmatic eclecticism that sought to obtain a maximum of physical relief in spite of the ultimate outcome of the sickness.

In many instances the sick poor avoided contact with rational physicians altogether, since the professional cosmology defied popular beliefs by implying a natural causation and possible mastery over events judged by the victims to be divinely inspired. Others sought to utilize all available and potentially useful measures regardless of their source, especially if they were free of charge, as in voluntary hospitals and dispensaries. Thus, despite ideological and social barriers, the poor gradually came into closer contact with the medical profession. Although at times it was indeed the last resource, to be reluctantly tapped under the threat of death, hospital care became increasingly acceptable for routine illnesses.

Following Enlightenment ideals, the assumption underlying most medical activities, including hospital treatment, was that human happiness and productivity could be promoted if health were protected or restored. This optimistic viewpoint considered fatalism and ignorance in health-related matters a barrier to be overcome. Replacement of religious and magical concepts of illness by biomedical models was imperative. Perhaps the very ambivalence of the masses toward professional care provided a basis from which to "medicalize" society. Claiming to possess better knowledge about the bodily processes occurring in health and disease, as well as experience with effective therapies, a new medical elite, whose purpose was to contribute to societal order and prosperity by controlling disease, assumed prominent roles in European societies. Henceforth professionals were to be widely employed to deal with sickness as experts. All other individuals claiming healing roles in the popular sector were branded quacks and seen as obstacles to better individual and collective health. As one writer recently noted, "Doctors were poised to become the new priests of the modern secularized world."[52] Promoting their ascendancy and indeed the process of medicalization itself was a new temple built to accommodate medical activities: the hospital.

Role of hospitals in British philanthropy

Britain's voluntary hospital movement shared its values and organizing principles with other contemporary reform efforts, such as the establishment of charity schools, orphanages, workhouses, and prisons. Religious and secular philanthropic motives combined with pragmatic attempts to protect the social order while also providing opportunities for personal rewards to charitable patrons. For centuries poor people "impotent to serve" society because of sickness were among those considered worthy of relief. Part of this help was directed toward an amelioration of their physical sufferings, so that they might return to their chores. Supported by Scripture and a long list of theological writings from St. Augustine to Thomas Browne, almsgiving and assistance to the sick remained one of the most visible aspects of Christian charity.[53]

Given Britain's lack of institutional frameworks in which to carry out such medical assistance effectively, many localities organized systems based on home visits, systems that were later reestablished under new dispensary programs. In his account of the proceedings of the Corporation of Bristol, for example, one early eighteenth-century participant reported that to allow employment of poor people, "To such as were sick, we gave warrants to our physician to visit them; such as wanted the assistance of our surgeons, were directed to them, and all were relieved till they were able to work."[54] Sickness, then, was a barrier to the fulfillment of the Puritan work ethic. If allowed to establish itself, it would rob people of their means to work and to be self-sufficient, plunging productive persons into poverty and dependency, transforming them into public burdens. In providing relief, welfare officials were thus urged to assign high priority to health-related questions.

Fueled by mercantilist ideas and faced with governmental apathy, wealthy middle-class Britons launched early in the eighteenth century a number of voluntary initiatives designed to deal with some of society's most pressing ills. As pointed out by historians, it was a unique combination of methods and agendas that sought to further the "glory of God by promoting the usefulness of man."[55] This goal was clearly outlined by one typical representative of the movement, the pious Robert Nelson (1656–1715). Nelson, an influential Puritan and religious writer, defined charitable practices as "doing good to the souls and bodies of men." Among the benevolent deeds to be performed for the human frame he listed the visitation of the sick and relief of all "those wants the body labours under," meaning shelter, clothing, nourishment, and protection from as well as cure of sickness.[56]

In his 1715 *Address to Persons of Quality and Estate,* Nelson specifically considered the nation's urgent need for more hospitals. His proposals had two objectives in mind: attention to the sick poor, whom he characterized as "miserable objects perishing without medical help before their time," and the advancement of medicine through "useful experiments" made on hospital inmates. In addition to calling for a hospital to house those deemed incurable, Nelson also advocated the establishment of "hospitals for every capital distemper of the body," that is, ailments of the eyes, stone, gout and rheumatism, dropsy, asthma, consumption, and finally ailments of a "nervous" sort. Ironically, Nelson's seven categories of disease were, perhaps with the exception of rheumatism and consumption, health problems largely afflicting the middle classes in Britain and not the poor. The lower classes, in contrast, suffered from a multitude of febrile distempers, many of them linked to their social status in society. Yet erecting these special hospitals was an example of the good works Nelson so fervently endorsed. The utilitarian aspect of hospital foundations, however, was by no means neglected. Wrote Nelson: "There might be mighty improvements made in the art of curing, and with God's blessing, many thousands of lives might be preserved for the good of the public."[57]

Another typical representative of the British philanthropic movement was John Bellers (1654–1725), an important Quaker and London merchant who in 1714 published a work titled *Essay towards the Improvement of Physick.* Dedicated to the British Parliament, the book was based on Bellers's studies of London mortality statistics. According to his computations, almost twenty thousand persons died each year in London, about half of them from "an army of diseases" that could in his view be prevented or cured. When Bellers extrapolated his figures to the rest of Britain, it appeared to him that the whole kingdom lost about a hundred thousand inhabitants per year "for want of timely advice and suitable medicines." This figure, in Bellers's eyes, constituted a very significant drain of national resources according to the prevailing mercantilist criteria. In fact, he calculated that every lost worker was actually worth two hundred pounds to the British economy.[58]

To remedy the situation so dramatically illustrated in his work, Bellers announced a twelve-point plan for legislative action. Like Nelson's, his program included the construction of hospitals for the destitute, the blind, and those considered incurable, as well as the appointment of physicians and surgeons at the parish level to treat the sick poor. Moreover, Bellers also envisioned the creation of a national institute charged with the responsibility for obtaining new and effective medicines. For this purpose physicians were urged to travel abroad and gather all pertinent information about potentially useful remedies. Lastly, the author told Parliament that improvement of the healing arts should become a matter of governmental concern, with the College of Physicians in London reporting every year to the legislative bodies concerning "the state of medicine."[59]

Bellers's call for the creation of hospitals was linked to the concept that "experience makes the best physicians" and was meant to upgrade both the knowledge and the skills of contemporary healers. Physicians, he argued, could markedly improve their understanding of diseases and medicines through mass observations of sick people collected into hospital wards. "These hospitals," wrote Bellers, "will breed up some of the best physicians and chirurgeons because they may see as much there in one year as in seven anywhere else." This clinical knowledge was to be supplemented by postmortem examinations "for the better information of physicians" when the causes of illness remained hidden and no clear idea could be ascertained regarding the action of remedies. Finally, both clinical and pathological experiences were to be preserved for posterity and especially for medical education, using a recording system wherein "each patient be registered in a book, with the daily prescriptions that is made of them, and how they succeed."[60]

Such clear advantages suggested that the hospital should indeed become a kingpin in future medical and surgical instruction. Bellers saw hospitals as "great nurseries" and called for the construction of university-affiliated institutions at Oxford and Cambridge "with different wards for each distemper." Referring to courses of hospital training, he estimated that students would "learn more in seven years than in fourteen years without them." Moreover, such an institutional arrangement provided the needed bodies for anatomical dissection, drawing corpses from among the deceased patients and thereby avoiding the popular protests caused by grave robbing. Above all, Bellers believed that vital knowledge of a clinical nature was to be added to the traditional baggage of "aphorisms and theory" the better to equip future graduates for handling the difficulties of practice.[61]

Nelson's and Bellers's programmatic statements for the institutionalization of the poor soon became realities. The first voluntary hospital exclusively devoted to the care of the sick opened its doors in London during 1720. The Westminster Infirmary was the tangible result of lengthy deliberations begun in a Fleet Street coffeehouse on January 14, 1715. The "charitable proposal" drawn up after the initial meeting stated the intentions of the first nucleus of philanthropists: "to provide poor sick people with necessary food and physick during illness; to procure them the advice of physicians or assistance of surgeons and nurses when necessary." At the same time, following Nelson's holistic approach to caring also for the moral ills of the poor, the founding group went on record that "The Society designs to reclaim the souls of the sick."[62]

The new hospital in Westminster was soon followed by other similar establishments, such as Guy's Hospital in 1726,[63] St. George's Hospital in 1733,[64] London Hospital in 1740,[65] and finally the Middlesex Hospital in 1745.[66] With the exception of Guy's, which owed its creation to the generosity of a single donor, these London hospitals or, better, infirmaries were the result of philanthropic associations that included businessmen, bankers, lawyers, and teachers, as well as physicians and surgeons. In a 1739 sermon delivered to the governors of the Westminster Infirmary, the bishop of St. Asaph characterized these groups of civic-minded people as an "alliance against misery."[67]

Patrons pledged specific sums of money or stock, their payments made quarterly, annually, or even in the form of life memberships. In exchange, each donor acquired the right to recommend a specific number of patients for admission to the hospital. Most subscriptions entitled contributors to sponsor one to three patients annually as long as the charitable payments were made in time. Those who were delinquent and did not follow up their pledges received first friendly reminders and then warnings, including threats that their names would be published in the newspapers as persons who had reneged on their philanthropic responsibilities.

The latter alternative was the charity's ultimate weapon, seldom if ever employed by the governors of a voluntary hospital but highly effective in forcing the payments of alms. After all, subscribers through their actions acquired prestige among their peers and in city circles. Because of their support, donors were entitled to attend general meetings of contributors and had a chance of being elected to the board of directors or managers of a hospital. Membership on hospital boards often became a source of social and economic rewards, bringing the benefactors into contact with other community leaders, aristocratic patrons, and prominent physicians and thus expanding their social networks. It also allowed the display of political and administrative skills.

While London's philanthropists were springing into action in response to the deplorable health conditions generated in their crammed metropolis, similar groups devoted to charity throughout the provinces banded together to erect hospitals in various British cities. The first voluntary institution to open its doors outside London was the Edinburgh Hospital for Sick Poor founded in 1729. Other local and county establishments were created in Winchester (1736), Bristol (1737), York County (1740), Liverpool (1749), and many other places.[68] By the end of the eighteenth century Britain boasted thirty general infirmaries in the provinces. The voluntary hospital movement claimed a total of four thousand beds, half of them located in the larger facilities of the five institutions already operating in London.[69]

Hospital medicine: advantages and drawbacks

After several decades of experience with voluntary hospitals various medical writers began to publish works on this subject, both extolling the virtues and criticizing the shortcomings of Britain's new system of health care. Though most were enthusiastic about what they judged to be accomplishments, a few questioned the very existence of these institutions and proposed alternative methods for delivering medical care. For example, as exemplified in the writings of Francis Home (1719–1813), professor of materia medica at the University of Edinburgh, and his student Thomas Beddoes (1760–1808), medical professionals expressed a variety of conflicting opinions concerning the utility of the new infirmaries. Home wrote that "nothing at present more distinguishes civilized from barbarous nations than the institution of hospitals for the relief of the sick";[70] on the other hand, Beddoes in 1791 flatly advised against the erection of such an establishment in Cornwall.[71] These judgments reflect, at least in part, the divergent experiences of those who practiced in the large, crowded wards of London hospitals and military outposts and those who worked in small, well-run provincial infirmaries. In London it soon became obvious that hospitals, far from being places for the recovery of the sick poor, could instead become agents for the dissemination of new sickness. Wrote the physician John Aikin (1747–1822), a prominent critic: "There cannot surely be a greater contradiction in the nature of things than a disease produced by a hospital."[72]

Most medical men writing during the period 1770–1800 chose to help British hospitals fulfill their "benevolent designs" by first analyzing and exposing the most important problems that beset them and then offering possible solutions. Aikin himself was very explicit about the advantages he saw for the sick who availed themselves of hospital treatment: "Whoever has frequented the miserable habitations of the lowest class of poor, and has seen disease aggravated by a total want of every comfort arising from a suitable diet, cleanliness and medicine, must be struck with pleasure at the change on their admission into a hospital where these wants are abundantly supplied."[73]

If sick people could recover after their transfer to a better environment in hospitals, removal to institutions also lessened opportunities for contagion affecting family members, friends, and even "idle or officious" neighbors, as another Edinburgh graduate, William Buchan (1729–1805), characterized them. In his book *Domestic Medicine* (1769), Buchan expressed concern about the effects of hospitalization on public health, especially the threat of contagious diseases for the upper classes. In fact, he urged masters to remove sick servants swiftly to infirmaries lest these people infect the entire household they were serving, since "most of the putrid fevers and other infectious disorders break out among the poor and are by them communicated to the more cleanly and the wealthy."[74]

Although many medical professionals had played a secondary role in the early voluntary hospital movement, they were quick to recognize its advantages for the improvement of medical knowledge. Before the proliferation of hospitals, most physicians and surgeons had been able to acquire only a limited knowledge of medical matters. Dependent on sporadic house calls or visitations from willing private patients, they exerted at best a partial control over their recommendations and treatments. Moreover, restricted by poor roads and long distances to a few daily consultations, practitioners could hardly expect to gain the wide clinical experience necessary to manage the diseases they were entrusted to heal.

The situation in hospitals was fundamentally different. Here medical men acquired a considerable authority and control over their hospitalized patients. This shift of power in the doctor-patient relationship, accentuated by social class distinctions, allowed for more complete follow-ups of individual cases and disease processes than the fragmented glimpses of private patients had previously permitted. Shifting to public practice also ensured greater patient compliance with prescribed therapeutic regimens and thus at least allowed for the opportunity to assess drug effects.

Aikin concurred that the sick poor were ideally suited for "experimental practice." "Hospital patients," he declared, "are on several accounts the most proper subjects of an experimental course. Accustomed to obey orders, and the confinement to strict regulations of diet and regimen are advantages not to be had in an equal degree in private practice." Aikin went on to explain that the healing art was by its nature rooted in experiment. The institutional setting provided a vastly expanded number of cases on which to conduct "all those gradual steps and minute observations which contribute to render an experiment both safe and decisive."[75]

The advantages envisioned by Bellers decades earlier made hospitals into what the founder of the London Hospital Medical School, William Blizard (1743–1835), called "the principal pillars of a rational system of instruction in the healing art."[76] Surgeons were the first to realize fully the hospital's potential for clinical instruction, undoubtedly because their diagnostic and operating skills were clearly linked to practical experience.[77] Yet physicians soon followed suit. Surrounded by retinues of eager students, those who attended the sick made their appointed hospital rounds with a feeling of enhanced status and confidence. Even a contemporary writer critical of the medical profession admitted, "I know of no better method of adding to your notoriety and consequently to your practice than that of becoming a physician to some public institution as a dispensary or hospital."[78]

However, there was a dark side to hospital care. In certain places the problems were appalling. To their credit, health professionals were quick to recognize the deleterious effects of crowding in hospital wards, as well as the importance of personal and environmental hygiene in the epidemiology of several infectious diseases. Among those creating such an awareness was John Pringle (1707–1782), a Scottish student of Boerhaave and a military physician who in 1750 published a monograph on "hospital and jail fevers." In his work Pringle described a fever frequently breaking out in confined places such as army hospitals, barracks, transport ships, and jails. The cause of this ailment was believed to be a specific poison produced by emanations from the sick housed in them. Once swallowed or drawn in through the breath, this poison caused a "slow" or clinically lengthy type of fever also called *"typhus,"* in which the bodies of those affected often adopted a tendency toward internal putrefaction. Although he advocated conservative therapeutic measures to deal with the problem, Pringle mainly stressed preventive steps designed to purify the air in all institutional settings – chiefly numerous methods of ventilation.[79]

Because of their crowded conditions, many hospitals shared in the genesis and transmission of slow fevers, and contemporary authors writing about infirmaries explained at length the dangers lurking in the wards. In a letter dated October 1, 1771, the prominent physician Thomas Percival (1740–1804), who attended the Manchester Infirmary, outlined some of the prophylactic measures needed to prevent the spread of hospital diseases. Besides adequate cross ventilation, Percival advocated daily sprinkling or washing of wards with vinegar as well as frequent fumigation of rooms, linens, and clothing, using tar-water steam.[80]

Aikin, on the other hand, proposed a number of architectural and procedural reforms. He was critical of large hospital wards that could not be properly ventilated, suggesting smaller rooms and insisting that all ambulatory patients spend as much time as possible in the halls and outdoors. Since hospitalization meant a possible trade-off between getting rid of the original ailment and acquiring in the wards another one of perhaps greater virulence, Aikin recommended new criteria for admission. His guidelines advocated acceptance only of patients who could be helped quickly and promptly discharged, since "the inbred disease of hospitals will amost inevitably creep in some degree upon one who continues a long time in them."[81] Persons affected by contagious diseases such as smallpox and measles were to be accepted only if the air surrounding them in the ward could be diluted through extensive ventilation, possible with the help of open windows and active fireplaces drawing out the poisonous particles generated by the victims.

Preoccupation with proper ventilation and cleanliness because of the threat of "hospital distempers" came to dominate most discussions about the virtues and faults of hospital care. If recipients of medical charity were felled by new disease in the hospitals where they sought relief, the "benevolent designs" of both philanthropists and health professionals would come to naught. Haunted by the specter of hospital-based epidemics, reformers went to work hoping to prevent them, and their efforts had two important consequences. First, they made hospitals the ideal laboratories for testing the tenets of a new hygiene already formulated on the basis of observations carried out in army camps, ships, and prisons. Once accepted as harbingers of disease and death, environmental factors such as polluted air, filth, crowding, and lack of food were targeted for removal and prevention, acquiring a hitherto-overlooked importance in the pathogenesis of fevers.

The second result of these efforts to prevent institutional contamination was a gradual sharpening of the criteria for selecting persons who were "proper" objects of hospital care. As Aikin remarked, "I would wish to enforce as much as possible the idea of a hospital being a place designed for the *cure of the sick.*" Only those suffering from maladies believed to benefit from medical treatments were to be admitted. All others, especially patients affected with contagious fevers, consumption, or incurable health problems, were viewed as "burdens on the house."[82]

However, if such criteria were to be universally enforced, the most needy objects of charity would be barred from admission to the infirmaries. This policy was agreeable to Beddoes, who took exception to the notion that hospitals were superior to home care in his argument against the establishment of one in Cornwall, but his ideas were extreme. What the majority was saying, nevertheless, was that hospital care was clearly not for everyone. Institutionalization was dangerous; beds were scarce and their maintenance costly. "Very great and extensive good may be done by dispensing advice and medicines to the poor in such cases as do not require admission into a hospital," observed Aikin, suggesting the establishment of outpatient departments to provide ambulatory care suited to cases deemed "improper" for in-house treatment.[83] The subsequent rise of the dispensary movement in Britain owes much to the restrictive admission policies of voluntary hospitals, and in contrast to the situation today, those patients seen but not admitted to the hospital often suffered from more severe and protracted ailments than those who managed to gain entrance.[84]

Finally, some eighteenth-century critics pointed to the inherent inhumanity of the voluntary hospital system. A prime target was the avarice and insensibility of the staff, from the penny-pinching behavior of administrators and the despotism of "Lady Matron" and "Lord Steward" to the greed and brutality of nurses or other servants who dispensed their services only to those willing to bribe them.[85] Other complaints ranged from insufficient or badly prepared food to unnecessarily restrictive visiting hours: "Shall a parent be denied the satisfaction of seeing a child, more dear on account of its misfortune, and shall not the child receive parental comfort?" questioned Blizard; "shall a son or daughter be driven cheerless from the door, uncertain of the state of a loved father or mother?"[86]

Another source of criticism was the payment of a burial security, demanded from incoming patients by the authorities of most infirmaries. The sum was meant to defray interment expenses in the event of the patient's death while hospitalized, and it terrified most newcomers to the institution. The request seemed to confirm patients' worst fears about the outcome of their stays in these establishments, compounding the anxieties caused by symptoms and separation from family. Aikin strongly objected to what he characterized as the "spirit of penurious economy which makes charity to appear so unlike itself," but most hospital managers, proud of their fiscal responsibilities, remained unmoved, even if the sums were trifling, given the low mortality rates in most voluntary institutions. Lack of proper complaint procedures also hampered the airing of grievances, since patients almost never dared to utter criticisms because of fear that the staff would retaliate.[87]

Physicians and surgeons were not immune to the charges of cruelty. "Gentlemen who arrived to the highest pitch of eminence in their profession use exceedingly harsh language and apparently unfeeling treatment to their patients," asserted one author.[88] Another, writing under the pseudonym "Mac Flogg'em," sarcastically suggested to physicians that "you must manifest your authority by being as rigidly severe and contumacious as possible and exert every endeavor to render the situation of the afflicted poor as irksome and miserable as you can." The proper "pomp and hauteur" could only benefit the institution by driving from the hospital burdensome patients "who had rather leave it half cured than to submit to your insolent and barbarous behavior."[89] Surgeons, in turn, were criticized for their apparent propensity for attempting operations, especially amputations, without the necessary consultations. "Experiments of this desperate nature are made on the poor that they may be practiced with more probability of success on the rich," asserted one critic, adding that "though this is a harsh imputation, yet I conscientiously believe it to be true in various instances."[90]

One of the basic premises underlying the charges of coldheartedness and mistreatment of patients by hospital staff members was an awareness that the sick were adversely affected by it. Buchan noted that he had frequently sensed in the poor a reluctance to seek admission to an infirmary, owing to preconceived fears and anxieties. Once inside, the sight, noise, and smells of disease as well as the "horrid assassinations of death" could only create further alarm and shock.[91] "To effectuate a cure in the body I hold it absolutely necessary to maintain peace of mind," concluded one medical writer. The remedy for all abuses was to appoint a "Humane Committee" acting as a hospital ombudsman and patient advocate. The proposals envisioned a group of people endowed by hospital authorities with sufficient discretionary powers to suspend or dismiss staff members found guilty of irregularities or violation "of the sacred obligations of the institution."[92]

Paradoxically, many of the insights into environmental hygiene and humanitarianism obtained from or proposed for hospital practice were shelved as Britain was engulfed in the Industrial Revolution. Because of late eighteenth-century population growth and reduced philanthropic aid, voluntary hospitals in most urban centers experienced degrees of crowding, dearth, and contagion similar to conditions prevailing among the poor. Greater incidence of hospital-acquired diseases contributed to increased in-house death rates.

THE ROYAL INFIRMARY OF EDINBURGH

Foundations and early development

I could not but admire the Royal Infirmary of Edinburgh. Few hospitals in England exceed it in airiness and cleanliness. Great attention is paid to the patients, and their complaints are very accurately minuted. The success of this institution is evident from the few that die in comparison with the number admitted.[93]

So wrote the famous English philanthropist John Howard on the basis of extensive hospital visits throughout Europe between 1778 and 1783, including three stays in Edinburgh. There the so-called Infirmary or Hospital for Sick Poor had opened its doors on August 6, 1729, to admit the first patient, Elizabeth Sinclair from the parish of Caithness, who suffered from chlorosis. Thus began the history of the earliest voluntary hospital in Scotland and the first institution of its kind outside London. Realizing the plight of the sick poor, Edinburgh's College of Physicians, the local Incorporation of Surgeons and Apothecaries, the Church of Scotland, noblemen, merchants, and the city's magistrates all cooperated in the venture. Since 1682 the College of Physicians had provided free ambulatory care to some of the poor living in the city. Two fellows of the college attended the institution in turn, and dispensed medicines purchased in part from fines levied against members who failed to minister to the sick. By the early eighteenth century this system was clearly considered insufficient, as the population of Edinburgh expanded.

Reasons for the erection of a voluntary hospital and proposals for raising funds were set forth in a 1729 pamphlet issued and distributed by "some gentlemen," probably including Alexander Monro primus (1697–1767), a surgeon recently elected professor of anatomy at the university.[94] Arguments developed in the document followed closely the tenets of contemporary British philanthropy and were thus a typical amalgamation of religious, humanitarian, economic, and medical considerations. For example, the religious justification in the pamphlet read: "As men and Christians we have the strongest inducements and even obligations to this sort of charity as it is warmly recommended and injoined in the gospel." A lay humanitarian statement followed: "Humanity and compassion naturally prompt us to relieve our fellow creatures when in such deplorable circumstances." The economic purposes were not neglected: "As the relief is a duty, so it is no less advantage to the nation, for as many as are recovered in an infirmary are so many working hands gained to the country." Finally, the document also included the medical goal "that students in physick and surgery might hereby have rather a better and easier opportunity of experience than they have hitherto had by studying abroad."[95]

Although this initial appeal failed, members of the College of Physicians persisted in their efforts. In 1725 they received a suggestion from George Drummond, who had just been elected lord provost in Edinburgh, that the owners of a fishery company that Drummond had managed were about to dissolve their business but could be persuaded to sell and sign their stock certificates over to a newly established fund created for the specific purpose of opening a voluntary hospital. With approval of city authorities and the Bank of Scotland, physicians of the college were ultimately successful in getting 352 subscribers, who pledged the necessary sum of two thousand pounds to purchase the stock.

The donors represented a cross section of the upper and middle classes of Scottish society and included the earls of Buchan, Hopetoun, and Leven; senators of the College of Justice; advocates; physicians; and surgeons. Further gifts came from David Spence, secretary to the Bank of Scotland, ministers, university professors, writers and booksellers, merchants, military authorities, and even the commander of a ship from the nearby port of Leith. Most contributors lived and worked in Edinburgh proper, but many other Scottish towns were represented. Even several merchants and physicians from London gave money to the new fund.[96] Such a diversity of contributors and the substantial amount of money collected point toward a number of motives operative among those who sought to establish a hospital. Not the least of these was national prestige and local civic pride, with patrons trying to imitate London's "charitable proposal," which, as noted, had already culminated in the foundation of the Westminster Infirmary in 1720.

On January 13, 1728, a general meeting of the donors was called and a set of "rules for the management of the Infirmary or Hospital for Sick Poor in the City of Edinburgh" approved. The new procedures allowed the annual election of twenty "extraordinary" managers, among them several prominent advocates; nine physicians, including Francis Pringle, president of the college, and Andrew Plummer and John Innes, professors of medicine at the university; and three surgeons, among them Alexander Monro primus. The managers made preparations to lease a house from the university in Robertson's Close, "made more agreeable and convenient by the professors of medicine granting liberty to the patients to walk in a garden immediately adjacent."[97]

The rules also provided for the selection of twelve "ordinary" managers from the larger group, "whose residence and business will best allow them to look after the affairs of the hospital." Two of them were to be "visitors" charged with touring the hospital by turns at least once a month and closely inspecting its management, "the treatment and dyet of the patients, the conduct of the housekeeper or mistress, the behavior of servants and patients and the whole economy of the house."[98] Two annual meetings in early January and July were to bring together all the managers for the election of a treasurer, a hospital clerk, and a housekeeper and for setting salaries for all the personnel.

Ordinary managers, in turn, would meet four times a year in February, May, August, and November. They had to examine, accept, and sign the treasurer's trimestral reports and make decisions about investments of the hospital's capital. Additional tasks included the ordering of repairs and supplies and supervision of daily activities by the professional and housekeeping staffs. Lastly, at a general meeting on the first Monday in July, the ordinary managers were required to lay before all extraordinary managers the records of their administration, including lists of patients admitted to the house.[99]

Hospital regulations allowed physicians and surgeons specific functions regarding the admission, management, and discharge of patients. The College of Physicians promised to staff the new hospital with some of its members, or as the advertisement in a local newspaper read, "Oblidge yourselves that one or more of their number shall attend the said hospital faithfully and freely without any prospect of reward or salary." This pledge, designed to encourage further subscriptions, was repeated on the eve of the hospital's formal opening. The physicians' visits were arranged in order of seniority on the roll of the college, and each rotation was to last two weeks.[100]

The Edinburgh Incorporation of Surgeons and Apothecaries was also willing to arrange a system of free attendance at the new hospital. Since their corporation act could not force all fifty of its members to participate, the leadership of the incorporation and the infirmary managers negotiated with Alexander Monro primus and five other surgeons, each of them agreeing to attend the sick for one month at a time and to dispense gratis from his apothecary shop all the medicines prescribed by physicians in the hospital. All of the six surgeons would also be available for consultations and would assist each other in the event of surgery.

After hiring a housekeeper to run the establishment with her maid and a clerk to record all administrative transactions, the authorities were ready to open the new infirmary. The "Little House," as it was soon called, was remodeled with the help of an architect. The two-floor structure contained five rooms and a kitchen, allowing at any given time the hospitalization of only four to six patients. One of the chambers on the ground floor functioned as a consulting or admission room and another housed the matron. The bedsteads were made of wood; the mattresses contained straw and were covered with cotton sheets and a quilt. Blue-striped curtains around the beds provided some privacy. As the newspaper announcement read, "A physician and surgeon will attend from 3 to 4 after noon in the Infirmary at the head of Robertson's Close, near the College, to receive such persons as shall be judged proper objects of this charity and to give advice and medicines during their sickness."[101]

In its first year of operation, the hospital admitted a total of only thirty-five patients. Just one of them died while being attended in the institution. A few additional people were seen in the consulting room on an outpatient basis and given medicines to take home. Compared with the 350 subscribers, 20 extraordinary managers, and several hospital staff members, the entire operation seemed almost ludicrous. It provided endless meeting opportunities for the administrators and considerable visibility to all charitable sponsors, but limited help to patients. In a sense the sick poor seemed merely an excuse for the social comings and goings of the infirmary's patrons. From a cynical point of view the contributions to the hospital fund could be viewed as initiation fees to some exclusive communal organization guaranteed to foster social recognition and advancement.

The new facility immediately attracted a number of medical students and surgical apprentices working with the professionals who were responsible for attending the sick. Given the physical limitations of the Little House, the managers were forced in November 1730 to adopt a series of regulations designed to avoid unnecessary overcrowding. Students were barred from the consulting room and allowed to witness surgical operations only if they had tickets issued by the attending physician or surgeon, who could not hand out more than two passes at one time. These measures were ostensibly taken "to safeguard the comfort and interest of the patients," but it is unclear whether they were strictly enforced. Managers also established a fee of two guineas for an admission ticket, issued by the treasurer, which entitled the student to "walk the Infirmary," presumably to follow the teachers on their appointed rounds.[102]

The early success of the Edinburgh Hospital for Sick Poor prompted managers to seek a royal charter and convert the hospital to a corporation. The scheme was designed to increase public interest and financial support for this new venture in health care. A committee that included the solicitor general, Charles Erskine; the commissioner of customs, George Drummond; and several physicians and surgeons petitioned King George II in 1731. Five years later, on August 25, 1736, the royal signature was finally secured at court in London and the charter of incorporation approved for what henceforth was to be called the Royal Infirmary of Edinburgh. Running the corporation were twenty managers, three of them permanent ex-officio positions belonging to the lord provost of the city of Edinburgh, the president of the Royal College of Physicians, and the deacon convener of the crafts.[103]

New building

Under pressure from the Incorporation of Surgeons to expand its facilities, the infirmary negotiated in 1736 the acquisition of a tract of land on which to erect a larger building. For a time between 1736 and 1738, a group of surgeons actually operated their own small hospital in College Wynd near the Little House, but the two charities managed to patch up their differences. In 1739 they finally merged resources in expectation of a significant expansion of the Royal Infirmary. Anticipating future growth, planners decided on a new building capable of accommodating a maximum of 228 patients, although at the outset the managers felt that their resources would allow them to care for only about 60 to 100.

New subscriptions from parishes belonging to the Church of Scotland were solicited. "Jesus Christ descends from his throne on his Father's right side, lays aside his robes of light, and clothing himself with rags, assumes the various diseases incident to humankind," preached one minister in Stirling, adding, "The Lord begs to build him a house to reside in while some of his faithful servants, eminent for their skill in physick, minister to his cure."[104]

With additional help from Episcopal congregations in Edinburgh and private donors, the treasurer submitted a budget that included construction costs for a new building. The donations were supplemented by projected hospital revenues: interest earned from the present capital investment and income from the sale of admission tickets to students. Other sums came from pledges by the Faculty of Advocates and Writers to the Signet and a tax that freemasons extracted from their members. Final approval of plans presented by the famous architect William Adams called for the construction of a wide U-shaped building with a central structure 210 feet long ending in two wings, each 70 feet in length. The new hospital was to have four floors, the top to be known as the "attick story." Many voluntary hospitals exhibited similar patterns of organization and were also constructed according to a series of contemporary criteria that stressed environmental purity, institutional order, and adequate ventilation. Like some of their medieval ancestors, these hospitals were supposed to be built on high ground and dry, gravelly soil to ensure optimum drainage. They were sited away from stagnating waters and polluting industries such as smelting houses and limekilns. To facilitate a good circulation of air, the building needed to be surrounded by an acre of land in which a garden could be laid out.[105]

The two-acre site selected by the managers of the Royal Infirmary of Edinburgh amply fulfilled all these criteria. The land was located in the southeastern part of the city, surrounded by gardens. The future building would overlook the Cowgate valley and face the crowded east–west ridge on which the city had settled for centuries. Location near the center of town and the university became key factors in its subsequent success as a center for both medical care and education.

After the foundation stone was laid on August 2, 1738, construction of the new hospital proceeded briskly, aided by donations of building materials, complimentary use of carts to transport them, and free work by masons and laborers who once a month returned one day's wages to the charity. Although the entire building was not finished until 1748, the first patients were able to move from the Little House into a section of the infirmary on December 1, 1741. Shortly thereafter, thirty-five beds arranged into a male and a female ward came into use, a number that increased gradually as the physical facilities were completed and additional financial aid was secured.

After its completion in 1748, the Royal Infirmary became a city landmark, "undoubtedly the most noble of the institutions in Edinburgh reared by the hand of charity."[106] Built of stone and lime, it resembled large aristocratic townhouses or hotels. Hospital structures, after all, were "meant to inspire with all the pomp of capitals and quoins, friezes and architraves."[107] Yet the Edinburgh infirmary was also a very functional building, "the whole laid out in a judicious and commodious manner."[108]

From surviving floor plans, the various rooms can be easily located.[109] On the ground floor, the central body of the house had an ample hall to receive visitors, patients, and healers and their students. This hall was surrounded by a number of vaulted rooms that housed the kitchen, pantry and larder, laundry, apothecary shop, and living quarters for the matron, keeper, and nurses. A second vaulted kitchen in the west wing was often used after 1755 by William Cullen (1710–1790), then professor of chemistry at the university, for carrying out the necessary experiments in connection with his "college of chemistry."[110]

Twelve separated cells on the ground floor were initially designed to shelter an equal number of "lunaticks," upper- or middle-class individuals judged to be "mad." The west wing contained two rooms for nurses, four cellars including two for storing coal, and a so-called deadroom for the temporary storage of recently deceased patients. The east wing, in turn, had a large consulting room for physicians and surgeons, the so-called governor's room, where decisions about admissions to the house were made during the day; it also served as a meeting room for the managers. A chamber for taking hot and cold baths, reserved for the patients, completed the first floor's arrangements.

The second story was reserved for medical cases housed in four wards. Two twenty-four-bed rooms located in the central building measured eighty-one by twenty-six feet and were adjacent to the central stairway emerging from the first-floor lobby. These stairs provided the main access to all four floors of the infirmary and were wide enough to accommodate the sedan chairs in which the patients were carried to their rooms. Passing through these wards to the wings, visitors would encounter on each side a smaller twelve-bed chamber, fifty by twenty-six feet, initially designated to house sick servants.

Both the third and fourth floors had similar arrangements, with the two larger wards on each side of the stairs and the smaller rooms in the wings. Surgical cases were kept on the fourth or attic floor in two wards built on each side of the amphitheater occupying the central area over the main stairway (see Figure 1.1). The domed room was described by a contemporary historian as "in the shape of a theatre, with benches rising on the three sides thereof from the floor, and galleries above, so disposed, that two or three hundred students and apprentices may conveniently see any operation performed."[111] Rooms located on both wings of the attic housed female patients who suffered from venereal diseases. Later, the managers temporarily authorized a lying-in ward for instructional reasons. On all floors, male patients were placed on the east side of the stairs and theater and females on the west.

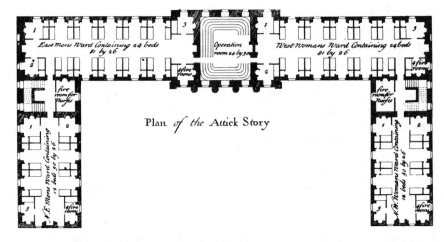

Figure 1.1. Floor plan of the infirmary, fourth story, 1740. From [John Stedman], *The History and Statutes of the Royal Infirmary of Edinburgh,* Edinburgh: Balfour & Smellie, 1778, n.p.

Beds were initially made of wood and replaced only in 1775 with iron bedsteads on casters. Each of them was large enough for just one patient and was, for ventilation purposes, located next to one of the large, eleven-foot-high windows. In the attic, where the ceiling was eight feet high, the windows were smaller. Another measure designed to avoid contagion was the distance of about six feet between beds and the strategic placement of fireplaces in the corners of rooms, to facilitate the circulation of air. All floors were tiled, using seven thousand unglazed paving tiles imported from Holland "to guard against fire, vermin, and stench," and the walls properly sashed and plastered to allow periodic whitewashing with limewater.[112]

A cupboard containing some of the patients' belongings and certainly a chamberpot was placed at the head of each bed, and curtains could be drawn around the bed "to form a kind of room." Each ward had two separate "fire rooms" with an open hearth and space enough to put up a single bed. In 1750 the back stairs of the building were converted into closets "for holding foul water and chamber pots that come out of the wards," a move that gained the hospital some welcome storage space and removed a major obstacle to the "sweet and clean" rooms envisioned by the managers.[113]

Two years later the hospital authorities approved the construction of a public bathhouse or "bagnio" featuring one cold and two hot water baths with their respective dressing rooms. This bathhouse, to be located on the ground floor of the west wing, was exclusively "intended for people of the city" and thus had its own independent entrance. The new enterprise was clearly intended to provide the hospital with additional revenues, since the prospective users of the facility had to pay a fee for bathing and being massaged by a retinue of "rubbers." Plans for the baths were originally proposed by Alexander Monro primus in 1748, after a similar venture organized first by the Royal College of Physicians and then by the Incorporation of Surgeons had been forced to close (in 1740) because of insufficient business. The managers, however, were counting heavily on the publicity generated by the activities of the infirmary to make their risky investment pay off. In 1754 they hired an architect, solicited subscriptions from future patrons, and then figuratively took the plunge.[114] The infirmary bagnio copied in part the marble splendor of its Roman and Renaissance predecessors, "finished in the neatest manner in all the other parts of its furniture." Regulations for the bathhouse were approved in 1756, stipulating the hours of business and fees to be charged.[115]

The grounds around the hospital allowed convalescent patients to breathe fresh air and get some exercise. South of the building were two public gardens at each wing, linked after 1768 by a gravel walk erected at the suggestion of the attending physicians.[116] To further ensure their privacy from the adjoining high school, patients were shielded by a high fence built a year later to discourage students from climbing into the infirmary property.[117]

Staff expansion

In the two decades preceding 1770, the hospital operated under a revised set of statutes approved in 1743 by the General Court of Contributors.[118] The increased complexity of its finances made it necessary to give the treasurer a small annual salary and hire a full-time accountant, who was entrusted with preparing the books. Given the influx of patients, the managers also created a new medical position, the "clerk of the house," a salaried house officer living on the premises and responsible for providing care in the absence of the attending physicians and surgeons. His responsibilities extended to include several administrative chores performed by the original clerk, such as keeping medical records. He now also inspected the students' tickets and dictated clinical cases to them.

In 1747 the hospital opened its own apothecary shop and employed an apothecary to prepare and dispense drugs for in-house and outpatient use. Medicines had hitherto been donated by the surgeons, who owned their own shops, but the financial burden became intolerable to those few attending the hospital in rotation. Another important innovation was the selection in 1751 of "two fixed physicians for the constant and daily attendance on the patients." The new "physicians in-ordinary" replaced the former clerk of the house, who went to occupy the post of apothecary. Both physicians had to live in the hospital, and they received their assignments and salary from the managers. The decision to create these jobs was prompted by the ever-expanding number of in-house patients in need of continuous supervision; they were not meant to replace the fellows from the College of Physicians, who continued to visit on rotation "once or twice a week, giving advice and assistance to the ordinary physicians." David Clerk and Colin Drummond, two young graduates of the local university and also fellows of the college, were the first to fill the new positions.[119]

The house doctors and visiting physicians and surgeons were aided by a number of newly appointed clerks who took up the administrative duties of the previous clerk of the house while also assuming responsibilities for the collection of fees from patients. The clerks were chosen from among the medical students who had already completed two sessions at the university; the jobs were limited to periods of two years, and the clerks had also to live on the premises.

With the hiring of a porter, a cook, and several nurses, the hospital acquired by 1770 a staff large enough to handle all the patients admitted to the house. The new appointees also took care of the expanding contingent of medical and surgical students who sought entrance to follow their teachers on rounds while also attending clinical lectures based on infirmary cases. Admissions between 1760 and 1770 nearly doubled, from 712 to 1,170 patients, and judging from the sale of tickets, so did student access to the wards.

Finances, 1770–1800

Voluntary hospitals depended largely on subscriptions, which in most cases accounted for 50%–75% of their total income. The rest was usually obtained through legacies, benefit performances, and a poor box. Fund-raising functions, such as the annual anniversary dinner, with its uplifting sermon, or special church collections were frequent. Some institutions even issued annual reports, printed pamphlets designed to project a favorable image to the public at large. These publications were crammed with favorable statistics and testimonials, contained a list of all subscribers, and made further appeals for money.[120]

In Edinburgh the minutes of the managers' meetings contained only occasional references to certain aspects of the infirmary's finances. In contrast with similar contemporary institutions, the Royal Infirmary did not initially rely on a large number of small contributors for its income. Only after 1796 did economic conditions in Britain and particularly Scotland force the authorities to broaden their appeals. In the infirmary's early years, most subscribers pledged and donated rather large amounts of money, often in the form of stock certificates in commercial enterprises, which became part of the hospital-owned capital yielding interest.

Not surprisingly, it was the interest received from commercial shares, beginning with stocks in the fishery company, that made up the largest source of hospital income (see Table 1.1).[121] Additional sums were received from the city of Edinburgh, which had borrowed the Scots Invalid Fund.[122] Until the last years of the century these interest payments yielded between 30% and 40% of total infirmary earnings, a welcome and regular source of money that helped cushion the fluctuating revenues from private philanthropy.

Because of their variable character, individual legacies and donations given to the infirmary were categorized by officials as extraordinary income. Among them were one-time bequests left by prominent Scottish aristocrats or merchants and some continuous benefactions, such as a fund established by the earl of Hopetoun for the care of incurable patients. Another endowment, initiated by a Mr. James Hunter, provided for the admission of servants.[123]

Of special interest was the legacy of Dr. Archibald Kerr, a Scottish physician who had died on the high seas during a voyage to England in 1750. In his will Kerr bequeathed to the infirmary his 420-acre estate on the island of Jamaica. The plantation, known as Redpen or Redhill, was carved out of valuable timberland and operated with twenty-five black slaves; it was located on the southern coast in Morant Bay, at some distance from Kingston.[124]

The managers were excited about this quite unexpected gift, and the minutes of their meetings during the next fifty years contain lengthy references to the property and a voluminous correspondence with the executors of the estate. In 1750 the plantation was apparently worth about £3,412, which included the value of slaves (about £2,115). It could be leased for about £218 per year, a sum that then represented close to 10% of the infirmary's earnings.[125]

Even after protracted negotiations with the proper authorities in Kingston, the managers actually received their rent only sporadically in the next decades. The long sea voyage delayed all official correspondence, while bureaucratic obstacles further aggravated the wait. Growing impatient, the officers of the infirmary finally decided in 1772 to negotiate a new lease for their property. The lengthy bargaining eventually succeeded in February 1774, when a Mr. Trecothrick signed a twenty-one-year lease by which he would pay a rent of £260 per year.[126] In 1798 the hospital advertised for a new lease but was forced to settle for a yearly rent of £300 offered by the former tenant. The Kerr estate remained in the possession of the infirmary for almost another century, providing a modest but predictable source of funds.

The infirmary gradually became an Edinburgh landlord through the purchase of properties located near the hospital. In the eighteenth century the procedure of buying dilapidated houses cheaply, repairing them, and then renting them out was already a profitable enterprise. Among these acquisi-

Table 1.1. Income of the infirmary, 1770–1800 (in pounds and shillings)

Income	1770	1775	1780	1785	1790	1795	1800
Interest	857.11	909.11	959.11	1,001.15	964.5	828.1	870.11
Legacies and donations	105.2	15.10	196.2	94.19	15.16	30.2	349.1
Rents	163.18	168.8	160.9	146.9	200.15	144.12	0
Jamaica property	218.11	258.14	260.0	260.0	260.0	260.0	409.13
Payments from soldiers and supernumeraries	287.17	169.7	193.13	297.19	193.1	218.0	357.17
Dividends from Edinburgh Assembly	150.0	183.5	105.11	97.5	0	0	0
Collections for sick servants	204.7	117.14	195.11	266.15	0	150.0	0
Ticket sales to students	412.13	356.9	387.19	740.5	831.1	720.16	800.2
Collection from baths	0	37.5	36.14	21.15	17.10	30.18	77.15
Charity box	74.4	4.4	11.9	0	20.5	0	0
Sick and wounded seamen	0	0	0	0	0	313.17	644.11
Dividends, bank stock	0	0	0	0	0	0	252.19
Subscriptions from contributors	0	0	0	0	0	0	260.18
Miscellaneous	113.3	10.10	19.10	9.3	334.5	79.10	58.12
Total	2,587.6	2,230.17	2,526.9	2,936.5	2,836.18	2,775.16	4,081.19

Source: Treasurer's Accounts, 1769–1795, 1796–1804, MSS Collection, Medical Archives, University of Edinburgh.

tions was Roehead's Brewery on Robertson's Close, which supplied the hospital with a product of somewhat inferior quality, if one gives credence to the patients' complaints. Not only did the managers seek income from their real estate transactions, but they simultaneously intended to control the immediate neighborhood and prevent construction of new buildings. Although the point was not expressly mentioned in their deliberations, the officials considered a higher population density around the hospital detrimental to proper ventilation and cleanliness, since tall buildings would hinder the free flow of air to the wards while their crowded inhabitants would produce dangerous filth and consequently miasma.

The rent collected from these properties was combined with money derived from leasing unused portions of the hospital itself. In fact, several unoccupied rooms were rented out at one time to a local apothecary, and in 1750 an entire ward on the top floor was converted into a printshop and warehouse.[127] The surviving documents remain silent about the impact on hospital routines of the new tenants, but it seems obvious that the infirmary managers were determined to use all available hospital space with profit and were even willing to put up with the inconveniences caused by such commercial dealings.

In 1755 the hospital decided to transfer the entire sum of £8,723 belonging to the Scots Invalid Fund to the city of Edinburgh and merely receive interest on this amount from the city fathers. Originally, the royal endowment was meant to help pay for the admission of soldiers, but now the hospital agreed to subsidize part of the cost. Accordingly, infirmary officials accepted a new arrangement whereby soldiers "certified to be proper objects by their Commander in Chief of his Majesty's forces in Scotland" were accepted into the house. While hospitalized, however, each soldier had to pay the sum of fourpence daily, the amount to be deducted from his pay by the army. Hopeful that they could thus admit a sizable number of paying customers, the managers authorized the use of sixty beds for sick soldiers and demanded from the government a supplemental salary for the two attending physicians, as reward "for the additional troubles."[128]

During that same year, 1755, the hospital authorities also petitioned the Town Council and the Presbytery of Edinburgh to authorize an annual collection "defraying the expense of twenty beds to be provided for the like number of servants belonging to families in town." Clearly the previous voluntary contributions subscribed for this purpose had proved insufficient, and more funds were needed. The money was to be collected at all the church doors of the city and suburbs on a prearranged Sunday, and ministers were urged to make the pertinent announcements, including strong pleas for donations, in their sermons.[129]

The first special collection brought £194 15s. Almost yearly thereafter similar appeals were made with equal success, each one specifically authorized by the Town Council and the church. In the 1770s the "Infirmary Sunday" was generally scheduled in the summer, during the middle or end of July, but by 1782, for unknown reasons, the date shifted to the end of February, and the event was soon neglected. Only two more collections were authorized before the end of the century, during 1788 and 1793.[130] In the early years, however, the cash obtained from these Sunday collections was as important as the income derived from the soldiers and other paying patients.

The sale of admission tickets to medical students and surgical apprentices became an increasing source of funds for the hospital. The practice began as early as 1730 and expanded in 1756 after courses of clinical lectures began to be delivered at the infirmary by university professors. An ordinary ticket costing 2 guineas allowed access to the wards for a period of three months to hear the lectures and to follow attending physicians on their prescribed rounds. "Perpetual" tickets, costing 7½ guineas to medical students and 5 guineas to surgical pupils, provided entrance to the institution for a whole year.[131] Income from the passes rose steadily in the century, especially after 1783, when the clinical course became a requirement for graduation from the medical school. In those last decades the tickets accounted for about 25% of the total hospital income, virtually doubling from £412 in 1770 to £800 by 1800 (see Table 1.2),

In January 1791 the managers received a letter from the commissioner of sick and hurt seamen asking permission to bring on shore in the neighboring port of Leith a number of ailing sailors, for the purpose of having the men conveyed to and treated in the infirmary. This event and similar later petitions finally resulted in a long-term agreement negotiated between hospital leaders and the British Admiralty.[132] By 1795 the Royal Navy stationed a permanent squadron in the Firth of Forth, and regular admission for sick and injured seamen became a reality. After some initial reluctance, the naval authorities paid per diem expenses and transportation costs to bring the men from Newhaven and Leith to Edinburgh.

Since substantial numbers of patients were involved, the managers first considered renting a nearby facility to house these sailors. Instead, they decided to build a new hospital wing with two wards while requisitioning beds in other parts of the hospital for additional admissions.[133] As in the case of hospitalized soldiers, infirmary officials were quick to realize the advantages of receiving regular payments from the government to cover all costs instead of trusting their revenues to the more uncertain flow of charitable subscriptions – particularly in a period of dwindling donations and growing deficits. In the war years between 1795 and 1800 the income derived from the Admiralty more than doubled, accounting at the turn of the century for 15% of total hospital earnings.[134]

Finally, two small items need to be briefly mentioned. One was the char-

Table 1.2. *Infirmary revenues*
from the sale of admission
tickets to medical students and
surgical apprentices, 1770–
1800 (in pounds and shillings)

1770	412.13	1786	660.19
1771	324.9	1787	737.2
1772	470.8	1788	707.14
1773	420.10	1789	669.18
1774	425.15	1790	831.1
1775	356.9	1791	702.19
1776	410.11	1792	916.2
1777	467.5	1793	906.13
1778	460.8	1794	838.8
1779	397.19	1795	720.16
1780	387.19	1796	856.16
1781	495.12	1797	877.5
1782	586.8	1798	846.16
1783	622.13	1799	852.0
1784	731.17	1800	800.2
1785	740.5		

Source: Treasurer's Accounts, 1769–
1795, 1796–1804, MSS Collection,
Medical Archives, University of
Edinburgh.

ity box, made of oak with iron fittings, placed inside the hospital to attract donations from grateful patients and their visitors. The other entry in the accounting ledgers was the revenues obtained from the public bathhouse completed in 1756. In spite of the previous failure of public baths, the bagnio at the infirmary became a successful enterprise that more than doubled its contribution to infirmary revenues between 1780 and 1800.[135]

During the last three decades of the eighteenth century expenditures recorded in the accounts appeared under eight separate categories (see Table 1.3). A brief study of the figures reveals that the cost of two items actually declined: the apothecary shop and the "incidents" or incidental expenses incurred in running the hospital. The former is noteworthy, since the infirmary significantly increased its yearly admissions, and thus its practitioners dispensed for a larger number of patients. In 1770 drug-related expenses amounted to 22% of the total hospital outlays for that year. Yet thirty years later the cost of running the apothecary shop had drastically fallen and constituted only 8% of all expenditures. The decrease cannot be ascribed to a hospital decision to stop issuing free medicines to outpatients, because these

Table 1.3. *Expenses of the infirmary, 1770–1800 (in pounds and shillings)*

Expenses	1770	1775	1780	1785	1790	1795	1800
Building and repairs	111.15	115.0	151.6	95.2	197.9	99.10	293.1
Maintenance	938.19	1,073.5	1,103.12	1,585.6	1,622.4	1,944.17	3,319.12
Apothecary shop	517.10	542.16	441.14	349.6	409.19	450.10	410.0
Plenishing and utensils	134.10	244.18	165.18	154.3	255.19	247.2	264.9
Coal and candles	204.3	183.8	226.18	110.0	287.7	214.16	369.13
Salaries	236.1	252.8	224.11	248.11	277.7	309.17	302.7
Incidentals	133.8	61.8	96.14	164.16	81.15	101.17	114.11
Public burdens	7.0	5.19	5.19	6.0	6.0	6.0	5.19
Totals	2,283.9	2,479.0	2,416.14	2,713.7	3,137.17	3,374.8	5,079.16
Surplus	304	249	110	223	301	599	998
Deficit							

Source: Treasurer's Accounts, 1769–1795, 1796–1804, MSS Collection, Medical Archives, University of Edinburgh. The figures and the addition are as reported in the original document.

restrictions were already implemented in the late 1750s, together with more meticulous dispensing procedures for inpatients.[136]

Staff salaries constituted between 6% and 10% of the total expenditures and actually increased very little during the period under study. From 1768 on, for example, day nurses received £3 per year and those working night shifts got twice that amount. These remunerations were increased in the 1790s after reports of frequent bribes and forced "gratuities" reached the managers. Nurses working regular hours during the day obtained £5 per year, and 6d per night was given to those attending the sick after sunset. By way of comparison, the attending physicians collected £50 yearly, the senior man getting a supplement from the Royal Army commander that boosted his total hospital income to £90 in 1789. The infirmary apothecary got a raise in 1790 that lifted his yearly salary from £40 to £60.[137]

In the decades before 1800 two other entries registered only moderate increases: "coal and candles," that is, fuel and light; and "plenishing," outfitting the hospital with the needed utensils, furnishings, and equipment. Together they accounted for 12%–15% of the total disbursements. Probably included under the latter rubric were a portable electric machine purchased in 1771 and the iron bedsteads ordered in 1775. Surgical items such as dressings, trusses, and prostheses may also have been included. During the 1750s, for instance, the managers often mentioned in their minutes the provision of wooden legs for amputees who had survived the surgical ordeal and were ready to be released from the hospital.[138]

The greatest increase between 1770 and 1800 was in the general category of "maintenance," which more than tripled during that period, virtually doubling in the last decade of the century. By 1800, indeed, 65% of all hospital costs were included under this entry. Presumably "maintenance" meant food and clothing, described as "the necessaries of life which do not admit of retrenchment," and all other supplies and services necessary to run the hospital with the exception of those specifically itemized by the accountant. Perhaps among them were the provision of water,[139] waste removal, laundry, bedding supplies, taxes and insurance premiums, and proper upkeep chores, such as painting and whitewashing the wards and surgical amphitheater. Certainly wine and beer occupied a prominent place among these rapidly escalating costs. Alcoholic beverages, the subject of repeated attempts to keep their consumption "within proper bounds," seemed to have occupied a special position, and their gradual restriction coincided with budget deficits experienced in the early 1790s.[140]

Expenses incurred in remodeling and repairing the building almost tripled in the three decades under scrutiny. However, these disbursements remained a fairly small and fluctuating item in the budget, never exceeding 6% of the total outlay. Among the possible projects included under this rubric was the refurbishing and enlargement of windows in the stairways in the interests of proper ventilation. Examples of other new ventures were the conversion of space under the back stairs into closets, a new gravel walk behind the infirmary ordered in 1768, and the construction of a higher wall to separate the hospital from the adjoining high school.

Finally, although consistently a negligible expenditure, the category "public burdens" deserves a brief comment. Included under the term were nonrefunded charges for transporting patients to and from the infirmary, as well as burial costs for people who had died in the hospital without having previously posted deposits to cover for such an eventuality. In 1791 the managers became concerned about the cost incurred in conveying a number of sailors by coach from their ships moored at Newhaven to Edinburgh; ship commanders were promptly provided with directions to deliver the sick directly to the hospital at navy expense to avoid further escalation of these "burdens."[141]

Under the careful supervision of its officials, the hospital managed to operate fairly well within the constraints imposed by its income. The hospital finances, aided by increasing ticket sales to students, regular government payments for the care of sick soldiers, and a steady income from interest and rents, remained in sound condition despite an occasional small shortage of funds. By 1790, however, the cost of running the institution produced the first significant deficit – about three hundred pounds, a figure that doubled the following year.

Hospital officials were quick to assert that the financial difficulties were not the result of poor management or extravagant spending. Rather, the mushrooming problems were rightly blamed on the "advanced charge of housekeeping" that every family experienced in those troubled financial times.[142] In response to the difficulties, such economies as a decrease in the consumption of wine and bed linens were instituted. Moreover, the authorities agreed to house a new contingent of paying patients – the sick sailors – and authorized two courses of clinical lectures per year designed to augment the sale of student tickets.

Conditions did not improve in spite of these measures. At an extraordinary meeting held on June 15, 1795, the managers of the infirmary seriously considered the possibility of curtailing hospital services by limiting new admissions and closing down several wards.[143] The move was supported by physicians such as James Gregory, himself a manager and university lecturer at the hospital. The mission of the institution was to serve a limited number of sick persons well rather than to admit indiscriminately all those who sought entrance, thereby straining the available resources and bed capacity. If the finances were insufficient, Gregory reasoned, it was more humane to keep many of the sick poor out of the hospital altogether than to provide them with inadequate care and to create a greater danger for them through hospital-acquired infections.[144]

To alleviate the deepening financial crisis, the commander of the army was contacted and asked to increase the per diem payments made by hospitalized soldiers. In addition, hospital officials finalized their contract with the Royal Navy. But these measures were not enough. Faced with the crucial decision to "abridge the benefits of this institution," the managers unanimously resolved to hold off on closing any part of it; first they would "publicly state its situation and give an opportunity to the opulent and humane to contribute to its support."[145]

The infirmary initiated a "scheme for the subscription of small sums of money to be annually contributed for this purpose." The proposed rate, "without meaning to set bounds to benevolence," was to be "a sum not less than half a guinea nor higher than one guinea yearly, to be continued during the pleasure of each subscriber." The first official subscription was apparently opened in 1796, but a list of contributors was not made available until the year 1801. Published as part of an annual report in the following year, the list contained 226 subscribers of one guinea each and an additional 61 persons who gave half that amount. In thanking the donors, the managers stated that the new source of funds "enabled them to meet all the increased expenses without restricting the number of patients or diminishing the benefits of the institution in any instance whatever."[146]

The new century presented the hospital authorities with a major challenge: increase income or sharply reduce services. "I do not believe the charity of the people is diminishing," argued James Gregory, concluding that "for their sake I hope it is increasing too, as it will cover a multitude of their sins."[147] Whether more wealthy Edinburgh "sinners" decided to atone for their wrongdoings is not entirely clear, although the hospital seems to have muddled through the difficulties. Public subscriptions were clearly not the panacea they were made out to be in the various appeals. In 1800 the collected monies represented only 6% of total income, equivalent to the rent being collected from the Kerr estate in Jamaica. Like similar institutions in London and the provinces at the turn of the century, the Royal Infirmary of Edinburgh experienced financial difficulties as competition for charitable donations and wartime austerity predictably exacted their toll.[148]

Registration system

In his writings, Bellers admonished physicians to collect and preserve hospital experiences with the help of casebooks. A contemporary, Francis Clifton, member of the Royal College of Physicians of London, suggested a similar record-keeping device "as the plainest and surest way of practicing and improving physick."[149] Clifton's "general medical table" contained columns in which to record the age, sex, temperament, and occupation of the patient, followed by a description of the presenting symptoms listed in the form of a diary. Another column registered the various treatments given in response to "morbid phenomena," and a final line summarized the outcome. The author was convinced that if physicians adopted such a log instead of trusting their experience to memory, "in time they will come to know diseases so perfectly that it will be impossible for them to miss of their reward."[150]

The voluntary hospital movement, for its part, greatly encouraged registration systems. One reason, of course, was that infirmaries were accountable to their subscribers and therefore kept accurate records of all their activities to justify investments and expenditures. Most boards of governors or managers were partly composed of lawyers and businessmen who were proud of their administrative sophistication and prudence in working for the public good. To carry out their mandate, these administrators hired an army of clerks whose mission it was to list all transactions and resolutions, respond to petitions, write letters and reports, copy writs, and set down the minutes of frequent meetings.

The number of patients admitted, the percentage of those cured or relieved, and mortality figures were important components of the data being generated. Managers could use them to illustrate their charitable works and promote further donations. Thus among the earliest rules enacted for the management of Edinburgh's Hospital for the Sick Poor in 1728 was a provision that "a register or record be kept in the hospital, in which is to be entered the names of all patients that shall be taken in, the parish of their birth or residence, their age, disease, when taken in, when dismissed, and whether cured or dead."[151] This *general register,* to be known later as the General Register of Patients, was used at the end of the year to prepare a report containing the total number of patients cured, recovered, dead, or dismissed for other reasons.[152]

According to infirmary rules the General Register was supplemented by another ledger "in which the physicians are to write all their prescriptions and directions concerning the patients."[153] This *prescription book* was intended to be one of the key documents for the internal administration of the hospital, since the medical orders were executed by the housekeeper and her nurses. Moreover, the items so ordered had to be copied onto lists for purchase from local drug shops or compounded by the in-house apothecary. A contemporary source described this daybook as formed "of a few sheets of paper stitched together, in which under the name of the patients and number of their bed, he daily writes the prescriptions and the directions as to diet and regimen."[154]

A third document not mentioned in the original rules was an *admissions' book.* As will be seen later, physicians were required to decide whether an individual patient was a "proper" candidate for hospital care, and the managers wanted to make sure that each subscriber did not exceed his allotment of sponsored admissions. Therefore the book listed "the dates or times when persons applied for admittance, the name of the petitioners, names of distempers, names of recommenders, cause of non-admission, and the times of admission."[155]

The basic clinical record at the Royal Infirmary of Edinburgh was the *ward journal*. This large volume was always kept on a desk that moved on casters, and "the clerk inserts every circumstance of the patient's case as dictated to him by the physicians, whom he attends for that purpose from bed to bed." This journal was apparently divided into seventeen columns:

The first contains the dates of the year, month and day; the second, the number of the bed wherein the patient lies; third, operation of the medicines; fourth, intervening symptoms; fifth, pulse; sixth, thirst; seventh, appetite; eighth, spittle; ninth, tongue; tenth, sweat; eleventh, urine; twelfth, faeces; thirteenth, ordinary symptoms; fourteenth, supervening symptoms; fifteenth, food; sixteenth, drink; and the seventeenth, medicines.[156]

Such a comprehensive management record of individual patients was supplemented by a *ward ledger* that summarized information from the ward journal. "Every patient has an opening left for them," commented the contemporary informant, "with the number of their bed and their name at the head." From the time of admission, when "an exact description of the patient's case was entered," the clerk added "daily from the Journal all that happens and the prescriptions for them while they continue in the house." On the last page, the ledger also had "an index of the several patients and diseases mentioned in it."[157]

Together with investment transactions and inventories of household items, purchase of provisions and payment of salaries, all medical records were available for inspection. The infirmary rules specified that "every donor to the hospital shall have free access to, and inspection of the books and records of the hospital, that they may offer their advice to the managers if anything occurrs to them, for the benefit and advantage thereof."[158] Subscribers had the right to check on the fortunes of their favorite charity; it remains unclear, however, whether many of them exercised such a prerogative. The privilege even disregarded medical confidentiality, although most of the donors seem to have been content with hearing or reading the reports prepared by the managers.

As the hospital expanded, the registration system became more complex and thus frequently broke down. The proliferation of wards, including those for servants, soldiers, and venereal and country patients, increased the num-

Table 1.4. *Official statistics of the infirmary, 1760–1800*

	1760	1761	1762	1763
Total no. patients	840	868	754	744
No. admissions	712	735	645	606
No. inpatients Jan. 1	128	133	109	138
Total no. discharges	685	736	571	594
No. cured	557	554	358	460
% cured	81.3	75.2	62.6	77.4
No. relieved	68	137	74	54
% relieved	9.9	18.6	12.7	9.0
No. dismissed by desire	50	31	98	48
No. dismissed incurable	10	14	26	21
No. dismissed for irregularities	0	0	16	11
No. ordinary patients	—	—	350	477
No. supernumerary patients	—	—	—	18
No. servants	—	—	158	127
No. soldiers	—	—	242	119
No. died in hospital	22	23	45	36
Hospital mortality (%)	3.1	3.0	7.3	5.7

	1770	1771	1772	1773	1774	1775
Total no. patients	1,302	1,599	1,590	1,882	1,884	1,962
No. admissions	1,170	1,454	1,447	1,709	1,696	1,795
No. inpatients Jan. 1	132	145	143	173	188	167
Total no. discharges	1,100	1,390	1,363	1,615	1,655	1,717
No. cured	791	1,071	1,078	1,392	1,410	1,560
% cured	72	77	79	86.1	85.1	90.8
No. relieved	188	206	180	158	146	101
% relieved	17	14.8	13.2	9.7	8.8	5.8
No. dismissed by desire	91	90	84	39	87	40
No. dismissed incurable	7	12	10	21	8	8
No. dismissed for irregularities	23	11	11	5	4	8
No. dismissed as improper	—	—	—	—	—	—
No. dismissed with advice	—	—	—	—	—	—
No. ordinary patients[a]	938	1,042	1,086	1,150	1,157	1,344
No. supernumerary patients[a]	45	27	41	99	87	80
No. servants[a]	93	125	133	184	193	204
No. soldiers[a]	226	405	330	449	447	334
No. died in hospital	57	66	54	79	62	61
Hospital mortality (%)	4.3	4.1	3.4	4.1	3.3	3.1

1764	1765	1766	1767	1768	1769
822	832	858	910	1,094	1,259
708	705	738	780	975	1,104
114	127	120	130	119	155
655	671	687	739	897	1,066
529	528	495	565	666	793
80.7	78.6	72.0	76.4	74.2	74.3
38	56	75	68	91	85
5.8	8.3	10.9	9.2	10.1	10.7
63	68	86	88	120	161
16	7	13	4	7	14
9	12	18	14	13	13
559	507	562	618	721	872
33	33	28	20	37	39
114	174	110	125	102	99
115	117	157	146	234	249
40	41	41	52	42	61
5.7	5.7	5.6	6.5	4.4	5.4

1776	1777	1778	1779	1780	1781	1782	1783	1784	1785
1,851	1,730	2,066	2,112	2,268	2,206	2,192	2,141	1,897	1,907
1,668	1,595	1,936	1,961	2,100	2,025	2,023	1,987	1,735	1,737
183	135	130	151	168	181	169	154	162	170
1,659	1,548	1,803	—	2,011	1,963	1,944	1,894	1,640	1,651
1,375	1,260	1,582	—	1,358	1,514	1,353	1,339	1,173	1,274
82.8	81.3	87.7	—	67.5	77.1	69.5	70.6	71.5	77.1
146	157	122	—	255	222	252	224	171	170
8.8	10.1	6.7	—	12.6	11.3	12.9	11.8	10.4	10.2
118	116	86	—	235	129	161	127	139	76
11	2	5	—	2	28	69	93	67	—
9	13	8	—	33	11	9	13	10	14
—	—	—	—	128	59	100	98	80	70
—	—	—	—	—	—	—	—	—	47
1,160	1,122	1,082	—	—	—	—	—	—	—
72	64	148	—	—	—	—	—	—	—
186	196	200	—	—	—	—	—	—	—
433	348	636	—	—	—	—	—	—	—
57	52	87	—	76	74	94	85	87	103
3.0	3.0	4.2	—	3.3	3.3	4.2	3.9	4.5	5.4

Table 1.4 *(cont.)*

	1786	1787	1788	1789	1790	1791
Total no. patients	1,986	1,922	1,874	1,977	1,896	1,685
No. admissions	1,822	1,768	1,730	1,830	1,768	1,543
No. inpatients Jan. 1	164	154	144	147	128	142
Total no. discharges	1,748	1,672	1,624	1,769	1,684	1,417
No. cured	1,354	1,242	1,269	1,328	1,185	992
% cured	77.4	74.2	78.1	75.0	70.3	70.0
No. relieved	166	226	219	230	274	220
% relieved	9.4	13.5	13.4	13.0	16.2	15.5
No. dismissed	105	89	39	82	109	94
No. dismissed incurable	—	—	—	—	—	—
No. dismissed for irregu- larities	11	16	—	5	7	9
No. dismissed as improper	46	52	59	63	53	64
No. dismissed with advice	66	47	38	61	56	38
No. died in hospital	84	106	103	80	70	103
Hospital mortality (%)	4.2	5.5	5.4	4.0	3.6	6.1

a These categories were not distinguished after 1778.
Note: Dashes indicate no data.
Sources: Scots Magazine; Infirmary Minute Books; patient registers.

ber of journals and ledgers to be kept. Total admissions to the house in the 1750s fluctuated around five hundred patients per year, a far cry from the thirty-five accepted into the Little House two decades earlier. Still, the information abstracted from all journals and ledgers needed to be periodically presented to the managers for their analysis and for transmittal to the court of contributors and the public at large. The latter task was assigned to the *Scots Magazine,* a popular monthly publication covering political, social, and literary events (see Table 1.4).[159]

By 1753 the managers demanded that ward journals "be laid upon the table" for inspection at their monthly meetings, and two years later the clerks were even barred from furnishing the abstracts directly to *Scots Magazine* without a prior audit by the managers.[160] Though the minutes of the meetings remain silent about the reasons for this new interest in medical statistics, it seems likely that fear of clerical errors and omissions was at the root of the revised procedures. In fact, on January 4, 1762, one of the hospital clerks was fired for not having transferred information from the ward ledgers to the General Register. Henceforth, the latter document had also to be presented to the managers at their monthly meetings.[161]

The task of generating accurate medical records grew more complex in the ensuing decades as annual hospital admissions soared near the two thousand mark. Already in 1770 the managers had exposed a series of delays in

1792	1793	1794	1795	1796	1797	1798	1799	1800
1,734	2,060	1,920	1,766	1,727	1,768	—	1,928	2,005
1,569	1,909	1,788	1,620	1,560	1,606	—	1,789	1,836
165	151	132	146	167	162	175	139	169
1,498	1,843	1,670	1,504	1,485	1,500	—	1,652	1,724
1,012	1,277	1,206	1,062	1,042	1,103	—	1,243	1,305
67.5	69.2	72.2	70.6	70.1	73.5	—	75.2	75.6
263	236	204	173	187	163	—	210	128
17.5	12.8	12.2	11.5	12.5	10.8	—	12.7	7.4
115	163	115	83	114	90	—	47	81
—	—	—	—	—	—	—	—	—
11	42	29	65	16	29	—	50	50
63	102	79	98	83	89	—	62	119
34	23	37	23	43	26	—	40	41
85	85	104	95	80	93	—	107	117
4.9	4.1	5.4	5.3	4.6	5.2	—	5.5	5.8

the transfer of cases to ward ledgers and decided not to accept the clerks' excuse that they were overwhelmed with "too much business."[162] Then, in the abstract prepared for the year 1775, the clerks publicly admitted that "there were besides about forty other patients admitted last year whose names were not inserted because the admission papers were lost."[163] Another significant gap in the reporting took place in 1779, when the clerks omitted all diagnoses and discharges and later abandoned their task of writing up the General Register. No further entries were made until January 1, 1780.[164]

Availability of the infirmary's Minute Books after 1789 allows a further glance at the registration woes. At an extraordinary meeting of managers held November 9, 1789, it was revealed that records for all surgical cases between January and May of that year had been lost. In addition, ward journals for several male sections on the medical floor were also missing, and the transcript of cases into the ledgers had fallen significantly behind schedule. "We regret much the loss of the several journal books," declared the managers in their minutes; "this is an evil from which it may be difficult to derive a remedy." One of the attending physicians, presumably Henry Cullen (son of William), was put in charge of a committee charged with investigating the deficiencies of the registration system. An amanuensis was hired to relieve the busy clerks and "insert cases which remained uncopied."[165] Monthly reports on the conditions of ward journals and ledgers were demanded by the managers throughout the 1790s, but judging from transcriptions to the General Register, matters continued to deteriorate until the end of the century.

General Register of Patients

Surviving volumes of the General Register suggest that its composition was a two-step procedure, using information obtained from the admission book as well as from the ward journals and ledgers. Clerks responsible for copying the data would first inscribe the patient's name, entrance date, and institutional destination. Each patient received a number reflecting the order of admission. The clerks would periodically return to the register, perhaps in anticipation of a managers' meeting, to fill out for each patient the diagnosis, date of release, and discharge status from information contained in the ward ledgers.

By 1770 the General Register routinely omitted the parishes of origin, substituting for them information about the type of patient admitted as well as institutional destination. Under the heading "quality" the clerk indicated whether patients were servants, soldiers, seamen, or medical and surgical "ordinary." Servants were generally entered together with their masters; foreign sailors of Russian nationality in the late 1790s were listed simply as "Russian"; and paying patients admitted into the ordinary ward were recorded as such.[166] Another category, "clinical," was reserved for persons assigned to the teaching ward. Finally, there were from time to time "surgical accidents," emergency admissions destined for the surgical ward (see Figure 1.2 and Tables 1.5 and 1.6).

In the early 1770s the register employed a very large number of diagnostic categories (see Table 1.7), but gradually many of them fell into disuse or were replaced by others.[167] By contrast, the number of discharge categories expanded. Patients could leave the hospital either "cured" or "relieved," "by desire" or as "irregulars" (meaning expulsion for violation of hospital rules). There were also "incurables" and of course a few listed as "dead." Beginning January 1, 1774, the register added another category, "improper," indicating the dismissal of patients whose ailments were not considered susceptible to hospital treatment. On January 1, 1785, the category "incurable" was dropped and replaced by "discharged with advice," a measure possibly designed to bolster the favorable image of infirmary statistics, since it shifted emphasis away from the limitations of medical intervention.

The recording procedure outlined here would explain the omission of diagnosis, date of dismissal, and discharge status in about 10% of all entries contained in the General Register. Perhaps clerks simply could not retrieve the information, because of incomplete or deficient ward journals and ledgers, or perhaps they just did not have enough time to transcribe the information. Since clerical appointments were limited to two years, many clerks were involved in the discontinuous recording process, a difficulty that promoted further error. Registrations for the year 1800 were particularly defi-

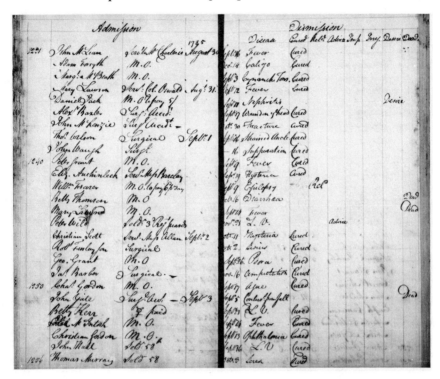

Figure 1.2. General Register of Patients: sample page, August 1785

cient, with over 30% of the entries lacking data about diagnosis and hospital discharge.[168]

Questions regarding the methodology employed in setting down the information must also be raised. At times diagnoses recorded in the register show a definite preference for certain categories, which became unusually frequent as if clerks simply assigned them almost at random, without checking the ward journals and ledgers. Between July and December 1775 the transcriber continually inserted "pains," "stomach complaint," and "erruption" in the appropriate diagnostic column, to the extent that these labels made up close to 30% of all the diagnoses listed.

One can only speculate about the deficiencies of the General Register. Were clerks so overworked that they were forced to place patient care ahead of registration tasks? Were the distortions simply a reflection of haste or actual indifference, since only the ward journal was relevant in the daily management of patients? Could some of the omissions have been deliberate, to suppress unfavorable information? The General Register was of great importance to the hospital. It brought together information needed by man-

Table 1.5. *General Register of Patients: sample of entries for the year 1770*

| Names | Quality | Admission | Disease | Date | Dismission | | | | | | Remaining |
					Cured	Relieved	Incurable	Dead	Irregular	By desire	Jan. 1771
Thom. Gascal	Soldier	Jan. 1, 1770	Venereal dis.	Feb. 1	Cured						
Sarah Mung	Medical ordinary	Ditto	Oedematous	Jan. 28							
Agnes Ritchie	Med ord	Jan. 2	Veneral dis.	Mar. 14						By desire	
Herman Samuel	Med ord	Do	Cancerous	Mar. 6							
Eliz. Anderson	Med ord	Do	Rheumatism	Jan. 19	Cured						
John Thomson	Chyrurgical	Jan. 3	Erysipelas upon his arm	Feb. 2	Cured						
John Reynolds	Soldier	Do	Veneral dis.	Feb. 20	Cured						
Wm. Coats	Soldier	Do	Peripneumony after measles	Jan. 6				Dead			
Eliz. Tait	Clinical	Jan. 4	Rheumatism	Jan. 9	Cured						
Don. Cameron	Med. ord	Do	Cough after measles	Jan. 26							
John Hamilton	Med ord	Do	Veneral dis..	Feb. 2	Cured						
Marg. Nicolson	Chyrur servt.	Do	Febrile complaints	Jan. 15	Cured						
James Harris	Med ord	Jan. 5	Fever	Jan. 24	Cured						
Andrew Tolmy	Clinical	Do	Ague	May 26	Cured						
Wm. Douglass	Clinical	Do	Nephritis	Jan. 22						By desire	
Euphemia Lees	Med ord	Jan. 6	Veneral dis.	Mar. 15	Cured						
Christian Stewart	Med ord	Do	Veneral dis.	Feb. 10					Irregular		

Table 1.6. *General Register of Patients: sample of entries for the year 1790*

				Dismission							
	Admission	Date	Disease	Cured	Relieved	Advice	Improper	Irregular	Desire	Dead	Remaining
Robert Burns	Surg accident	Mar. 6	Fracture	Cured							
Thos. Melbourne	M.O.	Mar. 9	Scrophula				Improper				
Thos. Holt	So. 35th	Mar. 10	Gonorrhea	Cured							
Sam Robinson	Do	Mar. 31	Lues	Cured							
George Taylor	Do	Mar. 23	Do	Cured							
Nath Gore	Do	Apr. 2	Do	Cured							
Robt. Gillespie	Svt. Mr. Drysdale	7 Mar. 11	Swelled testis	Cured							
Will Simons	So 10th	7 Mar. 31	Dis'd wrist			Advice					
Peggy Stuart	M/O	8 Apr. 16	Lues	Cured							
Will Jamieson	Clinical	8 Mar. 16	Dyspepsia	Cured							
John Balks	Clinical	8 Apr. 8	Ague	Cured							
Thos. Tweadale	Surg accident	9 Mar. 13	Fract cranium								
Jean Thomson	M/O	9 Mar. 14	Gonorrhea	Cured							
James Smith	So invalid	9 May 11	Ulcer of leg	Cured							
John Graham	M/O	9 June 1	Suppuration of testis	Cured							
Janet Reid	Surgical	9 Apr. 5	Hectica							Dead	
Isabel Ross	M/O	9 Apr. 2	Hydrothorax							Dead	
Duncan Robinson	M/O	9 Mar. 20	Ditto		Relieved						
James Smith	So invalid	9	Ulcer of leg	Cured							
Euphemia Sutherland	M/O	10 Mar. 17	Phthisis		Relieved						

370

380

Table 1.7. *General Register of Patients: disease categories employed in 1770*

Abscess in eye	Dropsy and pthisical	Hectic and foul ulcer	Pain of side and fever	Sibbens	Swelled arm from blood letting
Abscess on back	Dropsy ascites	Hemiplegia	Pain of stomach	Sinous ulcer	Swelled knee
Abscess on haunch	Dysenteria	Hemorrhoids	Pain of stomach and belly	Slight fever	Swelled leg
Ague	Dyspnea and dropsy	Hernia (inguinal)	Pain of stomach and bowels	Slow fever	Swelled testicle
Amaurosis	Dyspnea and sore throat	Haemoptisis	Pain of stomach	Slow fever and eruption	Swelling of eye
Anasarcous swellings	Dyspnea and stomach complaint	Hydrocele	Pain of stomach with cough	Smallpox	Swimming of head
Aneurysm	Epilepsy	Hydrops pectoris	Pain over whole body	Sore arm	Tertian intermittent
Angina	Eruption	Hypochondria	Palsy	Sore breast	Toothache
Ascites	Eruption on face	Hysteria	Palsy and swelling of ankle	Sore eye	Tumour on belly
Blind	Eruption on legs	Hysteria and cough	Paralysis	Sore foot	Tumour on neck
Bruise	Erysipelas	Incontinent with urine	Pectoral complaint	Sore knee	Tumour on side
Bruise on head	Exostosis	Inflammatory fever	Peripneumony	Sore leg	Tumour on thigh
Bruised arm	Febrile complaint	Intermittent fever	Phthisis; phthisical	Sore thigh	Ulcer behind ear
Bruised breast	Fever	Irregular ague	Phthisis pulmonalis	Sore throat	Ulcer of leg
Cancerous breast	Fever and cutaneous eruption	Irregular menses	Pleuratic complaints	Sore throat and headache	Ulcer on ankle
Cancerous lip	Fever and delirium	Ischuria	Pleurisy	Sore on ankle	Ulcer on arm
Carious jaw	Fever and diarrhea	Itch	Pleurisy and venereal disease	Sores on arm	Ulcer on finger
Cataract	Fever and pain of breast	Jaundice	Pneumatism	Sore on breast	Ulcer on head
Catarrh	Flooding after	Lethargy		Sores on eye	Ulcer on leg
Catarrh and fever		Lumbago		Sore on face	Ulcer on neck
Cholic and flatulency		Lust, constant and intense		Sore on foot	Ulcers
Consumption					Urinary complaint
Convulsive fits					

Convulsive paroxysms
Cough
Cough and breathlessness
Cough and diarrhea
Cough and dyspnea
Cough and fever after measles
Cough and rheumatism
Cough and slow fever
Cough and spitting of blood
Cough and stomach
Cough and swelling of belly
Diarrhea
Discharge from ear
Disorder of mind
Disordered imagination
Dog bite
Dropsy

miscarriage
Fluor albus
Flying pains
Fracture
Gonorrhea
Gravel
Gutta serena
Head and stomach complaint
Headache
Headache and cough
Headache and deafness
Headache and delirium
Headache and fever
Headache and ophthalmia
Headache and pain of joints
Headache and sore
Headache and tumour on thigh

Malignant ulcer
Measles
Melancholia
Nephritic complaint
Nephritis
Obstructed menses
Oedematous swellings
Ozaena
Ophthalmia
Pain in limbs
Pain in loins
Pain in shoulder joint
Pain of belly
Pain of bones
Pain of breast and rheumatism
Pain of breast with cough
Pain of head and back
Pain of joints
Pain of knee and stomach
Pain of side
Pain of side and cough

Profluvium mensium
Purulent disclosure by stool
Quotidian intermittent
Rheumatic complaints
Rheumatic fever
Rheumatism
Rheumatism and stomach complaint
Rose on face
Rose on leg
Schirrous testicle
Schirrous tongue
Sciatica
Scorbutic blotches
Scorbutic complaints
Scorbutic eruption
Scorbutic sores
Scorbutic ulcer
Scorbutus; scurvey
Scrophulous swellings
Serous eruption

Sore on hand
Sore on head
Sores on leg
Sore on nose
Sores on thigh
Cancerous sore
Fistulous sore
Scrophulous sore
Spina ventosa
Sprained ankle
Sprained thigh
Stiff hand from venesection
Stomach complaint
Stomach complaint and back pain
Stomach and bowel complaint
Stone
Stump after amputation
Suppressed menses
Swelled and discolored leg

Urinary and pectoral complaint
Venereal disease
Venereal disease and dropsy
Venereal disease and worms
Venereal pains
Vomiting
Vomiting of blood
Vomiting of purulent matter
White swelling
White swelling of knee
Worms
Worms and stomach complaint
Wound on foot
Wound on head
Wound on leg

agers, subscribers, and the public to support claims that the infirmary was indeed carrying out its benevolent function. Annual reports and, especially, favorable mortality statistics swayed opinion in important ways. Yet the increasing volume of patients played havoc with an accounting system devised decades earlier for a much smaller hospital population. There is no doubt that the managers were aware of the problems besetting the register. They tried, in a limited way, to correct them by further pressuring already overworked students, instead of changing procedures or hiring more clerks. However, having declared a fiscal emergency because of wartime conditions, infirmary officials were probably prevented from giving the problem a higher priority.[169]

Regulations

People hospitalized at the Edinburgh infirmary were subjected to strict regulations instituted "for better preservation of good order and harmony among the patients." In addition to being "precise and regular" in taking their medicines and eating the prescribed dietary items, inmates were required to keep their cupboards and beds in order. Tobacco smoking was prohibited.[170]

Apart from maintaining "general silence" in the wards while the attending physicians and surgeons made their rounds, patients were asked to avoid disturbances by talking in low voices to each other and the visitors. Yet there seems to have been quite a bit of "accidental" noise in the wards. Casebooks contain a number of reports about "furious" and "impetuous" delirium in patients suffering from high fevers. Constant screaming "in the night" and unruly behavior even requiring waistcoats were noted. One blind man became so violent that he had to be removed to the "iron room," meaning one of the cells on the ground floor originally reserved for lunatics.[171] Other patients were prevented from sleep by their own coughing and wheezing, as well as the epileptic or hysterical fits of their neighbors in the ward.[172] The hysterical attacks were often triggered by another patient's fit of a similar nature or, in one case, "induced by the crowd around her" after the physician's visit.[173]

There were few opportunities for social amenities at the infirmary, although in 1781 funds were obtained to erect a "set of rooms for the entertainment of the public," primarily to chat with other patients and their visitors.[174] Early bedtime plunged the wards into total darkness and the silence was interrupted only by whispers of patients in "friendly converse"[175] or shouts of those quarreling among themselves or with nurses.[176] Cullen commented to his students about a young boy hospitalized at the infirmary even though he was "of a condition above the vulgar, with more delicacy, attention and care, and had been bred a little better." Facing a ward full of strangers, the new patient was "struck with considerable dread and awe" and hid in his bed "not daring to look out from the chamber." A subsequent encounter with an armed soldier in the house only added to his terror.[177]

Violation of these rules was sufficient cause for immediate dismissal because of "irregularities." Some patients refused to take their medications, either by pretending to feel better or by bribing the nurses who dispensed them. Others balked at some of the physical healing measures, including enemas, insertion of catheters, electricity, cauterization, and head shaving.[178] Equally punishable were unauthorized visits into town to visit relatives. Although the infirmary granted temporary passes to convalescent patients, others took advantage of the privilege, especially for "convivial" reunions in nearby taverns.

A greater source of trouble was the constant smuggling of food into the hospital by well-meaning friends and family members. Addressing himself to John Hope, one of the attending physicians, a critic writing in 1782 remarked: "What is refused to your patients by the frugality of your temper, or your ignorance of the human system, is often supplied to them by the humanity and common sense of their friends."[179] Visitors brought tea, jelly, and biscuits to supplement the breakfast porridge. Apparently they did so "without trouble," meaning that both nurses and clerks tended to overlook the infractions if they could share the smuggled goods and likewise evade the scant institutional victuals. Problems generally started when less concealable items, such as bread, potatoes, and liquor, came to the attention of the matron and the smell of fresh herrings or their remains drew attention from attending physicians during rounds.[180]

Visitors also flocked to the hospital when patients were seriously ill or dying. "It is a custom in this country that people must not be allowed to die out of sight of their friends," observed Cullen, as he found "six or seven gossips in the room and as many candles lighted up."[181] Given the fears of insufficient ventilation and collection of contagion, such assemblies of friends expressing social solidarity were quickly dispersed in accordance with the new tenets of environmental hygiene.

All regulations were printed and posted on the walls of the admission room and in each ward. When violations occurred, managers generally ordered the rules read to remaining patients and nurses, pointing out the penalties applicable to those who disobeyed.

Complaint procedures

The infirmary's rules regarding patient behavior also contained an appendix listed as *nota bene* ("observe particularly"): "If any of the patients shall think themselves aggrieved, they are at liberty to complain either to the managers at their monthly meetings or the physicians and surgeons in their daily circuits."[182] Thus, to protect patients from abuse by hospital staff members, a system was established whereby inmates could present their grievances to the authorities. Since the infirmary also had statutes that prescribed monthly inspections of the wards by two ordinary managers elected official visitors, hospitalized patients possessed a number of opportunities to express themselves.[183]

Unfortunately, the official minutes of the meetings held by the managers between 1750 and 1800 (one volume from 1775 to 1789 is missing) contain only sporadic instances of such complaints – about articles of diet, abusive nurses, and dirty bedclothing. As pointed out by a contemporary observer, gratitude and awe hindered most patients from criticizing the conditions in the hospital. Perhaps more important was the fear of reprisal and the formalities necessary to document charges.[184]

Conclusion

The impressive development of the Edinburgh infirmary before 1770 and after owes a great deal to the ideology that guided the Scottish Enlightenment, concerned as it was with the social and economic improvement of society.[185] The provincial elite that was active in numberless literary and philosophical societies strongly supported the hospital building and development program. What began almost as an excuse to appear socially concerned grew over the decades into a complex enterprise that in a unique way embodied some of the most important goals pursued by the progressive Edinburgh leadership.

Among the donors and managers were the aristocrats, literati, lawyers, physicians, surgeons, and merchants associated with the Select Society, the Philosophical Society, and numerous less formal clubs.[186] As the Edinburgh Medical School reached new levels of popularity and recognition throughout Europe, the affiliated infirmary was not far behind. It was a city landmark, proudly admired by local citizens and foreign visitors, another Scottish achievement internationally recognized. Here then was a monument reflecting humanistic concerns for the lower sectors of Scottish society, an optional resource free of charge for the ill and injured. Never mind that its impact on local health conditions was virtually nil. Everybody knew that diseases were too formidable, the power of medicine quite limited.[187] Yet the very existence of such an institution, along with the efforts of the administrators and professionals who ran it, loudly proclaimed that the ruling oligarchy cared.

Despite temporary setbacks, the infirmary had also become an economic asset to, not a drain on, the financial fortunes of Edinburgh. For one, it began attracting royal funds for the care of soldiers and sailors. Students, to a considerable extent non-Scottish, paid substantial fees for gaining access to ward rounds and lectures. City government was the beneficiary of loans using hospital funds for its operations. Finally, donors and subscribers outside Scotland and a few paying patients also helped finance the establishment. Most important, on the educational front, the infirmary provided virtually all the local opportunities for the clinical training of medical students and allowed university professors to carry out limited research in the teaching ward.

With such an awareness of the philosophical roots of hospital philanthropy and knowledge concerning the administrative organization of eighteenth-century British hospitals, it is time to meet the main protagonists of the story: patients and healers.

2

Hospital staff and the admission of patients

WHO ATTENDS THE SICK? INFIRMARY PROFESSIONALS AND THEIR HELPERS

The crowded wards of a hospital open an admirable stage on which you [physicians] may exhibit your skill and exercise your genius; it is there that you will be furnished with a perpetual store and source of intellectual advancement.[1]

During the second half of the eighteenth century the infirmary operated with the assistance of various types of medical practitioners. In the first place there were the "physicians-in-ordinary," a pair of salaried doctors nominated and elected by the managers to take care of patients in the medical wards. Next came the attending surgeons, a pair of members from the Incorporation of Surgeons who rotated voluntarily through the hospital and treated incoming accident victims and people housed in the surgical wards. A number of fellows selected by the Royal College of Physicians, or "extraordinary" physicians, occasionally visited and consulted with house physicians. Finally, the infirmary welcomed professors of the Edinburgh Medical School, who were responsible for patients admitted to the "clinical" or teaching ward while the university was in session and who gave officially approved courses of clinical lectures based on hospital cases. All practitioners were assisted by a small staff of medical and surgical clerks, dressers, apothecary, nurses, and servants, the latter working under the direction of a governess.

Physicians-in-ordinary

On January 7, 1751, the managers of the infirmary reached a momentous decision when they decided to alter one of the mainstays of any voluntary hospital and hire their own physicians to take care of the patients. Under the guise of wanting to lessen the burdens of the local College of Physicians, which hitherto had graciously rotated its fellows through the institution, the administrators proposed to appoint "two fixed physicians for the constant and daily attendance on the patients."[2] The plan to shift responsibility for staffing the infirmary resulted from a growing realization that both quality and continuity of patient care were being jeopardized by the system of voluntary attendance organized by the college members. The managers had no control over those practitioners who consented to donate their time and visit patients at the hospital. In a period of institutional expansion, infirmary authorities sought to gain the necessary power to make their own selections of attending physicians and pay them for their services without alienating the college and forcing the cancellation of visitations by its members. In fact, the decision to create the new positions of physicians-in-ordinary was accompanied by a letter to the College of Physicians profusely thanking its leaders for their past charity and encouraging them to continue the practice.[3]

Having quickly won approval for the new scheme from hospital contributors and met with "cheerful agreement" from the College of Physicians, the managers proceeded to appoint the first two physicians for the posts. Not surprisingly, they were recent graduates of the local university who had also qualified for fellowship in the Royal College of Physicians: David Clerk and Colin Drummond. Clerk had received his degree in 1749 and had subsequently taken courses at the University of Leyden; Drummond had just graduated the year before. Both were hospital managers at the time of their selection and resigned from the board before taking the oath of allegiance and beginning their work.[4]

The shift from an exclusively voluntary to a salaried medical staff apparently occurred without dissent. Although relegated to a consulting role, the College of Physicians must have realized that the new arrangement would ensure the appointment of some of its best members. Rather than prodding all their active members, good and bad, into volunteering a month of service, the college could now look forward to being indirectly represented by practitioners whose livelihood depended solely on their hospital work. With ample medical representation on the hospital board, the house physicians in turn had little to fear about a lay "takeover" that would place nonmedical issues ahead of their professional concerns.

In conformity with the initial rules, the ordinary physicians had the option "either to visit all the patients of the house conjunctly or each to take half as his proper patients."[5] The second alternative apparently became the norm, although the physicians consulted with each other in difficult cases. "When a case proves so obstinate as to resist all the efforts of the physician for a cure, it will often be proper to throw the patient under the care of another physician that every charge of relief may be obtained," read one provision subjoined to the 1778 statutes.[6] In contrast to the situation in private practice, this withdrawal of one attending physician in favor of another apparently occurred often enough so as to cause no embarrassment to the practitioner forced to relinquish the case. As James Gregory noted, the substitution rule was "one of the oldest and most judicious regulations with respect to the medical practice in this Infirmary."[7]

This practice reveals a certain degree of reciprocal professional scrutiny or peer control, also operative between surgeons and university professors visiting the infirmary. With medical students glancing over their shoulders and often vocally expressing their disapproval while colleagues hovered nearby, hospital physicians had to be careful about their pronouncements and actions. Most of them seem to have adapted well to the institutional circumstances, and their candor often emerges from lecture and student notes. The hospital, according to James Gregory, was an embarrassing spot for "a dunce of a physician or surgeon," who in private practice "might long have escaped detection and enjoyed undeserved riches and honour."[8]

Ordinary physicians regularly made daily rounds at noon and again in the evening, and medical students were encouraged to follow them on their journeys through the various wards. During those visits, the attending doctors interrogated the patients and dictated their findings and prescriptions to medical clerks for insertion into the ward journal and transmission to the hospital's apothecary.[9]

Physicians-in-ordinary were also responsible for infirmary admissions, and the signature of one of them was required on all admitting slips, whether the patient went to a medical, surgical, or teaching ward. Even in emergency cases handled by the clerks, the admission had to be confirmed afterward by the signature of a physician. On certain occasions, the ordinary practitioners also authorized the transfer of patients from one ward to another. These transfers took place especially between the regular medical and the teaching unit, either to supply the professors with cases or to receive from them persons remaining at the end of the university semester.

Salaried physicians also ordered the patients' discharges from all medical wards except the teaching unit by signing the appropriate orders and indicating whether the patient had been cured or relieved. Suggestions regarding this admission and discharge process and the criteria employed in moving patients into and out of the hospital were repeatedly furnished by ordinary physicians to the managers. Control of these procedures enabled them to play a key role in shaping favorable statistics designed to bolster the public image for the institution.

Most regulations governing the duties of clerks, apothecary, and medical students were likewise drafted by the ordinary physicians before being submitted for approval to the board of managers. The increasing complexity of hospital functions, proliferation of wards, rise in patient admissions, and multiplication of student visits all required periodic reformulation of the rules, and the "in-house" physicians bearing the brunt of these growing pains shifted some of the new responsibilities to their already overworked clerks.[10]

Indeed, another duty of physicians-in-ordinary was close supervision of the medical clerks. Ward journals and ledgers inscribed by clerks had to be checked to ensure that the previously dictated information had been properly recorded. From flaws uncovered in the General Register of Patients and numerous complaints made by the managers, this function seems to have been neglected. The influx of patients in the last two decades of the eighteenth century probably left attending physicians with little time beyond that demanded by patient care and a new task: clinical lectures. The latter were officially sanctioned in 1791 by both the university and the infirmary as a course to be delivered during the summer months when no professor was available. For example, a surviving student notebook reveals that Daniel Rutherford, one of the physicians-in-ordinary, gave a three-month course between May and July 1799. University matriculation records indicate that the summer course of clinical lectures was very popular, attracting about seventy to one hundred students each year.[11]

Lastly, infirmary statutes stipulated that in treating their patients the ordinary physicians should consider using preparations listed in the hospital dispensatory containing a number of standard compounds stocked in the institution's apothecary shop. Arguing that similar therapeutical effects could be achieved with different types of medicines, the authorities asserted that "it therefore becomes the duty of an hospital physician to study frugality in prescription."[12]

If treatments failed and the patient died, ordinary physicians and attending surgeons could request permission for an autopsy. The procedure employed at the infirmary stipulated that relatives or friends of the deceased had to give consent before physicians applied in writing to the managers. The signature of at least three of the latter was required before a postmortem examination could be carried out.[13]

The initial salary paid to ordinary physicians was quickly supplemented in 1756 with government funds "for additional troubles with the care of soldiers."[14] Several years later this allowance helped provide the senior man with yearly earnings of ninety pounds; the junior physician apparently collected fifty pounds.[15] Thus being a physician-in-ordinary at the Royal Infirmary of Edinburgh during the decades between 1770 and 1800 became one of the most coveted positions within the local medical establishment. After Clerk's death in 1768, John Hope succeeded him while simultaneously holding the professorship of botany at the University of Edinburgh. Joseph Black, disciple of William Cullen and chemistry professor, briefly followed Drummond in 1773, and Cullen's own son Henry remained one of the physicians-in-ordinary from 1776 until his death in 1791. Cullen's successor was Daniel Rutherford, who also was a professor of botany for twelve years.[16]

Surgeons

From the inception of the infirmary, members of the local incorporation – later the College – of Surgeons rotated in their attendance at the hospital, often for brief periods of time not exceeding two months. Among their duties were the supervision and evaluation of clerks and dressers directly appointed by the hospital, responsibility for surgical instruments belonging to the infirmary, and inspection of the hospital's apothecary shop. Moreover, attending surgeons arranged the necessary consultations before all operations and scheduled all such procedures.[17]

As early as 1766 the managers considered this system of surgical rotation inadequate, since the brief succession did not allow surgeons enough time to get thoroughly acquainted with hospitalized patients or to discharge in a satisfactory manner their numerous responsibilities. In fact, hospital authorities charged that several attending surgeons had occasionally taken it upon themselves to send substitutes to the infirmary, thus contributing even further to fragmented patient responsibility and care.[18]

From 1769 on, surgeons were deprived of power to designate their own substitutes despite stiff opposition from the Incorporation of Surgeons. Hospital authorities appointed four men as "ordinary surgeons of the Infirmary," paid them each a modest salary of twenty pounds per year, and stipulated that they organize their own turns, attend jointly at consultations, and perform all the necessary operations. To some extent the new scheme was designated to create a surgical equivalent of the ordinary house physicians attending medical cases and to ensure the continuity considered essential for proper care and teaching. However, the hospital agreed to replace each year one of the four house surgeons, selecting the replacements from a list of candidates furnished by the incorporation and arranged in that organization by seniority.[19]

According to rules published in 1778, the surgeons also attended the hospital each day and made their rounds at noon. They had the power to admit and discharge patients but required a countersigned order from one of the ordinary physicians to make their decisions official. Moreover, surgeons were entrusted with the supervision of their clerks and urged to check the entries made in ward journals. A special evaluation of each dresser had to be provided in writing at the end of the month. Like physicians, surgeons were admonished to seek the proper authorizations before conducting an autopsy.[20]

Additional regulations specified that "in difficult, doubtful, or dangerous cases the surgeon in attendance is to call a consultation of the other surgeons."[21] No surgical intervention "of importance," however, could be carried out without a conference with the physicians-in-ordinary, a clear evidence of the subservient status of surgeons in relation to physicians in the infirmary. All operations were performed in the amphitheater, with previous notices posted in the consulting room to alert both the medical staff and students who desired to attend. The only exceptions were certain surgical procedures on women, which were to be conducted in private rooms with minimum assistance and no male spectators to avoid "doing greater violence to female modesty than consists with decency."[22]

Surgeons were judged to need specific qualities if they were to carry out their tasks successfully. "Undounted [sic] firmness of resolution capable of making him steadily persevere in his patient's good," was one author's prescription, "though to his unspeakable pain and torture to be staggered neither by tears, sighs, or groans, the sight of blood, or even death's pale image."[23]

Robbed of academic prestige by the physicians' refusal to institute a chair of surgery at the university and, after 1785, deprived by the infirmary of all previous input into the nomination process, many of the prominent Edinburgh surgeons resigned from the hospital roster in protest during the late 1780s. By the turn of the century only four of the twenty-three senior surgeons listed by the Royal College of Surgeons remained in attendance.[24] In the 1790s inexperience and lack of skillful operators were common. The managers responded by passing a resolution in 1794 that authorized the appointment of attending surgeons only from among those who had been members of the college for at least five years.[25] In 1792, Andrew Duncan, Sr., proposed to the managers a new system of attendance designed to correct the problems, but apparently his plan was ignored.[26]

Both infirmary managers and the College of Surgeons' leadership seemed to be deadlocked on any new schemes. James Gregory spoke of brawls among consulting surgeons. In one incident a dissenting member was summarily carried to the room's fireplace and given a "vigorous application of cautery to his tail." The heated discussions made Gregory remark that "they will conduct as little to the benefit of their patient as a congress of an equal number of game cocks turned loose in a cock pit."[27]

Conditions were apparently not any better in the operating theater. Instances of public drunkenness were witnessed by students when attending surgeons or their substitutes were suddenly called to the hospital because of emergencies. Surgery in those days demanded not only manual skills but a fair degree of mental fortitude. Thus alcohol seemed a welcome comfort, and the impulse "to moisten the clay" occurred even during the day: "I have seen several of them primed with a good dram of brandy just before they went to the theater, to the final consultation, and operation on some unhappy patient," revealed James Gregory in his polemical exposé of Edinburgh surgery, sarcastically adding, "I must do them justice to say that they drank their brandy most scientifically out of a cupping glass."[28]

Gregory's harsh critique of surgical attendance at the infirmary in 1800 generated a number of spirited replies and a protracted confrontation between the hospital authorities and the Royal College of Surgeons, including a number of legal actions. As a result of the various proposals and counterproposals from the contending parties, the infirmary finally prevailed in its efforts to appoint six surgeons, all fellows of the college, as official ordinary staff members. The first two on the list were to begin a two-year period of attendance, dividing among themselves the previously outlined responsibilities.[29] Greater continuity for the surgical rotation was ensured by the Town Council in 1803, with the appointment of a "Professor of Clinical Surgery," James Russell. Although the hospital managers refused to grant the new professor and his successors permanent teaching privileges, they nevertheless assured the university and Russell that they "would be most happy to give every accommodation in their power" to surgical teaching.[30]

Extraordinary physicians

Little can be said about the practitioners who were elected fellows of the Royal College of Physicians of Edinburgh. For over twenty-five years these men had been the only source of professional medical care in the infirmary, but the appointment of ordinary physicians in 1756 relegated them to a purely advisory role. Thereafter the college authorities selected their members for one-month rotations, and during that time the fellows came once or twice weekly to confer with the salaried staff about management of particularly difficult cases. As noted previously, consultations were always encouraged at the infirmary, and the availability of various physicians – ordinary, extraordinary, and teaching – was definitely seen as an advantage to hospital patients.

According to James Gregory, however, the practice of meeting with extraordinary physicians gradually fell into disuse toward the end of the century, since physicians-in-ordinary consulted frequently among themselves and at times with university professors and thereby lessened their need "to call for the assistance of their professional brethren" at the college.[31] The eventual departure of extraordinary physicians was symptomatic of gradual changes in the nature of services at the infirmary, from dependence on professional voluntarism to hired staff. It also attests to the growing self-confidence and prestige of ordinary physicians entrusted with the daily care of hospital patients.

University professors

The official infirmary statutes published in 1778 directed that "the profes-sors of medicine may have wards for male and female clinical patients,"[32] following a tradition begun in 1750. At that time John Rutherford (1695–1779), professor of the practice of medicine at the University of Edinburgh, had successfully petitioned the hospital managers and persuaded them to set aside for teaching purposes a small unit containing twelve beds. Over the next decades this ward gradually expanded, and toward the end of the cen-tury it was capable of admitting a total of thirty-two patients separated into equal numbers of men and women. The teaching or "clinical" unit re-mained open only during the academic year, stretching from early Novem-ber to late April; its patients were cared for directly by university profes-sors, who divided this duty among themselves in three-month rotations, November–January and February–April.

Hospital rounds were generally conducted between noon and one or two in the afternoon, at the same time physicians-in-ordinary and attending sur-geons were calling on patients in their respective wards. Usually one of the medical clerks assisted the visiting professor as he dictated the clinical notes and prescribed new treatments in the presence of medical students. Rounds were supplemented by two weekly "clinical" lectures, given at the hospital in the evening. These meetings, held in the managers' room, allowed pro-fessors to discuss the management of patients in more detail and with greater candor. Since clinical teaching was one of the most important functions of the infirmary, more detail will be presented in a subsequent chapter.[33]

In the late 1760s and early 1770s, John Gregory (1724–1773), then profes-sor of the theory of medicine, and William Cullen (1710–1790), professor of the practice of medicine, alternated in visiting the infirmary. Gregory generally attended from November to January 31, and Cullen from Febru-ary 1 until April 30. John Gregory was a distinguished physician from Ab-erdeen who had studied both at Edinburgh and at Leyden and who was the author of several publications on the mental qualities of man. In 1766 he succeeded Robert Whytt as professor; he was also elected first physician to His Majesty in Scotland. William Cullen had originally been a surgical ap-prentice and ship's surgeon who completed his medical studies at Edin-burgh and Glasgow. In 1755 he became professor of chemistry at the Uni-versity of Edinburgh, taking on the chair of medical practice in 1766. In fact, Gregory and Cullen agreed to switch their academic positions, giving courses in both subject matters in turn.[34]

Because of Gregory's illness and eventual death in 1773, Cullen had the sole responsibility of caring for patients in the teaching ward and delivering clinical lectures from 1772 until 1776, when the newly appointed successor to the chair of medical theory, James Gregory (1753–1821), took over these duties. James Gregory was a son of the late John Gregory and also a native of Aberdeen. He had received his education at Edinburgh and Oxford, and before returning to the Scottish capital, he spent a semester of clinical instruction at St. George's Hospital in London. Sarcastic and argumentative, James Gregory quickly gained notoriety for his outspoken comments in general and, in particular, for his feud with the Royal College of Surgeons and a public altercation with the professor of midwifery, James Hamilton, Jr., whom he struck with his walking stick. According to contemporaries, he was a popular teacher, generous with students and compassionate to patients, always wearing a cocked hat when he lectured.[35]

During most of the 1780s James Gregory shared his hospital duties with Francis Home (1719–1813). Home was originally an army surgeon who later received his medical degree from the University of Edinburgh. When botany and the knowledge of drugs were separated in 1768, Home became the first incumbent of a new chair in materia medica. His syllabus of drugs for the use of students appeared in 1770, and he was also widely known for valuable observations on diphtheria.[36]

In the early 1790s James Gregory and Home were joined at the infirmary by Andrew Duncan, Sr. (1744–1828). He became professor of the theory of medicine in 1790, by which time he was already a successful private teacher and author of several books on therapeutics. Founder of several Edinburgh medical clubs, Duncan is perhaps best remembered for his efforts in behalf of the mentally ill in Scotland, which eventually bore fruit with the opening of the Royal Edinburgh Asylum in 1813.[37]

Also participating in the clinical teaching were Thomas C. Hope (1766–1844) and Daniel Rutherford (1749–1819). Hope was the successor to Joseph Black in the chair of chemistry and the son of John Hope, former physician-in-ordinary and professor of botany. Also an Edinburgh graduate, he was described as one of the most popular science teachers in Britain.[38] Rutherford was also quite interested in chemistry but had succeeded John Hope in 1786 as professor of botany. A son of John Rutherford, who had established clinical teaching at the infirmary, Daniel was elected physician-in-ordinary in 1791, to succeed Henry Cullen. In accepting this position Rutherford changed his status from university professor taking care only of teaching cases to attending staff physician seeing patients in the ordinary wards. Like his predecessor, however, Rutherford was periodically authorized to give clinical lectures during summers when the clinical ward remained closed.[39]

Medical and surgical clerks

Following the resignation of Mr. Petrie in 1750 as clerk of the house, the managers decided to create a staff of house officers to replace him. The new elective positions, usually one surgical and two medical clerks selected among students "bred to medicine or surgery," were designed to provide a much more comprehensive and complete service for the infirmary patients. Clerks were nominated and appointed by the managers and could not be fired by attending practitioners. Candidates were generally medical students taking advanced courses at the university and young men completing surgical apprenticeships. They had to be unmarried and willing to live on the premises, where board and laundry were provided.[40]

During emergencies the clerks were allowed to admit patients and even prescribe if no attending physician or surgeon could be summoned. Their on-call status, however, sharply curtailed their outside activities. According to the rules, they could not "attend any medical or other classes or societies without permission from the managers," and they had to provide coverage for their necessary absences.[41] During their hospital tenure, clerks were exempted from paying the customary university fees.

The infirmary authorities also proscribed any outside medical activities "or any other business that may prove an avocation from their duties." Such "moonlighting" was expressly forbidden and punishable by dismissal; some clerks were indeed dismissed in 1775 "for practicing privately," because the furtive outings "took off the attention from the duties of the office."[42] Seeing patients in the city or suburbs was allowed only by official invitation and then only in the company of attending physicians and surgeons.

From the ever-expanding list of duties drafted for clerks by infirmary physicians it seems clear that most of the tedious tasks designed to ensure the accountability of hospital activities were borne by the weary students. In the 1766 and 1792 regulations, for example, one can divide all fourteen directives into three categories: clerical, medical, and financial. Among the essential clerical functions outlined in the documents were the listing of all patients in a general admissions' book and in separate ledgers for ordinary patients, soldiers, seamen, and servants. In addition, clerks wrote out admission slips, took dictation from attending physicians, and transferred all the information to ward journals, ledgers, and eventually the General Register of Patients. Prescriptions, in turn, were promptly delivered to the apothecary for processing.[43]

The clerks' medical duties consisted not only in accompanying physicians on their daily rounds but in visiting patients on their own in the morning and evening or "according to danger." Regularly scheduled visits took place between six and seven in the evening, and emergency cases were checked again before midnight. Progress reports based on such calls were given to ordinary physicians at their next visit. Finally, medical clerks were responsible for extracting payments from so-called supernumerary patients, a special category of individuals admitted but temporarily housed in small rooms because no beds were vacant in the ordinary wards. As agents of the hospital's treasurer, to whom they had to account for all monies obtained, medical clerks had the unenviable task of trying to collect sixpence a day from such patients or their relatives, a sum representing the stipulated cost of individual hospitalization. Being poor, many of the sick admitted in this category could not or would not pay; the situation placed clerks in a difficult position, since reporting noncompliance to the authorities often resulted in the patients' discharge. To motivate the clerks involved in the collections, managers often rewarded them at the end of their tenure with a special cash bonus for successful services rendered.[44]

From the 1770s onward, the medical clerks were classified by seniority and designated as the physician's first and second clerk. Money collecting was entrusted solely to the senior clerk, who also kept a daily account of the charges imposed for hospitalized soldiers and seamen so that managers could process their claims for reimbursement from the commander-in-chief of the army and the commissioner for sick and wounded seamen.[45] Finally, in 1792, the senior medical clerk became solely responsible for maintaining the General Register of Patients; the second clerk transcribed information from ward journals to ledgers.

The duties assigned to the surgical clerk also included purely clerical tasks, such as providing a list of surgical admissions, copying their case histories and progress into the ward journal, sending out written invitations for consultations, and keeping an inventory of surgical instruments belonging to the hospital. The surgical clerk, however, participated to a greater extent than his medical colleagues in the treatments administered to patients. He performed "lesser chirurgical operations," such as bloodletting, cupping, setons, and issues, and received permission to prescribe "in urgent cases when the surgeon is absent." Moreover, the surgical clerk assisted at operations scheduled in the hospital and was in charge of the electrical machine, attending "the patients when electrified or any other persons who shall come to the house for that purpose."[46] In the event of an autopsy, he usually carried out the dissections and prepared the postmortem reports for insertion into the ward journal. Finally, the surgical clerk played an important role in supervising the hospital-appointed dressers and instructing them in the art of dressing. He also prepared a book in which the attending surgeon evaluated the dressers' performance.

Given the numerous tasks assigned to the clerks, there were bound to be shortcomings in the performance of their multiple duties. The problems related to the registration system that have already been explained in detail led to the resignation and dismissal of several clerks. Worried about delays in transcription and faced with an increase in admissions, managers only reluctantly granted clerks permission to attend university lectures, forcing some of them to risk disciplinary action because of unofficial leaves. In the 1770s the clerks became more militant in voicing complaints about their working conditions, perhaps as a reflection of the changes occurring in the Edinburgh student body. In 1775, for example, clerks officially complained to the managers about the quality of hospital food ("their victuals also dressed in a very dirty manner"), demanding a cash allowance to purchase their meals elsewhere. Arguments about laundry privileges also surfaced. The confrontation ended with a reprimand of the senior medical clerk "for the spirit displayed" in these protests.[47]

Although the pay was small – ten pounds per year – the working hours long, and the tasks countless, the position of hospital clerk retained its attraction, even if it meant a temporary interruption of medical studies. A rigorous selection process by the managers lent status to the post. Working closely with physicians-in-ordinary, attending surgeons, and university professors in the infirmary was an experience unmatched elsewhere. Personal relationships forged with established practitioners during the appointment were invaluable in launching careers in private practice. Involvement with registration schemes fostered habits of record keeping and clinical case collecting, although clerks were denied permission to copy hospital records for their private use.[48] In the final analysis, the advent of a medical house staff composed of students decisively promoted the transformation of the Royal Infirmary of Edinburgh from a typical voluntary hospital into a first-rate teaching institution.

Apothecary

After establishment of the original infirmary in 1729, surgeons willing to donate their services to the hospital also pledged to supply free of charge from their apothecary shops all the drugs needed in the institution. This practice became increasingly costly to the volunteers as patient admissions rose, especially in the 1740s after "the family" had moved into enlarged quarters. Initially the managers gave additional responsibilities to the newly appointed clerk of the house, who was ordered to keep an account of the prescriptions used by both in- and outpatients. After firing the first clerk because of irregularities in 1747, the authorities replaced him with two men who were supposed to share clerical and dispensing functions, creating in effect a separate position of hospital apothecary. In that same year a "shop" or dispensary was opened in the infirmary to house the drugs, which henceforth were to be purchased directly by the institution or gathered from the "physic garden" adjacent to the university.[49]

The apothecary needed to be a person "well skilled in medicines as well Galenic and chemical as simple," possessing enough classical education "to read the contracted characters of a recipe in good Latin and to explain any directions given at the bottom of it without the help of a dictionary." Without this knowledge, the same source asserted, a physician's prescription would be "no more than a piece of hieroglyphics which he only understands as the ancient priests did theirs, without knowing the use of a letter." The writer seems not to have reckoned with the chronic problem of prescription illegibility that no amount of Latin could solve.[50]

Ideally, the hospital apothecary "should have served a sufficient apprenticeship to a regular bred apothecary" and have attended a course of materia medica at a college to enable him "to fully understand the virtues and qualities of medicines." The job carried substantial responsibilities in a period when there were still many substances employed in treatment and multiple ways of preparing them. It was felt that hospital apothecaries especially needed to pay careful attention to their compounding, since even "the smallest error may produce the most destructive consequences."[51]

By 1754 the infirmary took additional steps to organize the dispensing functions. Managers noted the casual manner in which medicines were being distributed to patients. A rapidly growing number of outpatients continued to receive complimentary drugs without proper prescriptions and signed releases from the apothecary shop. Worse yet, male inpatients got their remedies from the porter, the females from the clerk. Many simply did not bother to take the drugs, and nurses were usually powerless to enforce compliance because they remained ignorant of the physician's intentions. Volatile preparations evaporated on cupboards, and a similar fate befell many decoctions and infusions, to the point at which nurses did not trust the drugs at all.[52]

Faced with rapidly escalating drug costs and protests from physicians about dispensing irregularities, the managers demanded that the apothecary himself deliver and distribute bedtime medicines in the wards and administer all enemas ordered in male wards; nurses were charged with this task in female wards. Henceforth no medicines were to be taken from the shop without a properly executed delivery slip signed by the apothecary himself. All account books containing information about the donation, purchase, and allocation of remedies were to be laid monthly before the managers.[53]

According to the 1766 regulations, the apothecary was entrusted with the purchase of simple medicines and preparation of compounds listed in the hospital dispensatory. The acquired items were "set down in a cash-book," and those utensils and drugs available in the shop also needed to be registered in a warehouse book subject to yearly inventory checks. A third so-called shop-book contained "all the receipts of medicines prescribed for the patients of the Infirmary," inserted daily under the names of the patients for whom they were ordered. If minor surgical procedures or bleeding were included among the physician's orders, the apothecary notified the surgical clerk to ensure their execution.[54]

Every medicine prepared by the apothecary was required to have "the name of the patient for whom it is prescribed and the time and manner of using it affixed to the paper, box, pot, phial, etc. into which it is put."[55] All preparations were preferably completed in the forenoon and delivered in boxes to the nurses before six o'clock in the evening for distribution. No decoctions or infusions were entrusted to nurses in the wards; they were instead given directly to the patients by the apothecary himself, to ensure their administration before evaporation could occur. The same procedure took place with all nine o'clock in the evening or bedtime administrations.[56]

Finally, the apothecary was authorized by the managers to collect for his shop medicinal plants grown in the physic garden. He also participated in medical treatments with both medical and surgical clerks when the attending physicians and surgeons were absent or when an emergency dictated such an intervention. Because of these duties, he had to reside in the hospital and was barred from leaving the building except when officially authorized.[57]

The increased demand and accountability for dispensing functions forced the apothecary to seek an assistant who could help in the preparation of drugs and accompany ordinary physicians on their daily rounds. This position was not comparable in status to that of the medical and surgical clerks and was filled by an apprentice who also administered all enemas in the male ward. After 1766 the assistant was compelled to participate in the transcription of information from ward journals to ledgers for all female patients admitted between December 1 and May 1. This measure was probably designed to lessen the burdens of the clerks and allow them time to update the General Register. Unfortunately, it introduced another element of discontinuity into the already cumbersome registration system.[58]

In the beginning apothecaries received the same salary as the clerk of the house – ten pounds per year in 1747, a third of the sum paid to the physicians-in-ordinary. This compensation increased gradually to forty pounds yearly in 1790 as status rose and responsibilities expanded. In that year another increment, to sixty pounds per year, signaled the growing importance of the post, especially in view of the fact that the apothecary shop controlled the expensive supply of wine and liquor to patients, a source of anxiety in the economically troubled 1790s. By 1795, in fact, the consumption of porter was "placed on the same footing as the wine" and the apothecary directed to discontinue issuing both beer and wine unless he received each day a new prescription for these items from the attending physician.[59]

Dressers

The infirmary also hired another type of student help: the dresser. Each six months the managers selected and appointed six dressers and another six alternates or "supernumeraries" from a large pool of applicants who had submitted their requests in writing. All candidates had to have possessed a valid ticket of admission to the hospital for at least six months before the election, and the successful nominees paid to the "fund of the house" the sum of three guineas for the privilege of serving.[60]

The main function of this surgical assistant was periodically to examine the wounds and sores of medical and surgical patients housed in all wards, cleaning them and applying new bandages. Patients requiring the service were divided among the team of available students, and each dresser, wearing an apron and equipped with a box of clean dressings and a pail for soiled ones, slowly made the rounds under the direction of an attending surgeon or clerk. This routine generally took place between four and five in the afternoon; supernumerary dressers also attended and assisted with the chores, witnessed by authorized students. Written reports about the condition of the wounds of individual patients were filed daily and delivered to nurses for transmission to the surgical clerk.[61]

Two members of the each dressing team reported for additional duties to the surgical clerk at five o'clock in the evening. This rotation lasted two weeks and obligated the dresser to assist with or execute bloodlettings, cuppings, or other minor surgical procedures ordered by the attending physicians and surgeons. A one-month period was spent dressing sores in the ward reserved for patients suffering from venereal diseases. Finally, dressers needed to be available to serve as assistants during surgical operations, "each having his particular charge assigned by the operator."[62]

At the end of their period of service, dressers who had "regularly and faithfully discharged the duties of the office" received a certificate. Their evaluation was carried out by the attending surgeons, who personally wrote their assessments about performance into a special book. The managers occasionally intervened, when certain dressers attended irregularly and failed to fulfill their duties. These and other violations of the statutes usually led to the dismissal of the responsible dresser and the appointment of an alternate to serve for the remaining term of office. In one case a dresser was fired after being "convicted of carrying on a criminal correspondence with one of the nurses."[63]

Being elected dressers at the infirmary was the first opportunity for medical students and surgical apprentices to become officially linked with the hospital and start careers as house officers. Their work was eagerly observed by other students and attending practitioners and often led to subsequent hospital appointments. According to the dispute between managers of the infirmary and the Royal Medical Society in 1785, dressers seem to have enjoyed substantial educational advantages. As unpaid employees with daily tasks to perform, they were allowed to go into the various units and carry out not only wound dressing but also bleedings, cuppings, and electrification. "A knowledge of the small operations which are performed by the dressers and the method of applying electricity is so necessary for every gentleman that it would be shameful to be ignorant of them," asserted the student committee in their answer to the hospital authorities.[64] Practical, on-the-job training was highly valued by students who otherwise were merely passive observers of infirmary practice, and the managers were deluged with applications for the official and alternate dressing positions.

Nurses

Little is known about nurses at the infirmary. Their "mean station" or low status as unskilled servants was attested by the scant wages paid to them and repeated complaints about their brutality and neglect of duties. Indeed, most of the women hired for the job in the last half of the eighteenth century in Edinburgh were domestics who probably could not find employment elsewhere and took on the task of nursing as a last resort. Given the considerable scarcity of servants in the city at that time,[65] this qualification generally meant that the hospital attracted women who through their past behavior and actions had been found "unsuitable" for private service.

The unattractiveness of the situation may have prevented the hiring of "trusty, careful servants whose faith can prevent their abusing the confidences reposed in them and whose humanity can keep them from trifling with the lives of their fellow creatures."[66] After all, the position of nurse was already recognized in the eighteenth century as "one of considerable importance in the complete establishment of the institution" and one requiring considerable skills. Unfortunately, it was also correctly perceived that learning those skills while simultaneously attending to a large number of patients was quite impossible and a constant source of frustration and hostility. Yet all these insights meant little in a real world governed by the forces of the Edinburgh marketplace.

The infirmary had two types of nurses: ordinary and "supernumerary." The former could function either as day or as night nurses. So-called supernumerary women were hired for modest fees to act as private-duty nurses and provide around-the-clock attention to particular patients who were able to pay them their wages. Most if not all of the eight nurses employed by the hospital worked during the day, and the occasional nocturnal nurse and her supernumerary sister were the only help available at night. Physicians' orders occasionally specified "a night nurse" in addition to diet and medications,[67] especially if the patient was restless or delirious and needed to be restrained. Female relatives of patients often acted as supernumerary nurses with the consent of attending physicians and surgeons.[68] All nurses were hired and dismissed by the matron. Half of them stayed for only a year or less.

In 1768, as a result of a grievance filed by the house clerks against one of the nurses, the matron was authorized to increase the salary of day nurses to £3 per year; those working at night received double the amount.[69] These wages, raised again only in 1792, to £5 yearly for day nurses and a flat rate of 6d. per night for those working that shift,[70] were extremely low at a time when ordinary domestic servants got between £7 and £15 per year in addition to tips and "vails."[71] The only male nurse, employed in the soldiers' ward, received £7 10s. in 1790, when all female nurses still received a yearly salary of £3 10s. It was no wonder, then, that a nurse might be open to the accusations of "accepting money, for conniving at this irregularity of the patients, and of her inhuman behavior to the patients at night."[72]

According to the infirmary rules published in 1778, one ordinary day nurse was assigned to each ward. Her main responsibilities were to "remove all dust and nastiness" out of her unit before nine o'clock in the morning, presumably with the assistance of some of her ambulatory patients. She also had to maintain proper ventilation ("Keep windows open between 9AM and 4PM," read one order written by the attending physician) and clean the tainted air lingering about by steaming vinegar. Mattresses previously used by patients considered contagious needed to be removed and exposed to the open air. Ideally, all blankets and bed linens had to be taken away and washed before reuse by newly arriving patients. Linens were frequently changed if the patients were incontinent or sweating profusely.[73]

A most important duty was to "give to the patients under her care their food whenever it is brought from the kitchen." The distribution needed to be carried out according to a list prepared in the kitchen and based on dietary instructions from the physicians. Moreover, the nurse was in charge of "giving and applying the medicines" to patients, "in the manner marked on the signatures of each."[74] "As apothecaries cannot be supposed to be present at the swallowing of every dose of medicine that patients should take," nurses were also compelled to assume the responsibility for patient compliance with the therapeutic regime.[75]

Each day after dinner, nurses collected all the "boxes, pots and phials" from every patient, placed them in a labeled box, and conveyed all of them from the wards to the apothecary shop for exchange with an updated set of medications. The move was probably designed to keep a minimum of drugs in the individual patient's cupboard while also establishing an important system of checks on the actual dispensing and consumption of drugs. Alcohol was one of the most popular items prescribed, and the authorities tried to keep a careful eye on its in-house administration. James Gregory reported an incident during which infirmary nurses got drunk with wine prescribed for patients and got into a scratchy fight with each other.[76] Other intoxicated nurses were discovered during evening rounds by attending practitioners.

Ironically, nurses were held accountable for enforcing all regulations pertaining to patient behavior while in the wards. They had to make sure the prescribed diet and medicines were consumed, maintain discipline in their units, monitor the movement of patients inside the hospital, and check on the visitors, confiscating any food or other items brought in from the outside. All violations were to be immediately reported to the matron or clerks as "irregularities" that could justify the expulsion of transgressors.

Such power vested in the nurses produced conflicts and abuses. In the best Scottish tradition of offering gifts to servants as a form of gratuity to get better service, patients and visitors to the hospital attempted similar ploys to secure favors. If bribes were not spontaneously offered, the nurses might pressure patients or their relatives into providing them under the threat of mistreatment. "Sometimes the contributions of benevolence have been forced from the friends of the sick and even the sick themselves to gratify the palate and pride of one of those humane animals you entitle nurses," protested one Edinburgh observer in 1782.[77]

The minutes of the managers' meetings illustrate several problems with nurses that occurred in the 1790s. In 1794, for example, in spite of a recent boost in salary, new complaints surfaced that several infirmary nurses were taking money from the patients while deliberately neglecting those who could not or would not pay the bribe. The authorities reacted by again posting all regulations pertaining to patient and nurse conduct in the wards and threatening offenders with instant dismissal.[78]

Similar allegations surfaced in 1800. At an extraordinary meeting of the managers in January 1799, Margaret Hill, the nurse in charge of the women's surgical unit, was reinstated after expulsion by the attending surgeon for suspected misbehavior. In this instance, the charges could apparently not be substantiated. Such decisions were usually made because of the extreme shortage of potential new nurses, even when the physicians and surgeons demanded dismissal. Nurses "unfit for the situation" or "of bad description" were quietly shifted to another ward, preferably from a medical to a surgical one or vice versa. The matron usually lent a deaf ear to the professional complaints and forced attending practitioners to take their protests in writing to the managers.[79]

Finally, nurses were supposed "to be attentive to the state and symptoms of the patients" and report them to the physicians, the surgeons, or their respective clerks. Whether they were capable and willing to provide such assistance remains unclear, but various sources report assistance in ferreting out patients who feigned illness. William Cullen found nurses useful in his sometimes obsessive drive to rid the hospital of malingerers. "I have employed the nurse to let me know whether the patient made me a fair report," he revealed to his students during a clinical lecture in 1772.[80]

Like all other hospital personnel, nurses showed great variation in their "dispositions." At one extreme was the permissive type, described as "too sympathizing, disposed to palliate faults of patients which ought to be reported," while at the other end was the nurse who "from a natural impatience can hardly tolerate the caprice of patients."[81] Perhaps nurses of the latter kind were the majority and were responsible for the contemporary stereotype of intolerance and brutality.

With their want of proper training, meager wages, and long working hours in an atmosphere that inspired fear and revulsion among ordinary people, these illiterate women were asked to perform a variety of unpleasant tasks for which they often lacked enough time and the most elementary skills. It is no wonder that diets were incorrectly assigned, medications omitted or given to the wrong patient, orders for bloodletting ignored, dressings and linens left unchanged. As he discussed the treatment of a patient suffering from rheumatism, who needed to sweat, Cullen grumbled: "The feet were allowed to be cold and the sweat did not continue half of the time owing to the negligence of the nurse or her want of skill, and here I must observe that a little mismanagement not only disappoints us in the cure but renders the disease worse."[82]

In their frustration nurses frequently became irritable and hostile, "a fury in human shape," as one contemporary patient characterized them, whose "tongue kills more than ablest doctors cure," insulting "poor wretches she was placed to cheer, and sharpen sorrows she was bound to succour."[83] Overworked and underpaid, bewildered and disparaged, unfit for all the duties required of her, the eighteenth-century nurse cut a tragic figure among members of the hospital staff.

Ancillary personnel

From its inception, the infirmary operated like an upper-class household, with a "mistress" or "matron" in charge of the "internal economy of the family." According to early rules, this governess had to be "a woman free of the burden of children and care of a separate family," living on the hospital premises.[84] "Her sobriety, prudence, temperance and chastity should have so entirely divested her of their opposites that nothing can be feared," wrote one Edinburgh graduate.[85] The matron was in charge of a small staff of "inferior" servants that included the nurses together with chambermaids, cooks, and a porter. "To her all the servants and patients within the hospital are to be submissive and obedient," read one of the regulations.[86]

From her office on the ground floor, the governess directed all the purchases of supplies necessary to run the hospital, following directives issued by the treasurer after consultation with the managers. Her instructions required her to be "particularly attentive that the vivres, especially those intended for the patients, be sound and of the wholesomest kind." Every year in August she also made "an inventory of all the furniture and utensils then in the house" for submission to the managers.[87]

The matron went on rounds of all wards at least twice a day "to examine their state and correct what is amiss," the morning call set for ten o'clock, after the nurses were supposed to have cleaned the premises and before the visitations by physicians and students. She also was authorized by the managers to admit patients, "whether hurt by accident or suddenly or dangerously taken ill," in the event that the attending physicians or their clerks were not available.[88]

Little is known about the performance of the "mistress of the house." In the early years there were disagreements between her and the first clerk of the house, Robert McKinley. In 1746 McKinley accused Mrs. Waldie, the second governess, of "speaking harshly to the patients," watering the milk, preparing bad rice puddings, and frequently having her friends over for tea. The first complaint was apparently verified by the managers and the matron reprimanded.

The growing financial crisis, especially in the 1790s during the war with France, taxed the governess's managerial skills. Furtunately, at a time of escalating food prices, shortage of linens, and dwindling income, the infirmary relied on the services of Mrs. Rennie, apparently an able and durable housekeeper who also made great efforts to keep her best nurses. After her departure, however, the post of matron changed hands every four or five years. Repeated protests about the quality of institutional food and inadequate bedding were laid at the matron's doorsteps, as well as escalating disciplinary problems with underpaid nurses and porters.[89]

The porter, like all other servants, had to be unmarried and reside in the hospital. His major responsibility was to "keep the court, lobby, staircases, managers' room, and consulting room, theatre and cupola, with all the passages to the offices and wards, always clean and neat."[90] In addition, the porter controlled the access of visitors to the infirmary by checking all passes issued to the attending medical staff, students, and relatives of patients. Every day, about fifteen minutes before medical rounds, he locked the side doors of the building and opened the main entrance, "which is to be shut again when the physicians and surgeons are gone from the house."[91]

Porters also received low salaries by servants' standards – about six pounds per year, but double the wages given to nurses – and were therefore susceptible to the same temptations as the latter. Students without proper admission tickets or borrowed ones would try to bribe them to gain access. Visitors loaded with forbidden food would offer gratuities to pass the contraband prepared for their starving in-house relatives. Hospital regulations published in 1778 expressly stated that the porter "is not to accept of vales or drink money from strangers who come to see the house."[92] The rule was probably based on experiences with incumbents during the 1740s and 1750s. Predictably, John Forbes, the very first porter hired by the infirmary, was promptly fired for accepting tips "from curiously-minded persons whom he admitted to the theatre to see operations." The main fear of the managers was that such gifts would be "of great prejudice" to the charity box placed at the entrance to the institution, diverting income used for incidental expenses.[93]

Finally, the hospital hired a cook and several washers to work in both kitchen and laundry. The cook was required to check daily with the matron and receive from her the cards containing dietary instructions for each patient in the house, as well as the bill of fare and necessary provisions to prepare it. Before the food was actually sent up to the wards, samples of the meals had to be presented to the matron for inspection. As will be seen later, the hospital rules prescribed three different kinds of diet for its patients: low, middle, and full. Special orders for fruits in season were sometimes attached to the physicians' instructions.[94]

There were no separate laundry facility or washing house in the infirmary until the early nineteenth century. Most of the bedsheets were sent out to a private facility several miles away from the city. Maids made use of the patients' bathing facilities to clean the rest of the linen. Since it could only be dried outdoors, immediate shortages occurred during foul, wintry weather. The washing women only partially bleached sheets and clothes, a procedure that left the linens stained. As more surgical cases were admitted during the 1790s and early 1800s, additional bedsheets were stained and damaged by discharges from sores and contact with caustic medications, including silver nitrate. Given the unfavorable economic position of the hospital at that time, a severe shortage of bedding occurred, forcing patients to remain in their own dirty clothes, often lying for days in bed without any sheets.[95]

As noted before, the infirmary had a special category of servants who were attendants in the public bath or "bagnio." These male and female "rubbers" reported to the governess and received salaries as well as room and board in the house. They seem to have worked under the immediate supervision of a "keeper of the bath," who was responsible for maintaining "the baths and adjacent rooms constantly clean and in neat order." This man needed "to learn by means of a thermometer, the proper degrees of heat both of the air and water" of the public bath and to have an ample supply of towels, sheets, and brushes in readiness for the paying custom-ers.[96]

Because they were attached to a seemingly profitable venture for the hos-pital, the status of both keeper and rubbers seems to have been slightly higher than that of other servants. Rules enacted in 1756 specified that the rubbers could enlist the help of other servants if clients in the bath required it and could "order food and other items users of the bagnio may need" to be prepared by the kitchen staff. Meals were served in the bath or changing rooms attached to it, with "wine or milk to be furnished from the stores of the infirmary."[97]

In addition to their specific duties outlined in the various rules governing hospital functions, all servants were required to be available for other tasks as ordered by the authorities. Enjoined to be "obedient to the matron," porters assisted patients in their climb up the stairs to the wards, while servants helped in restraining delirious and hysterical patients, all within a hierarchical system that governed the "downstairs" of the hospital.

Closing the list of staff members was the hospital chaplain. This man was expected to administer to patients "the lenient balsam of Christianity by infusing into the anxious, trembling, palpitating soul a conviction and hope."[98] Not only was he perceived as providing needed reassurance in the midst of despair, but he had an equally important mandate for moral regeneration and rekindling of religious fervor. Illness produced a "susceptible disposi-tion of the human mind," and "a wise and humane clergyman should avail himself of its situation . . . by visiting patients in such situations and ad-monishing them to refrain from a repetition of those irregularities, which perhaps laid the foundations of their present sickness." Indeed, disease could be "the consequent punishment, of their criminal neglect of the perfor-mance of religious duty," and just as metals were more malleable when heated up, so would souls afflicted by illness bend and be "congenial" to moral exhortations.[99]

Until 1756 several Church of Scotland ministers attached to parishes in Edinburgh attended by turns, each serving from two to four weeks. For some clerics, however, increased admissions made this additional obligation quite burdensome. The managers therefore obtained permission from con-tributors to appoint their very own "chaplain of the house" at a "moderate" salary of twelve pounds per year. His duties consisted in "preaching in the theater every Sunday, to say prayers twice a week, and to be ready upon a call to attend dying patients."[100] A Mr. Willis, minister of the gospel, was the first appointee, but the minutes of the managers' meetings remain silent about further developments until late in the century. There is a note that the current chaplain, Charles Ochilbree, was officially admonished on De-cember 1, 1794, "accused of entertaining principles and keeping company with persons inimical to the present happy constitution of this country," a probable reference to Jacobite sympathizing.[101]

In the "household" constituted by the infirmary, then, "upstairs" members were the managers, practitioners, and hospitalized patients, whose relations were structured along formal hierarchical lines. In the wards, salaried physicians-in-ordinary were at the top, with professors accorded the status of distinguished visitors. Communications among them were usually made in writing and officially presented at the monthly meetings. In turn, clerical personnel and servants under the direction of a housekeeper were part of the "downstairs" support staff in charge of furnishings, supplies, meals, and keeping the premises clean and ventilated. All activities were monitored and regulated by a complex accounting system that sought to ensure order and thrift.

"THE PATIENT COMES INTO OUR HANDS": ADMISSIONS PROCESS

His vehicle is borne within the gates
And now he finds himself amongst a crowd
Of wretched candidates to gain admission;
each recommended by some kind subscriber.[102]

Transportation and letters of recommendation

Once a decision to seek admission was made, the sick person or relatives and friends first made inquiries in hope of securing an official sponsor. Most subscribers authorized to send patients to the infirmary possessed printed "letters" in which the name of the applicant could be entered. The forms contained standard language absolving the hospital from any responsibility for conveying patients to and from the institution, as well as for payment of burial expenses. Over the years these documents were amended to clarify their meaning, since apparently "the public did not properly understand the method of application." Printed copies of subscribers' letters were inserted in local Edinburgh newspapers and also mailed to ministers of many parishes in Scotland.[103] Except for emergencies such recommendations were absolutely necessary. According to the infirmary's statutes, particular attention was given to endorsements from the most generous benefactors.[104]

In 1774 the infirmary's managers decided that subscribers sending patients from the country had "to subjoin to their recommendation an obligation to reconvey them when they are dismissed from the hospital to the respective places whence they came from."[105] The new directions also went

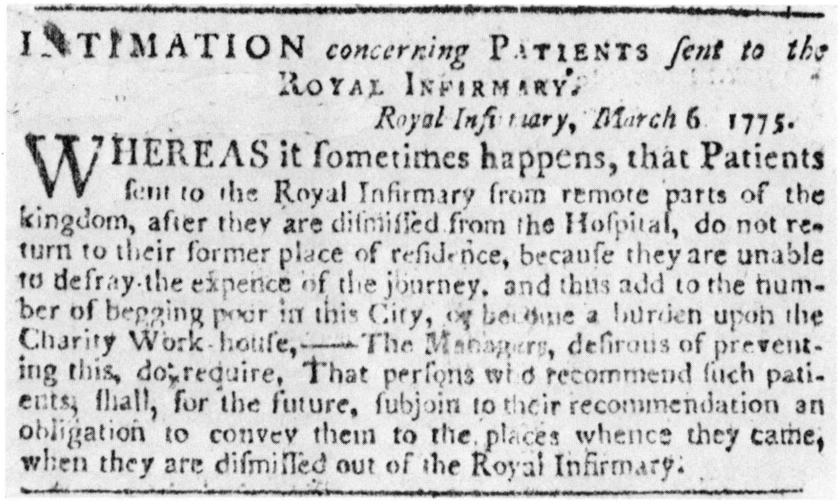

INTIMATION *concerning* PATIENTS *sent to the* ROYAL INFIRMARY.

Royal Infirmary, March 6. 1775.

WHEREAS it fometimes happens, that Patients fent to the Royal Infirmary from remote parts of the kingdom, after they are difmiffed from the Hofpital, do not return to their former place of refidence, becaufe they are unable to defray the expence of the journey, and thus add to the number of begging poor in this City, or become a burden upon the Charity Work-houfe,——The Managers, defirous of preventing this, do require, That perfons who recommend fuch patients, fhall, for the future, fubjoin to their recommendation an obligation to convey them to the places whence they came, when they are difmiffed out of the Royal Infirmary.

Figure 2.1. Advertisement from the *Edinburgh Evening Courant*, March 8, 1775

out to numerous Scottish kirks and were printed in a local newspaper, the *Edinburgh Evening Courant,* on March 8, 1775 (see Figure 2.1).[106] Later in the century efforts were made to curb the issuing of admission letters by unauthorized persons who were either not donors or presently in arrears with their subscriptions. For their part, patients traveling long distances were encouraged to provide advance notice of their arrival.

There is no evidence that the infirmary owned a sedan chair for the conveyance of local emergency cases, though other provincial hospitals generally did.[107] "However, street chairs," either private or rented, brought patients "affected with fractures, dislocations or dangerous wounds," who were carried directly up to the wards without spending time in the admission room.[108] Most sick people seeking admission actually walked to the hospital,[109] a practice that Cullen, for example, considered highly detrimental. In his lectures he occasionally mentioned how the exertions of "coming to the house" aggravated cases of fever and rheumatism or caused "fainting fits."[110]

Carts or wagons brought laborers returning from seasonal farm work in England. Others traveled by sea. Many suffered from so-called "intermittent fevers" contracted in the fens of Cambridgeshire. Weakened by their febrile fits and exposed to the elements, some of them died on the journey.[111] Accident victims were also adversely affected by extended travel to the infirmary. Following a fall, one man had to be "transported from above 20 miles distance" with a badly mangled leg. By the time he arrived at the hospital, the swelling of his limb was so extensive "as to prevent the state of the bones from being ascertained."[112]

Admissions room

Prospective patients arriving at the gates of the infirmary were directed by the porter to a waiting room on the ground floor of the hospital. Unlike other voluntary institutions, the Royal Infirmary accepted persons every day of the week. According to the General Register, Monday was the preferred day for reception, especially toward the end of the century, when it replaced Wednesday. Only half the average number of patients came on Sundays. January and March seem to have been the busiest months of the year, followed by June and April. Admittance dates for patients listed in student notebooks were influenced by academic schedules, and not surprisingly they reveal that November, December, and January accounted for 85% of all admissions to the teaching ward.

All persons "desirous of accommodation" gradually filled the waiting room each day, patiently biding their time until the ordinary physicians appeared at noon in the company of their clerks to ask questions before going on rounds. Most if not all people without letters of recommendation were turned away.[113] Others had only notes from "persons wholly unknown," who, the statutes warned, may "recommend a patient rather for the sake of subsistence in the hospital than for any disease to be cured."[114] One person fitting the latter description was a patient of Cullen's "who had been long accustomed to lodge in hospitals and expected to meet with good entertainment and to pass part of the winter with us."[115] Emergency cases, on the other hand, were usually accepted without letters of recommendation.

Although the infirmary had a total capacity of 228 beds, only about 180 were in use at any given time because of limited subscription funds. A "full" house was defined by the managers as whatever was consistent with funding levels received, not by the actual availability of beds and wards. Allowing for one or two wards that were usually empty in rotation for ventilation purposes, so as to eliminate any contagion, that meant an occupancy rate of about 70%. To avoid the specter of long waiting lists and utilize all available bed space, hospital officials authorized the admission of so-called supernumerary patients, accepted upon payment of one guinea as a security deposit to be used against the hospital's daily charges of sixpence.

Supernumerary patients remained in this category until beds became vacant in the free ordinary wards or they were discharged. As noted before, payment of the daily hospitalization costs had to be made to the senior medical clerk. A check of the infirmary statistics for the years 1763–1778 reveals that the number of supernumerary patients fluctuated from 30 to 40 per year in the early period and from about 90 to 140 per year in the late 1770s, representing on the average about 3.6% of all hospital admissions. Another requirement for entry was the so-called caution money, a deposit left with hospital authorities. The sum of ten shillings was to be used for return transportation or burial expenses in the event of death while in the hospital. For many out-of-town applicants the guarantee was posted by local relatives, friends, or a parish.

Physicians-in-ordinary were given discretionary powers to receive a few persons "who merit compassion" without payment, patients defined as those "who from the nature of their ailment and poverty together, could not be rejected without doing violence to the laws of humanity."[116] In the early years many applicants were treated solely as outpatients, receiving free medical advice and medicines. As economic conditions deteriorated in the 1790s the managers again tightened the conditions of admission, especially because letters of introduction were frequently sent by persons not authorized to grant them.[117]

Admissions depended on institutional economic and medical factors regardless of community needs, even if the demand for beds was increased because of a local epidemic. Such fiscal restraints were reinforced by medical fears of overcrowding, with its threat of hospital-induced diseases. Examples like that of the Hôtel-Dieu in Paris, where patients were "swept by the hundreds" because of what was judged to be "bad air," were presented to justify the constraints imposed on the acceptance of the sick.[118]

The Edinburgh statutes allowed "diseased people of all countries or nations" to be admitted, but in practice many came from the city of Edinburgh and surrounding villages. Some patients were Highland laborers returning north from seasonal work in England after the fall harvest. Sick and injured soldiers from the local garrison or regiments stationed in other points of the Lowlands were frequent applicants, joined in the 1790s by a growing number of sailors from vessels belonging to the North Sea Squadron. Local servants and artisans often applied, and in the early years a small number of "incurable" persons were received under the terms of a special fund established by the earl of Hopetoun, a prominent Scottish aristocrat.[119] The regulations suggested that preference be given to those arriving from distant places, "while others living in the town or neighborhood may wait till they can find access."[120] In the event that the "country in general is sickly" and the hospital full, convalescents living nearby were supposed to be discharged and followed up as outpatients in order to make room for the new arrivals.

The waiting room was a noisy and crowded chamber off limits to students; it was eventually also found "inconvenient and inconsistent with proper decorum for the physicians to consult there."[121] In the midst of chatter and confusion, physicians and surgeons (whom Joseph Wilde, in his long poem *The Hospital,* called the "Aesculapian board") checked letters of recommendation, asked questions "relating to the disease," and scrutinized "the manner and appearance" of the applicants before making decisions on admission. The statutes suggested that cases of acute diseases "where lives are in immediate danger" and sudden accidents such as "fractures, dangerous wounds, contusions" were to be admitted promptly, and even the clerks or matron were authorized to approve such entries.[122] Acuteness or chronicity were presumably judged on the basis of symptom duration and intensity.

By statute physicians were urged not to admit persons suffering from ailments considered "improper for hospitals." Among them were advanced cases of pulmonary consumption requiring fresh air not sufficiently available in the infirmary wards and chronic cases of scrofula, a form of tuberculosis in the neck, if it was not amenable to surgical excision. Moreover, palsies and dropsies, if they occurred in persons of "advanced age or debilitated habit," could not be expected to yield to cures. Yet the rules left physicians a considerable amount of latitude, and the proscriptions were never absolute. Physicians could admit such cases "for palliation," since the managers did not wish "to do great violence to humanity as to reject a patient in very necessitous circumstances."[123] The general guiding principle shared by managers and physicians was that of enhancing the benefits that could be bestowed on the sick poor in a hospital setting given the limitations of money, beds, and medical treatment.

Among other regulations governing entry to the infirmary was the principle that "women having young children are not to be received without first having their children provided elsewhere."[124] The rule had been formulated in part because of mounting apprehension that the children, especially those under five, would become permanent residents of the house if the parent died there while being treated. Thus the managers insisted on receiving deposits of money to cover transportation expenses as well as pledges from relatives willing to assume parental responsibilities in the event of death. Sick children, in turn, were in greater danger of dying than adults and could affect the institutional mortality rates.

The General Register listed a fair number of mother–child admissions, especially in the 1770s, but either the practice stopped in the 1790s or their registration was omitted. In most cases the child was not officially counted, and many mother–child entries occurred because both suffered from a similar ailment, frequently venereal disease. Other shared illnesses were ague and smallpox, with occasional admittance of an epileptic child or a mother affected with hysteria. Some fathers and their children also gained entry. Lastly, pregnant women were barred from the infirmary as "improper." Nonetheless, about forty of them came in every year from 1756 until 1793 to be housed in a special ward organized solely for teaching purposes. These women were not entered in the official hospital statistics, and their care was entrusted to the professor of midwifery and his students.

Thanks to information from the General Register and student casebooks, it is possible to reconstruct a partial profile of those persons who successfully applied for admission to the Royal Infirmary during the decades 1770–1800. For the total sample more men (61%) than women (38%) were admitted (the sex of the remaining 1% is unknown). A gradual shift toward more admissions of men was probably caused by an influx of soldiers and, in the 1790s, sailors. At the same time admissions of servants, predominantly female, decreased by almost 50%.

Information about age or "time of life" of those who entered the hospital is available only from the casebooks. Average age for the entire sample was 28.6 years, with males significantly older (32.7 years) than females (25.5 years). The youngest person accepted by the pl.ysicians was a 6-month-old girl suffering from hydrocephalus, who died a day after admission; the oldest was a vigorous eighty-two-year-old man claiming to have an attack of gout after completing a six-hundred-mile walk. More than 50% of all patients listed in the casebooks were 25 years old or younger.

Marital status was infrequently furnished in the student accounts – less than 20% of the time – and then only for women. Of those 20%, the unmarried constituted a slight majority (47.4%) over the married (43%), with widows making up the rest (9.6%). The average age for unmarried women admitted to the hospital was twenty-four; those listed as married were somewhat older, thirty-two, and the widows averaged forty-five.

In addition to soldiers, servants, and sailors, all listed as such in the General Register, the infirmary admitted a great variety of tradesmen as well as agricultural and industrial workers (see Table 2.1).

Once the brief interrogation was concluded, both ordinary physicians and attending surgeons quickly reached a judgment about the "propriety" of each application. If they decided to admit the sick person they signed a paper indicating the destination within the house. Then the medical clerks made an appropriate entry in the admissions book and "sent a list of daily newcomers to the matron for the provision of bed and linens."[125] "At length dismissed to his appointed ward / . . . / he quits, respectfully the healing senate / and seeks the destined place of his repose"; thus Wilde described this phase of hospitalization. A final task remained: "to ascend the lofty stairs that lead to rest," preceded by a guide, possibly the porter or a nurse.[126]

On their arrival in the ward, some patients were invited to hand over their tattered and dirty clothes in exchange for clean hospital garments. As the managers were informed, "many of the patients from extreme poverty have no change of body linen and even at their admission are frequently in a miserable condition from foul linen."[127] If it was prescribed by the physician, the patient also received a bath. "Safe at last, he casts his eyes around

Table 2.1. *Occupations of
infirmary patients*

Armed forces

Sailor	Soldier

Servants

Barber	Nurse
Coachman	Porter
Footman	Waiter
Gardener	Unspecified

Tradesmen

Basketmaker	Nailmaker
Blacksmith	Painter
Brewer	Papermaker
Butcher	Paver
Cabinetmaker	Plasterer
Carpenter	Printer
Carter	Saddler
Caskmaker	Shoemaker
Coachmaker	Silver refiner
Crystal cutter	Stonemason
Cutler	Tailor
Dyer	Weaver
Mason	Wright
Marble cutter	

Agricultural workers

Farmer	Laborer
Flax dresser	Miller
Flax dripper	Ploughman
Fowler	

Industrial workers

Copperplate worker	Leadworker
Glassworker	

Miscellaneous

Clerk	Musician
Excise man	Schoolmaster

the spacious ward," wrote Wilde about his admission, impressed by the new surroundings yet fearful of what the future would bring.[128]

Ordinary medical and surgical wards

The bulk of patients were destined for the "medical ordinary" ward; others, simply labeled "chirurgical" or "chirurgical accident," went to the third-floor units located around the amphitheater where operations took place. Often patients originally listed as medical ordinary were turned over to university professors for care in the teaching ward, especially if the teachers were unable to come to the waiting room to make their own selections. These transfers might take place days or even weeks after the original admission, if the nature of the ailment or its teaching value dictated relocation.

A study of admissions inscribed in the General Register between 1770 and 1800 reveals the following percentages for each ward:

Medical ordinary	41.5
Surgical	17.4
Soldiers' ward	18.8
Servants' ward	10.6
Teaching ward	9.0
Seamen's ward	2.0

Their distribution over the three decades shows that medical ordinary admissions decreased progressively from a peak of 53% in 1775 to a low of 31% in 1795. At the same time patients entering the surgical wards increased from 13% to 21%.

These changes are not indicative of a significant shift away from cases broadly considered "medical." Reductions in both the medical ordinary and servant categories were more than made up for by a new group of mostly medical cases arriving in the infirmary: sick seamen. By 1800 soldiers and sailors provided one out of every three admissions to the house. Further, the teaching ward, filled exclusively with medical patients, almost doubled its receptions between 1785 and 1800, a phenomenon that coincided with the University of Edinburgh's decision to require a course of clinical lectures for graduation.

In spite of problems associated with the infirmary's surgical staff, there was toward the end of the century a perceptible increase in cases destined for the surgical ward. Between 1790 and 1800, in particular, surgical cases constituted 20% of all admissions. In 1792 the Royal College of Surgeons requested the establishment of an additional ward for acceptance of patients fresh from the operating theater, possibly a sign of greater concern with postoperative hospital infections. In fact, the petition spoke of impure air in the ordinary surgical ward, especially during the summer months, as capable of "retarding the cure of patients" who had undergone surgery. In response, the male fever ward, located near the amphitheater, was removed to the upper floor of the newly constructed wing housing sailors, and the vacated room was turned over to the surgeons.[129]

Country ward

The so-called country ward made its first appearance in the General Register of Patients with a listing of nineteen women who remained in the hospital on January 1, 1777. A year later the register disclosed both a female and a male country ward, each containing patients admitted under the medical ordinary category. One can infer that the transfer to this new ward was ordered for patients from outside the city of Edinburgh who were suffering from health problems categorized as medical.

In subsequent years the number of patients hospitalized in the country ward fluctuated slightly, averaging about thirty men and twenty-two women, or almost 30% of the entire hospital population remaining at the end of each calendar year. In 1779, moreover, the women's country ward listed not only twenty-five adults but also seven children who accompanied their mothers and often shared the same diseases.[130]

A small student casebook containing fourteen entries from the women's country ward admitted between November 18, 1784, and January 27, 1785, provides more detail. The patients were under the care of Henry Cullen, at the time physician-in-ordinary at the infirmary. The average age of the women admitted was just under thirty years, and more than a third of them complained of fevers (see Table 2.2).

Clinical ward

After two years of successful clinical lectures by John Rutherford, the managers authorized in 1750 the establishment of a "clinical" or teaching ward "not to exceed ten beds," to be open during the academic year. The professor was placed in charge of this unit and given total responsibility for patient care. His daily rounds became an important part of clinical instruction and attracted a large number of students.[131]

Sustained demand by students and greater income through the sale of admission tickets allowed the teaching ward to expand, and by the 1780s it contained thirty to fifty beds about equally divided between men and women. The unit usually operated from November 1 until April 30, at which time

Table 2.2. *Country ward for women under the care of Henry Cullen, physician-in-ordinary, November 1784–February 1785*

Name	Age	Admission	Discharge	Days hospitalized	Diagnosis	Discharge status
Catherine McIntosh	41	Nov. 18, 1784	Feb. 13, 1785	87	Gonorrhea	By desire
Helen Bishop	60	Dec. 16, 1784	Dec. 27, 1784	11	Fever	Cured
Christy Watson	17	Dec. 20, 1784	Jan. 17, 1785	28	Fever	Cured
Janet Williamson	15	Dec. 27, 1784	Jan. 11, 1785	15	Vertigo	Cured
Barbara Murray	16	Dec. 27, 1784	Jan. 20, 1785	24	Amenorrhea	By desire
Betty Simpson	19	Jan. 5, 1785	Jan. 16, 1785	11	Fever	Cured
Christian McDonald	30	Jan. 9, 1785	Jan. 15, 1785	6	Psora	Cured
Agnes Brockey	22	Jan. 10, 1785	Jan. 18, 1785	8	Fever	Cured
Peggy Aikin	20	Jan. 14, 1785	Feb. 9, 1785	26	Pectoral complaint	Cured
Catherine Dagon	16	Jan. 18, 1785	Jan. 23, 1785	5	Amenorrhea	Cured
Helen Whyte	29	Jan. 20, 1785	Feb. 8, 1785	19	Eye infection	By desire
Margaret Campbell	50	Jan. 25, 1785	Feb. 11, 1785	17	Hysteria	Cured
Jean McLean	53	Jan. 26, 1785	Feb. 1, 1785	6	Fever	Cured
Ann Wright	26	Jan. 27, 1785	Feb. 15, 1785	19	Venereal disease	Cured

Source: Dr. Cullen's notebook of clinical case histories, Edinburgh, 1784–1785, MSS Collection, University of Edinburgh.

the remaining patients were sent to other wards and placed in the hands of ordinary physicians. After 1790 the managers encouraged further expansions of the ward. At peak months of the academic calendar up to one hundred beds provided a greater number of cases for study and discussion, since clinical lectures were by then required for graduation from the Medical School.[132]

It is difficult to assess the percentage of patients who actually ended up in the teaching ward, because professors frequently requested transfers from other units days or even weeks after the original admission. A check of the data available from the General Register for 1770–1800 reveals that about 9% of the new patients went directly into the clinical ward. For the decade 1790–1800 the figure was around 10%, so that this was the third largest contingent behind the medical and surgical ordinary groups. A check of those remaining in the house January 1 on between 1778 and 1787 (the period in which the register listed patients by wards) reveals that the clinical ward kept between 12% and 17% of all patients.

All 808 patients listed in student casebooks were treated in the teaching ward, among them several soldiers, sailors, servants, laborers, and tradesmen. As previously noted, their average age was 28.6 years. They were chosen by the professors because of their clinical peculiarities, the acute or subacute nature of their ailments, or, as Cullen demanded, their "ordinary appearance."[133] Although admission criteria varied among the professors in charge of the clinical rotation, almost 40% of all those accepted to the clinical ward claimed to have been acutely ill for ten days or fewer.

Soldiers' ward

During the 1745 Scottish rebellion, the infirmary prepared a ward containing twenty-four beds to be occupied by sick and wounded soldiers. An agreement between the commander-in-chief of the armed forces in Scotland and the managers stipulated that this unit was to be under the care of a visiting regimental surgeon who also promised to supply drugs, dressings, and bandages. For its part the hospital consented to provide nursing care and meals. The costs of hospitalization were borne by the soldiers themselves, who paid two shillings and sixpence per week, a sum deducted from their pay by the army's paymaster and turned over to the treasurer of the infirmary. Physicians and their students making rounds were allowed to visit the soldiers and use their case histories as illustrations in clinical instruction. During the conflict, the hospital virtually became a military institution, supplied by the army with "coals, candles, nurses, servants, clerks and loaves of bread" to help with the care of soldiers, who occupied most of the male wards.[134]

After the war the number of military admissions decreased significantly, but a special ward devoted to sick soldiers remained in operation, intended primarily for the six hundred members of the local garrison housed in Edinburgh Castle. In 1755 the infirmary reached a new agreement with General Bland, then commander-in-chief, whereby the city of Edinburgh received from the British treasury all monies assigned to Scotland by the king's Invalid Fund, an endowment designed to defray all expenses related to the care and subsistence of sick and invalided members of the armed forces. In return, Edinburgh's municipal government committed itself to pay an annual interest on this sum to the hospital. Assured of a steady income, the managers agreed to "fit up sixty beds for the reception of as many soldiers to be certified to be proper objects by the Commander-in-Chief of his Majesty's forces in Scotland, who are to be taken care of and dieted and to receive medicines at the expense of the house."[135] The soldiers themselves, however, were ordered to continue the practice of paying fourpence per diem, about half of their daily pay.[136]

In the following year new regulations governing the soldiers' ward also went into effect. Regimental surgeons were required to send along in writing with the patient "a particular state of the case," duly signed by the person responsible for the referral. Soldiers sent to the hospital could no longer carry their weapons with them, except in emergency cases or when they were stricken while on patrol. The commanding officer furnished a list of equipment and clothes brought by the patient to the infirmary to ensure that these items were returned to him at the time of discharge. Admission and treatment were placed in the hands of the ordinary physicians, who received a governmental subsidy for their efforts. The physicians consulted with the attending surgeons if the nature of the complaints justified it, or called the regimental surgeon residing in Edinburgh Castle, who was required to visit all hospitalized soldiers twice a week.[137]

Soldiers could not be discharged until they were judged cured or incurable, except for misbehavior or if they were in need of country air. A released soldier was given an advance on his salary to ensure that he had enough money for a return to his assigned military post, and was furnished with a certificate of dismissal for presentation to the regimental commander. This document also specified in miles the rate of daily marching allowed to him by the attending physician. Constables were required to billet the convalescents along their routes. The system was designed primarily to avoid desertion or unauthorized furloughs, common among hospitalized soldiers. Finally, if a soldier died in the hospital, the army also took care of funeral expenses, including the services of the chaplain.[138]

Unrest and occasional violence among hospitalized soldiers forced the managers in 1759 to transform a small chamber adjacent to the soldiers' ward into a "guard room" so that "good order may be kept among the

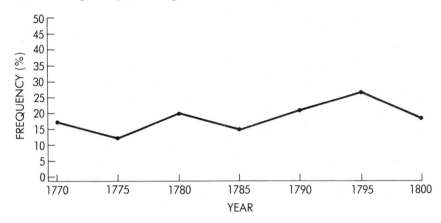

Figure 2.2. Admission of soldiers, 1770–1800, as a percentage of total hospital admissions, according to the General Register of Patients

soldiers who are patients here."[139] The success of this measure was questionable, since the General Register indicated that a considerable number of inmates continued to run away. Repeated fights broke out, and one soldier was said to have died of head injuries received from another soldier.[140] A military inspector was appointed to visit the ward regularly, a responsibility that hospital authorities in 1798 sought to transfer to the junior physician-in-ordinary. A male nurse was in charge of cleaning and dispensing drugs.[141]

In the early 1760s almost every third patient admitted to the infirmary was a soldier, as Scots disbanded after the Seven Years' War gradually made their way home. In tribute to their service, the managers accepted those who were sick and temporarily waived the customary per diem fee. According to published statistics, however, the percentage of soldiers fell rapidly, fluctuating between 13% and 25% for the next two decades, but no official figures were made available after 1778. A check of the General Register reveals that for the same period soldiers constituted between 11% and 25% of the total contingent remaining in the house each January 1.[142]

Three separate documents shed additional light on the type of man who was sent to the soldiers' ward. The General Register listed the newcomers simply as soldiers or added their regiment; most frequently cited were the First Royal Fusiliers, the First Royal Dragoons, the Third Regiment of Guards, and simply the term *recruit*. Soldiers were admitted singly or more often in groups of two, four, or more. Soldiers made up close to 19% of all patients accepted into the hospital between 1770 and 1800, but the rate fluctuated significantly over the three decades (see Figure 2.2).

The second set of data capable of shedding further light on patients in the soldiers' ward actually comes from students' casebooks. Since they recorded only admissions to the teaching unit, soldiers were underrepresented in the total sample (only 4%), but information obtained from these clinical histories is nevertheless instructive. The average age of soldiers admitted was 25.5 years, significantly below the mean for the entire male sample. Not only were soldiers younger than laborers and sailors, for example, but the casebooks also seem to indicate a more recent onset of illness prior to admission for soldiers than for any other group. According to the calculations, the soldiers were sick on the average about 34 days before seeking institutional assistance, virtually half the time (67.5 days) estimated for the entire group.

One probable reason why soldiers sought admission sooner than other people was orders from their superiors after they had reported being sick. Many were also a long way from home. Since the army had a contract with the infirmary, regimental commanders did not hesitate to send their sick men to the hospital if the military surgeons suggested such a course of action. Moreover, the proximity of the infirmary to Edinburgh Castle, where various troop contingents were stationed, made transportation easy and inexpensive. Yet because of the availability of care at military bases, half of the soldiers informed admitting physicians that they had already received some form of treatment before admission.

Among those accepted were quite a few guards from Edinburgh Castle who, while on duty in frosty winter nights, succumbed to chills and fever.[143] The casebooks also registered the onset of abdominal cramps, diarrhea, and inflamed eyes and bladders in men patrolling the military compound.[144] Just as frequent, however, was the acquisition of a venereal complaint while on furlough. A few soldiers were hospitalized in the teaching ward because they suffered from smallpox and incipient tuberculosis.[145] In 1799 Daniel Rutherford treated one soldier who had contracted an intermittent fever in the south of France after being captured during the Napoleonic Wars.[146] Soldiers' wives were not immune from the occupational hazards of army life. After much exposure to cold and wetness "while following her husband on his march," Anne McIntosh came to the hospital with rheumatic complaints.[147] Finally, traumatic events and their consequences were not uncommon, in war and peacetime alike. One man had received a head wound from a bombshell; another was injured in the chest during the revolutionary war in America; and an intoxicated castle guard fractured a leg as he plunged down over the east side of the city's promontory.[148] Further information about sick soldiers is available from a surviving ward ledger (see Table 2.3); there is also a body of data about Russian soldiers received in 1799 and 1800.[149]

Table 2.3. *Soldiers under the care of the physicians-in-ordinary, 1776*

Name	Age	Admission	Discharge	Days hospitalized	Diagnosis	Discharge status
Thomas Mowat	19	Jan. 9	Jan. 23	14	Vertigo–venereal disease	Relieved
James Aleson	20	Jan. 9	Jan. 29	20	Venereal disease	Cured
Thomas Rylie	41	Jan. 11	Feb. 8	28	Venereal disease	Cured
Michael Brien	19	Jan. 11	Jan. 26	15	Venereal disease	Cured
James Singleton	22	Jan. 13	Jan. 26	13	Venereal disease	Cured
Johathan Lee	42	Jan. 26	Feb. 1	6	Back pain	Cured
William Campbell[a]	20	Jan. 26	May 23	56	Pectoral complaint	Cured
Joseph Brightwell	23	Jan. 26	Feb. 2	7	Pectoral complaint	Cured
Thomas Powers	46	Feb. 2	Feb. 4	2	Pectoral complaint	Relieved
Cornelius Danvers	29	Feb. 2	Feb. 4	2	Venereal disease	Cured
James Murray	31	Feb. 14	Mar. 2	18	Pectoral complaint	By desire
David Haldane	56	Mar. 23	Apr. 18	26	Leg-cramps–venereal disease	By desire
John Scully	21	Mar. 28	June 10	74	Venereal disease	Cured
James McGlashan	39	Mar. 28	Apr. 27	30	Nephritis	Cured
Thomas Aiton[a]	18	Mar. 30	Apr. 19	20	Rheumatism & skin rash	Cured

Name	Age			No.	Disease	Outcome
John Taylor	18	May 16	June 3	19	Skin eruption–venereal disease	Cured
Francis Stevens	30	May 16	June 4	20	Venereal disease	Cured
James Taylor	16	May 17	July 21	65	Leg ulcers–venereal disease	Cured
William Dalgardner	19	May 24	June 18	25	Rheumatism	Cured
John Blenshot	19	May 29	June 27	29	Inflam Testicle	Cured
George Gambier	24	May 29	June 23	25	Swollen leg–venereal disease	Cured
Thomas Parret	32	May 29	Nov. 20	175	Leg ulcers	Relieved
Charles Mathews	23	May 29	Sept. 19	113	Paralysis	By desire
Allinus Wilkins	23	May 30	June 6	7	Pectoral complaint	Relieved
Walter McIntosh[a]	16	May 31	June 12	12	Pectoral complaint	Relieved
Jonathan Magilla	27	June 5	June 29	24	Pectoral complaint	Cured
Thomas Dutton[a]	20	June 8	July 22	44	Venereal disease	Cured
Samuel Wright	26	June 15	July 22	37	Venereal disease	Relieved
George Fleming	23	June 18	Aug. 19	62	Headache	Cured
William Gray[a]	21	June 21	June 28	7	Venereal disease	Relieved
Abraham Ankerwright	32	July 5	July 30	25	Venereal disease	Cured
Hugh Morrison	32	July 13	Nov. 21	131	Leg ulcers	Relieved
Ezekiah Page[a]	30	July 30	Sept. 5	37	Pectoral complaint	Relieved

[a] Not listed in the General Register.

Source: Ward journal, 1773–1776, MSS Collection, Medical Archives, University of Edinburgh.

Servants' ward

Domestic servants frequently sought admission to the infirmary. A majority of them were young women suffering from febrile or respiratory ailments considered contagious and therefore a threat to their employers.

In promoting his London dispensary, John C. Lettsom characterized servants as possessing "a degree of delicacy of body as well as sensibility of mind that renders them less able to undergo difficulties or exposure to the wide world." These tender frames and delicate constitutions were supposedly the result of "receiving indulgencies," being "accustomed to the plenty of their master's table," and "a continual intercourse with people of decent manners."[150] This was certainly not quite the case in Edinburgh during the later decades of the eighteenth century. The city was at that time afflicted by a "great penury of good servants," and employers were forced to put up with emigrants from the Highlands who were unwilling or unable to join the swelling ranks of the early industrial labor force. According to contemporary sources, these newcomers displayed few social graces and objected to wearing shoes and stockings, preferring instead to wander barefoot on streets and in houses regardless of the season. They also showed a propensity for indulging in whisky drinking and had a "tendency to the itch," a rather ambiguous condition ranging from lack of personal hygiene to scabies.[151]

The growing shortage of domestic servants had a gradual effect on their wages, which nearly doubled between 1750 and 1790. As their regular income soared, they no longer needed to depend on "vails" or tips from their employer's guests provided in the form of "card" or "drink" money.[152] Living conditions, however, remained primitive in spite of gains in salary. Lack of space in crowded Edinburgh flats forced maids to sleep on floors or in lower drawers of large kitchen cupboards.[153] The meager diet provided by penurious masters consisted more often of porridge and kale than of discarded "plenties" from the main table. Working hours were long and hard, conducive to fatigue, lack of sleep (excessive "watching"), and sickness.

The latter invariably set off a series of paradoxical attitudes in servants and masters. Concealment by the servants was frequent, owing to fear of dismissal and the ensuing vicissitudes of abandonment and pauperism. Being far away from supportive family networks, however, domestics at times shared their anxieties with employers and demanded help for their suffering. Certain masters, in turn, displayed genuine humanitarianism, prudent self-preservation, or a combination of both and called physicians, surgeons, or apothecaries to their dwellings to take care of sick servants as if they were members of the immediate family. Others simply sought to put distance between their families and the sick assistants by quickly removing them to special lodging houses or, if available, hospital wards.

Some of the servants admitted to the hospital worked for prominent Edinburgh citizens. The infirmary, however, was not always the final dumping ground for sick household workers slaving for callous or frightened masters; it also was seen as a reward conferred by subscribers on servants who were thus excused from their duties and sent along with letters of recommendation that ensured their admission.[154]

Some servants apparently welcomed the opportunity to get away from hard work. Several complained about excessive "confinement" in places of employment and blamed their symptoms on poor living conditions.[155] Others were outspoken about the bad food received from their masters. One woman with a scaling skin problem confided that her ailment had started after entering service because she was obliged to eat fish almost exclusively. Forced to quit her job, she speedily recovered on a normal fare of bread and vegetables.[156] Another similarly blamed her skin disorder on the steady diet of "herrings and haddocks."[157]

As early as 1738 the managers of the infirmary proposed to set aside twenty-six beds for the care of sick servants engaged by "well disposed families in town," provided that employers would pay for the costs of hospitalization. The offer was apparently ignored until 1755, possibly because of the financial obligations attached to it or the paucity of servants seeking admission. In November of that year a similar plan was unveiled, this time to be underwritten by a special "Servants' Fund." Monies were to be "specifically applied for servants in the city and suburbs" who could not easily gain admittance into the ordinary hospital wards because the beds were constantly in use.[158]

As already explained, negotiations with the Town Council and Presbytery of Edinburgh established a mechanism for annual collections at all churches in the city and suburbs to finance the hospitalization of a limited number of servants. The printed appeal began with the statement "that such is the poverty and too often the inattention of some families in this city, that when their servants are taken ill of fevers, or other acute distempers, many of them are left to shift for themselves without money and without friends." The document went on to the standard portrayal of those deserving charity: They were hardworking people who through no fault of their own became sick, and "after spending all their wages, they sometimes [are] obliged to pawn or sell their cloaths to procure lodging, medicine, and advice."[159]

To justify the charitable collection further, employers were depicted as kindhearted people forced to remove their sick servants to hastily rented rooms, placing them in the care of "ignorant people without remedies, diet or nurses." Such transfer was too expensive for many masters financially "straitened or ill-accommodated in their own houses." The predictable result of all this distress was that "hereby many useful lives are annually lost to the public."[160]

The first collection, on December 29, 1756, raised two hundred pounds, and hospital administrators proceeded to open two separate ten-bed wards, one for sick "men servants," the other for "women servants." A servant applying for admission had to furnish "an attestation or obligation" from the employer, certifying that the person was indeed in service and sick and that the master would pay for the necessary transportation to his home after discharge, or would be responsible for a burial charge of ten shillings in the event of death in the hospital.[161] The people sent into the servants' ward were "seized with fever and other acute diseases," a possible indication why many of them were perceived as dangerous to the other members of a household. The circumstances, as Lettsom frankly admitted, "may render it highly expedient to remove them to lodgings."[162]

According to an infirmary pamphlet, the servants' ward was "regularly attended and supplied with every mean of recovery, under the immediate inspection of the physicians and surgeons." Those who entered were registered in a separate ledger containing the name of each servant, the disease, the family to which the servant belonged, the day of admission as a patient, and when each was dismissed. This document was available for inspection by managers and subscribers. A committee of ministers from the local churches periodically visited the ward before authorizing further petitions to raise funds.[163]

Official infirmary statistics published in *Scots Magazine* listed the total admission of servants for the years 1762–1778. In the early years they made up close to 20% of all entries, but with a gradual increase in patient population and fixed funding for only a limited number of servants' beds, the rate gradually slipped to about 10% in the 1770s. According to data from the General Register, the servants' ward received 10.6% of all admissions during the decades 1770–1800. A high of 18% occurred in the year 1785; the rate steadily declined thereafter to reach its lowest point, 5.2%, in 1800. Servants were likeliest to enter the institution on Mondays and Wednesdays, and the greatest influx occurred during the months of February, March, and April.

The student casebooks disclose seventy-two servants among patients hospitalized in the teaching ward, about 9% of the entire sample. Of these patients 80% were women. The average age for men and women both was only twenty-two years of age, the lowest of any group admitted to the hospital, with over 90% under the age of thirty. The youngest hospitalized servant was twelve years old, the oldest fifty-three. Two-thirds of all these domestic workers had not been sick for more than a month prior to admission, a finding which reveals that they suffered predominantly from acute and subacute ailments. Perhaps because of the brief duration of their symptoms, servants also had the lowest percentage of treatment before entering the infirmary.

A separate analysis of fifteen female patients admitted to the servants' ward between December 30, 1784, and February 2, 1785, confirms some of the conclusions reached from the previous samples. These cases were under the care of Henry Cullen, physician-in-ordinary from 1776 until his death in 1791. The average age of this group was also twenty-two years (see Table 2.4).

Seamen's ward

As early as 1758 the infirmary minutes recorded a petition from captains of vessels docked at Leith belonging to the Royal Navy. These officers wanted the hospital to allow the admission of sick sailors "desirous of being taken care of on reasonable terms," since no other suitable local quarters could be found. In their response the managers went on record that they were "most willing and ready on every occasion to do everything in their power for the service of the government."[164] Thereafter, the Royal Infirmary became another institution participating in the traditional contracting system organized by naval authorities. Under this plan, the commissioner for sick and wounded seamen arranged for a number of beds in voluntary hospitals and rooms in private lodging quarters to house his personnel. Because of repeated financial abuses and insufficient concern for the affected crew members, this method of care was rapidly declining in the second half of the eighteenth century; it was replaced by governmental establishments such as Haslar Hospital at Portsmouth, which opened in 1754 and provided accommodation for about two thousand seamen. Similar foundations at Plymouth and Greenwich followed.[165]

Contributing to the failure of the contracting system were the methods hitherto employed in admitting seamen to the institutions. Since the expenses of transporting these patients to the hospital were not covered by the arrangement, the sailors were often unceremoniously dumped at the piers, so that nearby charities were forced to organize and pay for their transfer. To make matters worse, many crew members suffered from contagious fevers and venereal diseases considered "improper" or dangerous to other hospital patients.

An Edinburgh graduate, James Lind (1716–1794), the man who had discovered the usefulness of lemon juice in the cure and prevention of scurvy, condemned this abandonment of sailors in port. Writing in 1779, he labeled the practice irresponsible, as a lack of information about the condition of the men only promoted further in-house infection once they were brought

Table 2.4. *Servants' ward for women under the care of Henry Cullen, physician-in-ordinary, December 1784–February 1785*

Name	Age	Admission	Discharge	Days hospitalized	Diagnosis	Discharge status
Mary Wilson	17	Dec. 30, 1784	Jan. 10, 1785	11	Hysteria	Improper
Catherine Wilson	21	Jan. 7, 1785	Jan. 16, 1785	9	Anasarca	Cured
Elizabeth Manar	18	Jan. 8, 1785	Jan. 18, 1785	10	Cold	Cured
Janel Coote	23	Jan. 10, 1785	Jan. 24, 1785	14	Hysteria	Cured
Mary Thompson	19	Jan. 11, 1785	Jan. 25, 1785	14	Rheumatism	Cured
Mary Forbes	23	Jan. 14, 1785	Feb. 24, 1785	41	Anxiety	By desire
Nelly Wood	19	Jan. 15, 1785	Jan. 24, 1785	9	Fever	Cured
Janet Brown	23	Jan. 15, 1785	Feb. 1, 1785	17	Fever	Cured
Mrs. Robertson	45	Jan. 24, 1785	Mar. 22, 1785	57	Phthisis	Died
Ann Campbell	23	Jan. 25, 1785	May 9, 1785	104	Pectoral complaint	Cured
Catherine Duff	19	Jan. 27, 1785	Feb. 15, 1785	19	Leucorrhea	Cured
Jenny Grant	18	Jan. 27, 1785	Feb. 7, 1785	11	Fever	Cured
Peggy Bruce	23	Jan. 28, 1785	Feb. 26, 1785	29	Hysteria	Cured
Jean Henderson	20	Feb. 1, 1785	Feb. 5, 1785	4	Amenorrhea	Cured
Betty Sutherland	25	Feb. 2, 1785	Feb. 24, 1785	22	Toothache	Cured

Source: Dr. Cullen's Notebook, 1784–1785.

into the wards.[166] Problems of discipline, drunkenness, and desertion created additional burdens for hospital administrators already struggling to maintain order in the wards. Not surprisingly, most voluntary hospitals gladly terminated their obligations with the Royal Navy.

Early in the 1790s, however, the Edinburgh infirmary actually increased its commitment to admit seamen. As already suggested, financial considerations must have been a powerful inducement. At a time of declining private contributions, the commissioner of sick and hurt seamen paid a daily per capita sum of money to the exhausted hospital coffers. If only the ship captains could be persuaded to assume the responsibility of conveying the sailors to and from the infirmary, no additional "public burdens" would mar an otherwise attractive financial arrangement.[167] Apparently such an understanding was reached, and the managers went ahead with plans to house the sick seamen. They decided to divert some of their capital funds and in 1792 built an additional ward adjacent to the existing building, secure in the knowledge that the navy was to "compensate for any additional expense." The result was the erection of two extra wards, each capable of housing a dozen patients.[168]

The new arrangement was facilitated by the perception among government officials and hospital administrators that the infirmary already possessed valuable experience in handling members of the armed forces. No barriers existed to the admission of contagious and venereal cases, and soldiers were routinely admitted to their own ward. In fact, a committee appointed by the managers in 1791 to study the feasibility of further naval admissions recommended that incoming sailors be subjected to the military guard already in the house. To avoid disorders and desertions, all men were strictly confined to the hospital premises unless given special permission by the attending physician. As a further gesture, sick officers were encouraged to secure lodgings near the hospital and, if so inclined, to be "attended by Infirmary physicians and furnished with medicines of the house" for a fee of six shillings.[169]

Another factor that might have encouraged the naval authorities to continue sending patients to the infirmary was the quality of the surgery carried out there in spite of the problems surrounding the attendance of surgeons. Naval surgery remained largely undeveloped, but the Edinburgh hospital had an excellent reputation in wound healing and amputation.[170]

The naval presence near Edinburgh increased as a squadron belonging to the British North Sea Fleet was stationed in the Firth of Forth. By the spring of 1795 the French forces controlled the entire Continental shoreline facing Britain, and fear of an invasion brought more men into the area. Under those circumstances Sir Gilbert Blane (1749–1834), a former medical student in Edinburgh and new commissioner for sick and hurt seamen, inquired about the possibility of accommodating even more sailors in the infirmary.[171] The managers debated the issue at length, especially a proposal to rent a nearby dwelling to house the sick and wounded. Finally, they agreed to provide up to thirty-seven additional beds in the existing facilities through a judicious reshuffling of patients in other wards and the installation of additional beds.[172]

Following Lind's recommendations, seamen were sent ashore with a "sick ticket" or note expressing the nature of the disorder and in particular distinguishing those who were suffering from fevers. Ship surgeons had to be alert about "deceptions" among the sick wanting desperately to become "objects of invaliding" and thus to escape from a service into which they had been compelled by press-gangs. As the famous naval physician Thomas Trotter (1760–1832), another Edinburgh graduate, observed, some men employed caustics to produce ulcers, drank tobacco decoctions to bring on a fast pulse and sick stomach, or even went to the extreme of inflating the urethra "to give the scrotum the appearance of hernia."[173]

Before leaving his ship, a sailor received an additional set of clothing and bedding for use in the hospital, his worn set to be fumigated or destroyed at the discretion of the admitting physician. At Haslar Hospital, Lind claimed that "every patient, on his admission, is immediately carried to the bathing room to be well washed and cleaned," a procedure probably not routinely carried out at the Edinburgh infirmary. At Haslar a vessel with camphorated vinegar was kept constantly heated, spreading its vapor around the beds, "and the ward every night and morning [was] fumigated with gunpowder."[174] These and other measures ensured a low mortality there, about 5.5%; home station hospitals near small parts – a category that would have included the Edinburgh infirmary – registered rates of 8% in 1779, 4.9% in 1782, and only 2.6% in 1794.[175]

In the General Register, seamen appeared in significant numbers only after 1795. By 1800 they constituted close to 11% of all admissions, almost as many entries as recorded for the teaching ward and twice the number accepted in the servants' ward. Sailors were mainly admitted in midweek, especially Wednesdays and Thursdays, with the busiest months being January, March, and September. Medical problems vastly dominated in the diagnostic categories, constituting over 86% of all cases admitted.

The admission figures obtained from the General Register are confirmed by an analysis of seamen remaining in the house on January 1. In 1795 they represented only 4% of the patients still in the hospital, but this figure more than tripled in the following year, to over 14%; half of these cases were surgical. By December 31, 1800, the sailors made up over 12% of the in-house patients.

Student casebooks list only twelve seamen admitted to the teaching ward. Their average age was 32.4 years, slightly below that for the entire male sample but considerably older than the ages registered for soldiers and servants. The youngest patient claimed to be 19 years old, and the oldest said he was 56. When asked about duration of their symptoms, the sailors gave the longest history of troubles prior to admission of any group, averaging about 77.4 days, twice the length reported by servants and significantly longer than reported by soldiers. In fact, half of the cases were chronic (more than 30 days old), and about a third had lasted more than 3 months. Because of the duration of their symptoms, seamen had the highest rate of treatment before admission: 66.6%. Such lengthy histories of troubles were not surprising, given the sailors' inability to seek hospital treatment while serving on ships out at sea; application for entering the infirmary could be made only after the voyage was over and the vessels returned to their harbors for new supplies.

Venereal or "high" ward

During their meeting of February 20, 1749, the managers authorized the opening of "two small wards to be filled up in a warmer manner for such patients as are to undergo salivation."[176] Both units were reserved for women patients "infected with venereal distempers hitherto excluded by the statutes."[177] Located in the attic floor of the hospital – thus the designation "high" ward – the ward had by 1778 a larger room containing twelve beds and a smaller one, with four beds, reserved for women who had acquired the social disease "not by any fault of their own but by that of their husbands or from suckling infected children."[178]

Like other contemporary hospitals, the infirmary had initially excluded venereal cases from admission, but the growing influx of soldiers "tainted with the pox," and increasing medical confidence about curing the distemper, led to a relaxation of the rules without a compromise of the moral issues involved. The rejection of venereal patients had been socially justified on the premise that acquiring the sickness revealed a life-style not consonant with the ideals to be espoused by the "industrious" poor who were "deserving of charity." Medically, the venereal sufferers were blamed for corrupting the air about them through emission of "putrefactive effluvia" issuing from sores and inflamed mouths, the latter a side effect of mercurial treatments designed to curb the disease, which caused profuse salivation.[179]

Isolating these patients in a remote part of the hospital and avoiding escape of the vitiated air to other wards answered one kind of objection, although the moral stigma remained. As John Aikin wrote in 1771, "Persons most liable to receive this disease are such as are least accustomed to regulate themselves with prudence"; he concluded that "confinement and rules of the hospital cannot be more usefully employed than upon them." Such segregation had to be strictly enforced, and the inmates of the "lock" ward were continuously kept in their rooms except when the nurse was present, "so that these patients cannot have any intercourse with the other wards of the hospital."[180]

In a series of practical recommendations to physicians and students visiting the infirmary, the managers warned them about the dangers of the "salivation" ward, occupied by people described as being frequently more incorrigible and less correct in manners than other patients. Not only was the air tainted from the nature of ailment and treatment, but the lack of discipline made it necessary for the attending physician "to be peremptory in his orders with respect to the cleanliness of the ward and regular manners of patients." Nurses "of no less authority than prudence" were required to enforce the seclusion.[181]

While the 1778 description made a clear distinction between patients in the large and in the small ward, subsequent entries in the General Register simply listed one "lock" ward, variously occupied to capacity at the end of each year. An analysis of these listings, which are available only for 1774–1786, reveals that the ward generally had between six and twelve women patients, representing about 6% of the total inpatient population remaining in the house. Most of them were inscribed as suffering from lues venerea, but there was an occasional case in which another diagnosis was entered, such as rheumatism and cancer of the nose, no doubt concurrent with the venereal complaint.

For 1781 the high ward is recorded as "new room" in the General Register, populated by only four patients. Whether the women had been transferred to another unit cannot be ascertained, since the minutes of meetings held by the managers are missing for this period. From time to time the lists contain the name of a male or female child, who probably was admitted with the mother and subjected to similar treatments.

Other wards

A committee appointed by the managers approved in 1755 the creation of a "ward for pregnant women" to be located on the attic floor of the infirmary. The decision was taken in response to a petition by the incumbent professor of midwifery at the university, Thomas Young, who wanted his students to acquire practical experience in obstetrics.[182] Therefore the lying-in ward was kept open only during the six months of the academic year, November to April, and the women being admitted had to express in advance their willingness to have their babies delivered by students.[183]

The General Register omitted these admissions and only during the 1780s made passing references to their existence. The total number of pregnant women entering in those years fluctuated between thirty-seven and forty-one per year. Their condition was clearly deemed improper for care in a voluntary hospital, and managers barely tolerated the operation of this ward because of its teaching value and the revenues flowing from the sale of admission tickets to students. After much wrangling, the ward was finally closed in 1793 when Alexander Hamilton, then professor of midwifery, established by subscription the Edinburgh General Lying-In Hospital. Hamilton's final request to convert the infirmary unit into a female fever ward was approved.[184]

Indeed, the growing number of infectious cases being admitted to hospitals forced the creation of fever wards. In Edinburgh such a unit was probably established in the 1780s, but the loss of hospital minutes prevents further details. A male fever ward is definitely mentioned in the General Register under the list of patients remaining in the house on January 1, 1786. It contained ten patients and was located on the third or attic floor of the hospital until 1792, when it was transferred to the top floor of the newly completed wing housing the seamen.

When the infirmary first opened the doors of its new building in 1741, provisions had been made to admit up to twelve persons considered insane in an equal number of vaulted cells located on the ground floor. Admission to these units, unlike that to the other wards, was to be permitted to members of all social orders, preferably to upper-class persons who could afford to pay for their care and to bring their own servants to look after them. In many contemporary British hospitals, the caged insane were a source of entertainment for other inmates and visitors alike, but there is no evidence that the Edinburgh infirmary ever admitted such patients.

In a letter dated September 21, 1795, one of the university professors, Alexander Monro secundus, wrote to a friend who sought to admit a "lunatic" that "the managers of the Royal Infirmary have for many years past declined the admission of such persons."[185] A few years earlier the authorities had indeed rejected an application for the acceptance of a young man "with disordered judgment."[186] As Monro recognized, the alternative for Edinburgh citizens was admission to the city "Bedlam," a damp and unheated place with twenty cells attached to the old city wall and part of the local workhouse where the poet Robert Fergusson had ignominiously died in 1774. His tragic death and the refusal of infirmary officials to accept the insane led to the establishment of the Royal Asylum at Montrose, founded in 1779, and later the Edinburgh Asylum, which received its charter in 1807 largely through the efforts of Andrew Duncan, Sr.[187]

Finally, an incident early in 1791 prompted a petition to the managers to create a ward for the admission of sick children. As noted before, children were officially "improper" candidates for admission to the house, but some of them periodically gained access, mostly in the company of a sick parent or on special occasions as teaching cases. In April 1791 a child belonging to a patient under the care of the surgeon John Bell was left in the clinical unit after the parent was discharged, presumably suffering from an ailment or just simply abandoned there. For several months the authorities attempted in vain to effect the removal of this child, while efforts to create a children's ward continued. Later that year, however, the managers denied the request and the abandoned child was finally taken away.[188]

Except for making a rough judgment between medical and surgical cases, the infirmary not only admitttd but also distributed most of its patients according to social rather than medical criteria. Even the segregation of venereal cases into a locked ward was determined by moral considerations rather than medical guidelines, since more patients affected with this desease – including all the men – were housed in ordinary wards and in the units reserved for soldiers and sailors. Only late in the century, with the advent of so-called fever wards, did a process of ward selection begin that was partially based on diagnostic principles, although here again fear of contagion and hospital-acquired diseases played a major role.

"Giving a fair report": taking a clinical history

After their admission, patients were placed in the charge of nurses and clerks and, except in emergency cases, "not properly examined as to their complaints" until the next day.[189] "Now the awful moment is arrived / which must decide on all his future days," wrote one contemporary patient, referring to the arrival of an attending physician, "with a mixed sense of pleasure and of pain, / of hopes and chilling fears."[190] The purpose of this visit was the taking of a detailed clinical history from the patient. In a period when physical examination was minimal, its techniques largely undeveloped, physicians relied almost completely on the patient's own account of sickness. Symptoms were elicited by questioning the patient, sometimes extensively. "We never can with certainty know the cause if we are not acquainted with the previous history of the patient," emphasized Daniel Rutherford during his clinical lectures, adding with some frustration, "This is almost impossible in our hospital."[191]

Rutherford's pessimism stemmed from the fact that physicians interviewing the new infirmary arrivals found themselves in circumstances quite different from those surrounding their dealings with upper-class private patients. The central issue was one of communication, made difficult by differences in social status that led to intimidation and fragmentary accounts provided within popular frameworks of sickness. "The vulgar have no talents in describing their situation and add a great many fancies of their own," lamented Francis Home, concluding, "We are often at a loss for judging their ailment."[192] Home alerted his students to the pitfalls awaiting those who evaluated complaints by relying on language and meanings learned in private practice: "If we lean entirely on the distinctions made from those of higher rank we will often find ourselves deceived."[193]

Student casebooks frequently reveal the frustrations of hospital practitioners confronting patients who "seem dull and indistinct" in their answers, "giving confused and perhaps inconsistent accounts" of their ailments.[194] Vague and partial descriptions led physicians to implicate the wrong body systems, as happened to Cullen with a case of bladder stones.[195] At times the perceived "inaccuracy" was compounded by the mental state of persons admitted to the hospital. One "languid and dejected" woman was in no mood to answer questions. Others suffered from very high fevers. "Cannot give a satisfactory history because he is delirious" was not an infrequent notation made on the chart, prompting physicians to search for relatives or friends in the hope of extracting information from those who had brought the sick to the infirmary.[196] This method was not always successful, and its failure left those in charge of the patient ignorant of previous clinical developments and treatments, as in the case of Margaret ("Peggy") Carmichael.[197]

There were other difficulties in obtaining good histories from patients. Language barriers crept in from time to time, for example, when Russian soldiers or Danish and Dutch sailors were admitted. One mute Negro slave, Cullen explained, was in trouble because "from his want of language, we can't learn sufficiently to guide us with regard to the cure."[198] Similar problems arose with a hemiplegic patient, "his speech so much affected that when interrogated he is only able to answer yes or no,"[199] or with a "fortuitous" boy, insensible following an epileptic attack, whose mother came to the rescue and furnished "the best account that could be obtained."[200]

Another situation less likely to occur in private practice was exaggerated, misleading, or completely feigned reports given by certain patients to ensure hospitalization. Assuming that "falsehood prevails among men," Cullen seems to have been especially concerned about "unfair reports," as he called them, and repeatedly urged his students to adopt a skeptical attitude when taking a history from the sick poor. "We are disposed to believe the testimony of one another and perhaps he is a bad man who is too suspicious," he remarked, "but nothing is more necessary than some doubt with regard to testimony."[201] Cullen frequently used hospital nurses to confirm or disprove the veracity of presenting complaints, trusting that patients would be more candid with members of their own social class and assuming that nurses would function as informers. At times this was the only way to uncover true cases of venereal disease admitted as skin troubles or to rule out the presence of digestive complaints presented to gain shelter and food.

Cullen also warned students about the use of leading questions during history taking, which might get patients simply to admit what physicians thought were proper symptoms or clinical developments.[202]

"The accession of symptoms": recording the complaints

Most clinical histories included in student casebooks start with a brief enumeration of chief complaints communicated by the patient to the attending professor. "Disease begins to discover itself" was the contemporary phrase frequently employed to convey the idea that, from the onset of its first symptom, every ailment began to reveal its particular identity just as a budding plant would disclose such essential characteristics as shape and color of leaves and flowers. Often, practitioners mourned the fact that hospitalization generally prevented them from witnessing the early stages of a gradual unfolding of disease traits, but Cullen seemed resigned to such conditions: "This is what we are particularly exposed to in this house."[203]

A good interviewer with knowledge of specific symptomatic sequences was expected to be able to obtain the necessary information and recognize the disease. It therefore behooved the physician to take his time and conduct a thorough interview, lest he miss valuable cues. In Francis Home's opinion, this step was just as important in dealing with poor as with rich patients. Given the perceived difficulties of communicating with the former, "the vulgar should describe every feeling and complaint and here an ample time should be allowed them." Home insisted, "We ought to hear them with all manner of patience and deliberation."[204]

Regardless of individual circumstances, key symptoms were collected and then committed to paper in the form of stereotypical formulas and sequences. Bunched together in specific clusters, they disclosed the efforts of hospital practitioners to organize the information gathered at the sickbed. For purposes of analysis, 35 of the most important and frequent complaints have been studied with regard to overall frequency, sex and age of the patient, and duration of symptoms and treatment before admission. A total of 2,705 individual symptoms were extracted from the 808 available clinical histories. Not surprisingly, pain was the most frequent complaint, "striking" or "darting" through the body and limbs, feeling like a "stitch" or "load" in the chest. Pain was followed by "heat" (fever), cough, swelling, debility, chills, and dyspnea in that order. The duration of these symptoms prior to admission was also obtained from many clinical accounts and calculated in days. Three categories, *acute* (fewer than 10 days), *subacute* (10–30 days), and *chronic* (over 30 days) were employed to measure their extent before hospitalization. Finally, domestic or professional treatment provided prior to admission was also ascertained by the interviewer. In general, patients with subacute and chronic complaints had received some form of care before entering the infirmary.

The most common symptomatic cluster was composed of chills, heat, and headaches and occurred most often in young females (average age 25.3). The patients were "seized with shivering" or rigors and "pain in the head." The duration of the complaint was brief, the symptoms usually having lasted fewer than 10 days and therefore having received little or no treatment before the patient entered the infirmary. Generalized malaise, "disposition to syncope," or pain often accompanied the other manifestations, frequently associated with sweating or "weakness" or "falling into a faint."

A second group included cardiorespiratory symptoms, such as dyspnea, "breast uneasiness," "load of the precordia," cough, and expectoration. "The chest feels stiff, the air pipes whistle" was a common complaint. One weaver related that "he had been forced to sit up in bed for the past four years," a dramatic example of significant cardiopulmonary dysfunction. More men than women seem to have been affected; they were significantly older (average age 30.7) than other patients; and the complaints were of longer than average duration, most of them chronic. Paradoxically, these patients had received less medication than usual for their symptoms, despite the extended interval before admission.

A third set comprised upper digestive troubles communicated by the patients as anorexia or loss of appetite, nausea or sickness, vomiting, and indigestion. These symptoms were predominantly recorded from younger females (average age 26.8) and were mostly subacute and chronic, except for the nausea, which also often accompanied febrile complaints. Like respiratory afflictions, these gastrointestinal problems were not readily subjected to vigorous treatment, perhaps because they were perceived to be trivial, very common, and mostly chronic.

A fourth group combined pain, stiffness of joints, and swelling, symptoms usually brought together under the label "rheumatism" and almost evenly divided between the sexes (average age 30). These problems were also subacute and chronic but had received more outside medical attention than the average admission to the hospital. In several instances the symptoms were acute, combined with fever and sweating.

Another sequence prominent in casebooks involved the lower digestive tract, with symptoms such as abdominal cramps, flatulence, constipation, or diarrhea. These afflictions occurred predominantly in men (average age 29.4) and could be placed in the subacute and chronic categories; they also had received a fair amount of treatment before admittance to the infirmary. Jaundice was occasionally linked to these symptoms (average age 41), but was of short duration prior to admission.

Smaller groups of mostly male patients (average age 34) complained of numbness, vertigo, and paralysis, frequently associated with pain, reflecting several chronic neurological disturbances, many of them the outcome of infectious disease. By contrast, fits and convulsions occurred in younger women (average age 19.7) suffering from chronic ailments, mostly labeled "epileptic." A most colorful description of symptoms was furnished by patients "liable to globus," meaning that they suffered from what was believed to be hysteria. The characteristic complaint was invariably described as beginning with a "sensation produced by the creeping of an animal on hind legs from ankle to knee," followed by "balls rolling about the lower part of the abdomen," together with a "murmuring noise." These "balls" eventually traveled up toward the esophagus, causing "feelings of oppression" in the chest and, after reaching the throat, a choking reaction with inability to swallow.[205]

A canvass of the surviving clinical histories does not allow the reader to gain much insight into what patients actually said during the interviews and how they expressed themselves. All protocols were similarly organized and written in terse, somewhat technical language. First came the presenting symptoms, organized in specific clusters, followed by an enumeration of circumstances that could be seen as "proximate" or "precipitating" causes of the ailment in question. These were generally followed by a brief past history of health problems considered "remote" or "predisposing" causes, depending on whether the terms were used as a temporal or logical sequence.[206] For female patients a menstrual history occasionally noted regular, irregular, or suppressed menses.

The total duration of the symptoms before admission was usually ascertained by the practitioner, and it generally defined the temporal character of the ailment. According to infirmary regulations, diseases first needed to be characterized as either acute or chronic. The statutes prescribed that acute cases be visited daily and remain under strict and constant surveillance by clerks and nurses. Chronic diseases, in turn, received an initial regimen but did not require frequent attention, and if conditions remained unchanged, the patients were to be promptly dismissed.[207] Patients listed in the casebooks suffered from ailments categorized as acute (39.5%), subacute (23.6%), and chronic (36.8%).

Diagnostic procedures

"As many symptoms cannot be described by the patient himself," asserted Francis Home, "these we must discover by our senses so we can better judge the nature of the disease than from any description."[208] Clearly, the clinical history needed to be supplemented with other sources of information, preferably generated by the physician himself, since "reports by the vulgar" were untrustworthy. Perhaps it is not farfetched to postulate that one of the incentives for expanding the physical examination was the practitioners' growing dissatisfaction with the information received from unreliable and deceitful lower-class patients. Inspection of the patient, pulse evaluation, limited palpation, and some special examinations and tests were employed as "sticks" or aids "to distinguish the external or internal seat of disease."[209]

Certain clinical histories contained observations about the appearance and complexion of the patient. Phrases like "spare" or "full habit of body," "reduced in flesh and strength," "robust," "plethoric" or "masculine appearance," and "ruddy countenance" appear side by side with more traditional expressions based on the humoral theory, such as "sanguine temperament" and others.[210] One woman admitted during the rotation of Andrew Duncan, Sr., in 1795 was described as showing "evident marks of facies Hippocratica," a facial contour suggestive of impending death.[211]

After checking bodily habit and posture, the physician inspected the skin and the tongue, examining their color and degree of moisture because of the customary belief that the tongue was an accurate barometer mirroring events occurring inside the body. A look at the fauces to inspect the teeth and throat was followed by a scanning of the chest and abdomen. In a number of so-called pectoral complaints, the cardiac pulsation was described as sharp or very distinct, meaning that a cursory palpation took place. If the pulse at the wrist was imperceptible, practitioners tried to assess the heartbeat. In one case the observer remarked that "the stroke of the heart is felt between the 6th and 7th ribs, is unusually strong and gives the fingers a kind of jarring sensation."[212] In an instance of thoracic fluid accumulation, the clinical history contained the comment that "the sound of the breast when struck is obtuse"; the remark reveals the practice of percussion, presumably using the full hand to strike the chest.[213] A similar method was used in cases where the abdomen was enlarged and fluid was suspected as the cause of the swelling. In such cases the abdomen "was carefully examined to perceive a distinct fluctuation."[214] In a case of distended, paralyzed bowels, "the tension is so great that a tympany is produced when the abdomen is struck."[215]

A most important diagnostic step was the taking of a patient's pulse, generally at the wrist. Frequency was one variable duly recorded in most notebooks, perhaps using a sandglass or stopwatch; it was qualified by taking into account the person's posture and other circumstances surrounding the measurement. At times when the pulse "amounted" to more than 100 strokes per minute, observers remarked that such frequency was due not to disease but to previous patient activity, upright position, or resting near one of the fires burning in the ward. "Today he was sitting by the fire in an erect posture," commented William Cullen about one of his patients. "I felt his pulse and it was so feeble and frequent as to pass my power of numbering."[216]

Another factor quickening the pulse, "seemingly in consequence of accidental emotion of the mind," was the "approach of physicians" during clinical visits. James Gregory believed that the arrival of a practitioner could "make a difference of 10–20 [pulsations per minute] in very irritable patients when laying out their hands to let you feel the pulse."[217] The reasons were pretty clear. Observed another author: "How common is it for the physician feeling the pulse of his patient to be conversing with him all the while and on a subject naturally agitating to the latter."[218] In several instances a second measurement was demanded after the patient was more at ease: "Pulse fluttered at our approach but soon came to 72," read one clinical history.[219]

Perhaps more important than frequency was the assessment of the pulse's strength and fullness, both highly subjective judgments on which critical diagnostic and therapeutic decisions such as bloodletting were based. A strong pulse could be suggestive of an inflammatory fever, which would generally be subjected to bleeding and purging, whereas a weak one resulted in a diagnosis of "typhus" and called for a supportive regimen of tonics and wine.[220] In "corpulent" persons with arteries cushioned by layers of fat, the efforts of physicians to count and evaluate the pulse before ordering a bleeding were likely to be frustrated.[221]

The presence of "heat," "hot skin," or simply fever was qualitatively evaluated by the intensity of previous chills, the color and warmth of the skin, the state of the sensorium, and subsequent sweating. Distinctions such as "low," "moderate," and "excessive" heat, rather than precise computations, abound in clinical histories. Inaccurate thermometers and often a true lack of correlation between the patient's subjective complaints and instrumental readings did little to encourage the widespread adoption of this diagnostic aid. Thermometers were small, with their cylindric stems ending in bulbs about a quarter of an inch in diameter. They were generally placed under the tongue for several minutes.[222] On rare occasions an attempt at exact calculation seemed desirable. Cullen, for example, wanted in one instance to evaluate the effects of camphor in fevers. "I measured his heat by an inspection with the thermometer," he explained to his students, as if the rigor of a therapeutic experiment demanded such precision but not the daily management of febrile patients.[223]

On occasion, special observations were carried out to ascertain the nature of certain complaints. Surgeons were called in consultation to perform rectal inspections with the help of a "flexible probe" and a candle, and physicians or midwives carried out pelvic examinations to ascertain the condition of the cervix or the size of the uterus or to detect the presence of stones in the bladder.[224] In a case of a neck abscess labeled "scrofula," when he was fearful of an obstruction, Daniel Rutherford employed a probe to check the fauces and throat; he told students that he had "kept a patient alive for two years by means of a hollow instrument through which food was conveyed into the stomach."[225] Finally, a number of people were subjected to crude visual tests. One clinical history carried the comment that the patient, who was suffering from an eye infection, "can now read small print when held within three or four inches of the eye."[226] Another person perceived in one eye only "a faint glimmer of colored light both on looking at the window and at a candle," with "some confused perception of colors in the right eye when she looked at the window with her left eye shut."[227]

Bodily discharges such as sputum, feces, and urine were frequently subjected to inspection and analysis. "The spitting is thrown upon the water," was noted in some histories, meaning that patients were instructed to cough into water bowls and physicians then observed the general behavior of this sputum. Mucous discharges generally floated on the water, while all purulent matter quickly sank to the bottom in more or less cohesive chunks, to eighteenth-century physicians an important diagnostic sign suggestive of pneumonia or even tuberculosis.[228] Urine was measured both in quantity and in quality, with special attention to color, transparency, and sediment. In cases of generalized swelling and "diabetes," physicians immediately began calculations of urinary output to guide them in their dietary indications and drug prescriptions. The sediment was examined after evaporation in a flask, and in the case of diabetes the presence of sugar was ascertained by the addition of quicklime, which gave off an "exhalation of evident ammoniacal smell by evaporation of small quantities of saccharine matter." The blood serum was similarly agitated and evaporated to yield a "gelatinous mass" tested for its "fruitness."[229] It was also observed through a microscope to check on the size and shape of red globules.[230] In cases of presumed jaundice, a piece of white cloth was immersed in the darkly colored urine obtained from the patient and then checked for a "yellow tinge."[231]

Having answered most questions and submitted to additional examinations, the newly admitted patients anxiously waited for the final verdict: a diagnostic label that could spell the difference between prompt recovery and chronic disability, even life and death.

"Forming a judgment of the disease": classification schemes

Having obtained a more or less detailed history from the patient and searched for additional clues of sickness at the bedside, eighteenth-century practitioners came to a final conclusion and assigned a diagnosis to each case. The names employed in such a determination were obtained from elaborate disease classifications or nosologies published in profusion during the century. Believing that individual diseases were real entities, just like plants and animals, physicians endeavored to collect and classify them by borrowing methods and taxonomies used in botany and zoology.[232]

As early as 1676 the English physician Thomas Sydenham (1624–1689) had written, "It is necessary that all diseases be reduced to definite and certain species . . . with the same care which we see exhibited by botanists in their phytologies."[233] Following Sydenham's suggestions, various medical authors tried to introduce similar order into clinical medicine. Diseases were collected and arranged into families, classes, species, and genera on the basis of anatomical, clinical, and pathological criteria that reflected the judgment and experience of the particular physician attempting the classification.

During the eighteenth century, François B. de Sauvages (1706–1767), a professor of medicine at the University of Montpellier in France, presented the first comprehensive nosological arrangement. His work *Nouvelles Classes des Maladies* was published anonymously in 1731, with an official and expanded version titled *Nosologia Methodica* following in 1763. Sauvages, who also had strong botanical interests, conceived of nosology as a practical discipline providing practitioners with a compass to chart their voyages through the complex sea of symptoms. Classifications were to be grounded on clinical histories and phenomena observed at the bedside, rather than on the anatomical location of symptoms employed earlier. On the basis of previous reports and personal experience, Sauvages established 10 classes of disease, 44 orders, 315 genera, and approximately 2,400 separate nosological entities, an enormously detailed scheme blemished, however, with many inconsistencies and duplications.[234]

In Edinburgh practitioners replaced the nosology of Sauvages with a simpler arrangement worked out by William Cullen. Originally published in 1769, Cullen's *Synopsis Nosologiae Methodicae* was specifically designed to guide medical students and young physicians at the bedside. Rather than a cumbersome, all-encompassing taxonomy, the new classification scheme was a didactic and practical index of clinical reality as experienced by the author himself in his work as naval surgeon, private physician, and university professor in charge of hospital patients. In fact, Cullen criticized his predecessors for attempting comprehensive arrangements not entirely based on personal observations, because lack of firsthand knowledge made them include virtually every symptom as a separate disease. By contrast, his own system had only 4 classes, 19 orders, and 151 genera.[235]

For Cullen, nosology was not only a necessary effort to discern individual disease states and get a grasp of the entire panorama of sickness; it was likewise the key for an improvement of therapeutics: "It is well known to be necessary in order to successful practice," wrote Cullen, "that remedies be adapted not only to every genus, but to every species, and even to every variety of disease."[236]

In Cullen's view, as more patients were seen, especially in hospitals and dispensaries, new genera of disease could be established and a number of "imperfectly related" ones dropped or possibly reclassified.[237] For Cullen such categories were not chiseled into stone but were only temporary guideposts, with their diagnostic, prognostic, and therapeutic implications all subject to revision as clinical observations demanded it. Yet in spite of its temporary character, nosology was seen as central to the study and practice of medicine. The absence of a classification system "would make the study of physic absolutely impossible," Cullen feared, "for if we cannot arrive at some distinction of diseases, we must act at random."[238]

Thus culminated the admissions process at the Edinburgh infirmary, a procedure guided primarily by social and economic considerations instead of medical need. Consequently, certain occupational groups – servants, soldiers, and later seamen – made up a large percentage of the patients allowed to enter the hospital, because the authorities received specific sums of money to pay for the care. Such circumstances prevented the infirmary from being responsive to the changing health conditions in Edinburgh and its vicinity. At the same time, because of the contracts and special collections, the hospital dramatically expanded the geographical area it served and even brought a considerable number of foreign people into the wards. In the decades under study, the infirmary ceased to be just a local institution and became instead an establishment of national scope, at the end closely integrated into the war effort against France.

Such contractual arrangements, while decisively contributing to the economic well-being of the charity, also produced a number of problems. As noted, the influx of soldiers and seamen into the wards created frequent disciplinary problems requiring the presence of guards. A fair number of men simply used their hospitalization to desert; others protested about the food and care they were paying for. As shall be seen later, their prevalent ailment was venereal disease, a fact that not only influences hospital statistics – the ailment was believed to be curable – but also diminished somewhat the moral taint associated with it, a stigma that prevented many similar institutions from accepting such cases.

Another feature worth stressing was the switch from an institution dependent on volunteers to one providing medical employment. This change ostensibly occurred in the name of progress and efficiency as the hospital expanded its bed capacity and assumed additional responsibilities. In reality it meant more power for the administrators, who made all personnel appointments, established rules, and set wages, thereby ensuring that social and economic issues would take precedence over medical matters. At the same time, however, the expansion of the salaried medical staff created valuable training opportunities for students hired as clerks and dressers. These positions were integrated into a hierarchical system of full-time house officers who worked on the premises in exchange for room, board, and free admission tickets to university lectures.

A final comment regarding the diagnostic process employed at the infirmary: As noted, the clinical history played a fundamental role once the social and financial criteria were met and the patient was certified as eligible for admission. A brief interview in the waiting room determined whether people were "proper" candidates for hospital care – generally meaning that they suffered from acute but not life-threatening illnesses. More extensive interviews and cursory physical examinations followed before treatment was instituted.

Diagnoses assigned to hospitalized cases were based on a rather complex classification system adopted by William Cullen, after 1760 the most prominent member of the University of Edinburgh medical faculty. Like other eighteenth-century nosologies, Cullen's categories implied the existence of a large number of disease species. These entities, defined by purely clinical criteria and based on the characteristic unfolding of symptom sequences, were considered to be as real as plant and animal species and part of the natural world order.

Diagnosis at the Edinburgh infirmary, therefore, meant that hospital practitioners had to recognize the particular species of disease by its characteristic manifestations in the form of symptoms. Extensive history taking and examination of the patient provided most of the evidence. However, the challenge for these physicians was to gather the necessary information in spite of the sick poor's inability or unwillingness to provide it. Just as important, valuable clues about the onset and early "unravelling" of the disease were usually lost before the patient decided to come into the hospital. Even prior treatments could mask the genuine "markers" needed to place the illness in a specific category. Such concerns, typical of the contemporary "medicine of species," progressively forced practitioners to rely less on the clinical story and to pay greater attention to the physical conditions of the patient.[239]

3

Patients and their diseases

There is no country in Europe, whose inhabitants are more distinguished by their healthiness – their longevity, – or the inconsiderable number of diseases to which they are liable, than those of Scotland.[1]

Despite the optimistic assessment here quoted from John Sinclair, eighteenth-century Scotland imposed a significant burden of disease on the poorest of its inhabitants. Many of the prevailing ailments were results of environmental and social factors, some peculiar to the country while others stemmed from conditions common throughout Britain and Europe.

ENTERING DIAGNOSES IN THE GENERAL REGISTER

The General Register of Patients is the only document still in existence capable of providing an overview of the types of disease seen at the Royal Infirmary. Since it was designed to summarize to subscribers and the public at large the daily movement of patients, clerks inscribing these folios employed a diagnostic terminology based largely on English terms familiar to the laity. Categories such as "catarrh," "pectoral complaint," "fever," "gravel," "venereal disease," "bruises," and "rheumatism" fill the pages of the register, next to a few more technical names, including "amaurosis," "cynanche," "dyspepsia," and "hydrocephalus." Often the diagnosis written into the books was what we would in retrospect consider only a symptom, and therefore there were many cases labeled "cough," "diarrhea," "headache," "itch," "pain," "spasm," or "swelling."

Instead of employing a limited or standard number of categories, the clerks vastly expanded the list of diagnostic tags. The result was a plethora of names or phrases, inconsistently applied to the incoming patient population. For the approximately 1,000 admissions recorded in the register during 1770, 243 different terms appear in the diagnostic column, including such entities as "hurt from a fall," "disordered imagination," "lust, constant and intense," "swimming of head," and "stiff hand from venesection." If we consider 3,047 diagnostic entries randomly obtained from sur-

Table 3.1. *Frequency of the most common diseases recorded in the General Register of Patients, 1770–1800 (randomized sample of 3,047 entries)*

Diagnosis	1770	1775	1780	1785	1790	1795	1800	Total
Venereal disease & lues venerea								
No. of cases	85	60	54	62	65	65	56	447
% of total sample	2.78	1.96	1.77	2.03	2.13	2.13	1.83	14.67
Row %	19.01	13.42	12.08	13.87	14.54	14.54	12.52	
Col. %	27.68	13.33	11.02	12.92	14.16	15.40	12.73	
Fever								
No. of cases	25	72	32	102	47	31	63	372
% of total sample	0.82	2.36	1.05	3.34	1.54	1.01	2.06	12.20
Row %	6.72	19.35	8.60	27.41	12.63	8.33	16.93	
Col. %	8.14	16.00	6.53	21.15	10.24	7.35	14.32	
Pectoral complaint								
No. of cases	4	25	17	10	23	35	25	139
% of total sample	0.13	0.82	0.55	0.32	0.75	1.14	0.82	4.56
Row %	2.88	17.99	12.23	7.19	16.55	25.18	17.99	
Col. %	1.30	5.56	3.47	2.08	5.01	8.29	5.68	
Rheumatism								
No. of cases	18	12	20	23	15	24	27	139
% of total sample	0.59	0.39	0.65	0.75	0.49	0.78	0.88	4.56
Row %	12.94	8.63	14.38	16.54	10.79	17.26	19.42	
Col. %	5.86	2.67	4.08	4.79	3.27	5.69	6.14	
Stomach complaint & dyspepsia								
No. of cases	12	20	20	14	26	16	12	120
% of total sample	0.39	0.65	0.65	0.46	0.85	0.52	0.39	3.93
Row %	10.00	16.66	16.66	11.66	21.66	13.33	10.00	
Col. %	3.91	4.44	4.08	2.92	5.67	3.79	2.73	
Ulcers								
No. of cases	9	4	1	12	13	38	6	83
% of total sample	0.30	0.13	0.03	0.39	0.43	1.25	0.20	2.72
Row %	10.84	4.82	1.20	14.46	15.66	45.78	7.23	
Col. %	2.93	0.89	0.20	2.50	2.83	9.00	1.36	
Sores on legs								
No. of cases	3	23	28	8	5	6	0	73
% of total sample	0.10	0.75	0.92	0.26	0.16	0.20	0.00	2.39
Row %	4.11	31.51	38.36	10.96	6.85	8.22	0.00	
Col. %	0.98	5.11	5.71	1.67	1.09	1.42	0.00	

Diagnosis	1770	1775	1780	1785	1790	1795	1800	Total
Ague or intermit- *tent fever*								
No. of cases	9	4	23	10	7	3	2	58
% of total sample	0.29	0.13	0.75	0.33	0.23	0.10	0.07	1.90
Row %	15.52	6.90	39.66	17.24	12.07	5.17	3.45	
Col. %	2.93	0.89	4.69	2.08	1.52	0.71	0.45	

viving folios of the General Register between 1770 and 1800,[2] the eight most commonly employed headings were those shown in Tables 3.1 and 3.2.

THE SPECTRUM OF DISEASES AT THE INFIRMARY, 1770–1800

To obtain a general view of the nature and frequency of ailments seen at the Royal Infirmary, an attempt was made to divide the numerous categories employed in the register into a smaller number of diagnostic groups. Instead of trying to match the archaic labels with specific modern medical terms, the general scheme retained the eighteenth-century nosological terminology but redistributed disease entities according to their presumed contemporary nature and affected body systems. For example, the study placed a disease termed chlorosis – in modern terms possibly an iron-deficiency anemia but a genus among Cullen's adynamic neuroses – under diseases affecting the sexual organs, because Edinburgh physicians considered it a form of amenorrhea. Although far from perfect, the arrangement avoids doing violence to eighteenth-century names, explanations, and meanings. In fact, each disease category was defined on the basis of Cullen's nosology, the guide routinely used by infirmary practitioners in diagnosis and treatment. Retaining the framework that originally shaped the disease perceptions of Edinburgh patients and practitioners is, I believe, essential for an understanding of hospital care between 1750 and 1800.[3] (Throughout this discussion, the use of italics is restricted to introduction of the physicians' technical terminology.)

Medical and surgical diseases

According to guidelines used in the admissions room, a basic distinction between medical and surgical cases was made at the outset, taking into account the character of the disease. In our sample of 3,047 diagnoses entered into the folios of the General Register between 1770 and 1800, 76.1% of all

Table 3.2. *Sex distribution for the most common diseases recorded in the General Register of patients, 1770–1800 (randomized sample of 3,047 entries)*

Diagnosis	Males	Females	Total
Venereal disease & lues venerea			
No. of cases	337	110	447
% of total sample	11.06	3.61	14.67
Row %	75.39	24.60	
Col. %	18.01	9.40	
Fever			
No. of cases	188	184	372
% of total sample	6.17	6.03	12.20
Row %	50.53	49.46	
Col. %	10.05	15.73	
Pectoral complaint			
No. of cases	94	45	139
% of total sample	3.09	1.48	4.56
Row %	67.63	32.37	
Col. %	5.03	3.85	
Rheumatism			
No. of cases	80	59	139
% of total sample	2.62	1.93	4.56
Row %	57.55	42.44	
Col. %	4.27	5.04	
Stomach complaint & dyspepsia			
No. of cases	62	58	120
% of total sample	2.03	1.90	3.93
Row %	51.66	48.33	
Col. %	3.31	4.96	
Ulcers			
No. of cases	57	26	83
% of total sample	1.87	0.85	2.72
Row %	68.67	31.33	
Col. %	3.05	2.22	
Sores on legs			
No. of cases	52	21	73
% of total sample	1.71	0.69	2.39
Row %	71.23	28.77	
Col. %	2.78	1.80	

Diagnosis	Males	Females	Total
Ague or intermittent fever			
No. of cases	34	24	58
% of total sample	1.12	0.79	1.90
Row %	58.62	41.38	
Col. %	1.82	2.05	

patients admitted suffered from medical problems, 20.2% were surgical admissions, and the rest remained labeled "unknown." This ratio changed constantly throughout the years. In 1770, for example, over 82% of all the incoming patients complained of medical conditions, whereas twenty-five years later this category made up only 69% of the total. Hence surgical cases experienced a gradual increase that more than doubled their admission rate by the 1790s (see Figure 3.1), a phenomenon reported for other eighteenth-century hospitals and frequently associated with changes in the ecology of disease brought on by urbanization and the Industrial Revolution.

If we use the first name of the patient as inscribed in the register to determine sex, we find that the data also show a slight prevalence of medical disorders among women, with men proportionally more affected with surgical problems. Checking the few occupations routinely listed, we learn that 85% of all hospitalized soldiers entered with conditions considered medical, a proportion even higher among the sailors (87%) and servants (89%). The following classification was adopted and will be considered in further detail:

Medical diseases

1. Genitourinary
2. Infectious
3. Respiratory
4. Musculoskeletal
5. Digestive
6. Nervous–mental
7. Cutaneous
8. Circulatory
9. Eye
10. Miscellaneous

Surgical diseases

1. Infectious
2. Trauma
3. Tumors
4. Surgical procedures
5. Miscellaneous

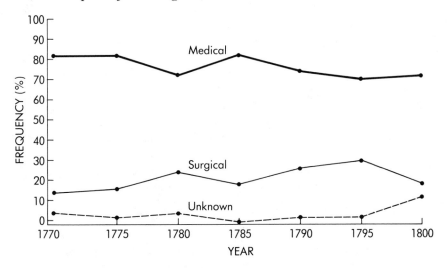

Figure 3.1. Distribution of medical and surgical cases, 1770–1800, as a percentage of total hospital admissions, according to the General Register of Patients

The diagnostic clusters derived from the 3,047 General Register entries in our sample were arranged in the following order of frequency (here and throughout, percentages may not total to 100 owing to rounding):

		No. of cases	% of total
1.	enitourinary diseases	628	20.61
2.	Infectious diseases	476	15.62
3.	Surgical infections	347	11.38
4.	Respiratory diseases	340	11.15
5.	Diseases of the digestive system	197	6.46
6.	Musculoskeletal disorders	181	5.94
7.	Neurological and mental diseases	162	5.31
8.	Traumatic conditions	149	4.89
9.	Diseases of the skin	125	4.10
10.	Circulatory disorders	79	2.59
11.	Tumors and cancers	75	2.46
12.	Eye problems	61	2.00
13.	Miscellaneous medical conditions	61	2.00
14.	Miscellaneous surgical conditions	37	1.21
15.	Surgical procedures	19	0.62
16.	Unknown	110	3.61
	Total	3,047	99.95

Genitourinary diseases

Twenty-four separate eighteenth-century diagnostic categories taken from folios of the General Register are included under the rubric "genitourinary diseases," with *lues venerea* most prevalent. Their relative frequency was as shown here:

Diseases affecting sexual organs		Urinary tract diseases	
Abortion	1	Anuria	1
Amenorrhea	9	Calculus	1
Chlorosis	4	Calculus urethra	1
Gonorrhea	48	Diabetes	2
Leucorrhea	8	Diseases bladder	1
Lues venerea	447	Dysuria	4
Menorrhagia	13	Enuresis	1
Phymosis	2	Gravel	2
Sibbens	15	Ischuria	6
Swollen testicles	16	Nephritis	13
Syphilis	15	Pain bladder	1
		Stone	3
		Urinary complaint	14

As can be readily seen from this list, the venereal diseases, lues venerea (71%), gonorrhea (7.6%), syphilis (2.4%), and swollen testicles (2.3%), together constituted more than 80% of all ailments in the group, and not surprisingly two-thirds of all cases occurred in men. One disease also considered venereal at that time was "sibbens," a condition apparently peculiar to Scotland.

At a time when many voluntary hospitals still regarded venereal cases as unfit for admission or allowed access only to "innocent sufferers" – women and children inadvertently infected – the Royal Infirmary of Edinburgh displayed a remarkable spirit of tolerance toward those afflicted by "the venereal taint."[4] One of the reasons was the high incidence of the disease among people guaranteed admission under a number of contracts. Having made those arrangements with the Royal Army and Navy, the authorities had little choice but to accept sick soldiers and sailors regardless of their ailments.

In spite of the stigma attached to those who contracted venereal disease, its frequency and ubiquity in all walks of life made it one of the inevitable risks of living and loving in the eighteenth century. It intruded into people's lives, often surreptitiously communicated to "infants, nurses, midwives and married women whose husbands lead dissolute lives."[5] Concealment was common, and transmission of the disease to others continued unabated because of fear of exposure and the dangerous effects of treatment. In Edinburgh visitors also reported that by the 1780s prostitution had become rampant in the city, the number of women in this trade having dramatically expanded in the previous decade. Fueling its spread in Scotland was what travelers perceived to be a somewhat more open view toward sexuality than that exhibited by its southern neighbors.[6]

However, the most important factor in the spread of venereal disease in Scotland and elsewhere was failure to seek proper treatment. William Buchan remarked that "not one in ten of those who contract it are either able or willing to submit to a proper plan of regimen." Given that the disease "assumed a variety of different shapes," many people remained unaware of their infections. Others, recognizing the symptoms and wishing to remain undetected, sought quick relief in popular remedies, but most clandestine cures were ineffectual and only masked the symptoms for brief periods of time. Unfortunately, the standard therapeutic regime required a protracted commitment few persons were willing to make. "This is the true source of nine tenths of all the mischief arising from venereal disease," concluded Buchan.[7]

Both physicians and surgeons accepted the influx of venereal cases in their wards. In fact, from their various publications one gains the impression that patients affected with venereal disease were welcome subjects for treatment, since practitioners were convinced that their medications could actually cure the ailment, a claim not easily made for most other diseases prevalent at that time. Here were splendid opportunities to demonstrate the beneficial effects of eighteenth-century therapeutics and to operate with a degree of certitude seldom possible in other clinical conditions.

Thus the prevalence of venereal cases in the infirmary – one must add to lues venerea at least another fifteen cases specifically labeled "syphilis" in the register and possibly a majority of those sixteen patients with "swollen testicles" – is not surprising, given the significant and steady arrival of soldiers, the presence of a "venereal ward" for women, and the coming of sailors in the 1790s. More than 75% of those labeled as having lues venerea were males and 54% were listed as soldiers, but as Andrew Duncan admitted in 1772, the disease was also frequent among the general population.[8]

In the General Register the terms "venereal disease" and "LV," an abbreviation for lues venerea, were employed side by side. The choice of terms probably depended on the clerk entrusted with the task of inscribing diagnoses in the books. Most medical authorities of the period subscribed to the idea expressed by one Edinburgh graduate, William Nisbet (1759–1822), that venereal disease was a generalized "constitutional" ailment resulting from the diffusion of a poison throughout the body. The effects were a "cachectic state of the body displayed in ulcerations of particular parts."[9]

Indeed, William Cullen in his own nosology placed the disease that he termed syphilis in the third class of so-called *cachexiae,* diseases neither inflammatory nor nervous in origin and affecting the entire human frame. For him syphilis was "a contagious disease after impure venery and a disorder of the genitals."[10] Cullen was convinced that sexual transmission occurred without the presence of open sores on genitals and that the infecting matter first lodged locally before being diffused throughout the body.[11]

All three terms, venereal disease, lues venerea, and syphilis, were used interchangeably by Benjamin Bell (1749–1806), a prominent Edinburgh surgeon attending the infirmary. In his famous treatise on the subject, published in 1793, Bell also stressed the contagious nature of the disease but remarked that on occasion the specific poison could be communicated from an open venereal sore to another person's wounds without sexual intercourse. At times midwives and surgeons who attended patients with such lesions were apparently infected in this manner.[12]

The first symptoms appeared three or four days later in the form of a chancre or "primary ulcer" on the genitals, spreading within a week or ten days to a nearby lymphatic gland in the groin and causing a localized swelling called a "bubo." Of interest is the fact that the initial lesions in adults were frequently located in the mouth and throat, forming what authors have described as "foul-smelling ulcers" of the tonsils, uvula, and tongue. These highly destructive sores often spread to the nose, larynx, and middle ear with symptoms of hoarseness, deafness, and swallowing difficulties. Whether these symptoms were the effects of kissing, oral sexual practices, or secondary infection remains unclear.

Practitioners differed in their explanations about propagation of the venereal "virus," as the postulated poison was often called. At this time, most of them were moving away from a purely humoral theory, arguing instead that the infective matter affected solid portions of the human organism at particularly vulnerable sites through changes in excitability. The major problem for those attending patients affected by lues venerea was to ascertain when the first phase of the disease, chancre or inguinal bubo, ceased to be a purely local problem, since during the next step the venereal matter "entered the system" and produced a "constitutional" disease with skin manifestations and later lesions in internal organs.

Bell, for example, believed that the swelling of an inguinal gland indicated the arrival of the poison there, to be diluted by a continuous flow of lymph through this structure. Success or failure in rendering the contagious matter harmless at the glandular site explained the great differences encountered in the onset of generalized symptoms, ranging from two or three weeks to eight and even twelve months.[13]

In 1770 venereal diseases accounted for 27% of the diagnoses recorded in the General Register, but from the mid 1770s onward until the end of the century the proportion dropped significantly, to 13%–15% of all admissions. By contrast, labels of "gonorrhea" gradually rose in the 1780s and reached their peak in 1790, but this shift does not explain the decline. Most physicians of the time, including Cullen, believed that gonorrhea was one of the initial local manifestations of lues venerea, an assumption buttressed by the publications of a Swedish physician, François Swediaur (1748–1824), in 1784[14] and especially by John Hunter's experimental conclusions of 1786.[15]

Yet in Edinburgh the theory that gonorrhea and lues venerea were two distinct diseases also had its advocates[16] and was forcefully defended by Benjamin Bell in his 1793 treatise.[17] Bell rejected the popularly held view that gonorrhea and syphilis were caused by the same venereal poison and differed simply in its localization, claiming on clinical grounds (experiments on medical students and therapeutic results) that they constituted two entirely separate entities with different causes.[18]

The gradual diagnostic distinction between gonorrhea and lues venerea in the General Register suggests that a number of medical clerks subscribed to Bell's theory. In fact, several entries for 1800 listed both LV and gonorrhea. Other instances of venereal disease could probably be found under labels such as "swollen testicles" and "ulcers." Owing to the practice of simply omitting diagnoses during the 1790s because of recording delays, it is hazardous to predicate a true decrease of venereal cases entering the infirmary. Given contemporary prejudices and stereotypes, a number of persons admitted with unexplained ulcerations, skin eruptions, throat complaints, or urinary difficulties were probably diagnosed as suffering from lues venerea and placed under treatment for this disease. Others with similar or unreported symptoms were almost certainly labeled differently, since syphilis has been known to simulate a vast number of other ailments because of its protean symptomatology. The Royal Navy fined each seaman contracting the "pox" the sum of fifteen shillings, a measure that fostered concealment and deceptions. Thus, with allowances for under- and over-diagnosis, the fact remains that venereal disease was by far the most common ailment seen at the Edinburgh infirmary during the final decades of the eighteenth century.

The "sibbens" or "sivvens" received this name in the Highlands because its principal skin lesions resembled the shape and color of raspberries, or *suibbean,* as they were called in Gaelic. In the Lowlands inhabitants used the term "yaws" for similar symptoms, a name obtained from sailors returning from the West Indies who linked this disease to an affection frequently seen in the tropics.[19]

The so-called Scotch pox, as it was popularly called in the eighteenth century, was a "loathsome and very infectious disease" not restricted to Scotland. According to local sources, its introduction to the region had occurred a century earlier and was blamed on the soldiers of Cromwell. Transmission of sibbens, however, unlike that of other venereal diseases, was believed to occur primarily through nonsexual contact, by "sleeping with, sucking, or saluting the infected," or through the use of such contaminated utensils as "spoon, knife, glass, cup, pipe, and cloth before they have been washed and cleaned."[20]

Most initial manifestations of sibbens appeared around the lips, mouth, and tonsils in the form of spreading ulcers; generalized skin eruptions followed, which developed spongelike pustules similar to raspberries in shape and color. Genital and perianal ulcerations with adjacent lymph node involvement were also frequent. If the nose was affected by the ulcers, widespread destruction of cartilage and bone would follow, transforming the face into a horrible and foul-smelling sore. Death was frequent, presumably brought on by a series of secondary infections.[21]

Contemporary observers made it clear that sibbens was a disease affecting the rural poor who lived in primitive conditions and lacked all forms of personal hygiene. The transmission was believed to occur when matter discharging from active ulcers came in contact with common utensils. It could also be passed from person to person or directly inoculated on contact with areas of broken skin, often excoriated by scratching for the "itch" or scabies.[22] Outbreaks were frequent in the countryside and affected entire families. The dramatic symptomatology, in turn, made outcasts of those suffering from it: "Whole families must perish, the infected being detested as lepers whom nobody would receive or go near," observed one Scottish surgeon.[23]

The General Register reveals that when individuals diagnosed as having sibbens entered the hospital, they often came in groups or families. In the sample studied, men and women were about equally represented, and with the exception of a single case, all were considered "medical" cases.[24] Both ulcerations and initial skin appearances were sufficiently similar to symptoms of lues venerea so that most physicians considered sibbens a special form of venereal disease in spite of repeated histories of nonsexual transmission, especially among children. The presence of genital lesions and the prompt response of the disease to therapy employed in cases of syphilis seemed only to confirm the close association. Sibbens therefore shared the moral stigma associated with the acquisition of a venereal disease, causing Bell to observe that "even those who get it in the most innocent manner are so much ashamed that they never speak of it as long as it can possibly be kept secret."[25] Needless to say, such an attitude obviously facilitated the dissemination of the disease.

So-called female complaints were rare because eighteenth-century physicians generally believed that a hospital setting would only perpetuate disorders associated with the menstrual cycle, since they were mainly brought on by pregnancy, confinement, and lack of exercise. However, some patients were admitted to the infirmary with diagnoses of *amenorrhea* or "suppression of menses" and *menorrhagia* or "immoderate flow of menses," because of disabling gastric symptoms, headaches, and general weakness. A related ailment, *fluor albus* or *leucorrhea,* also popularly known as "the whites," consisted of a whitish or yellow vaginal discharge frequently following but at times preceding excessively heavy or irregular menstrual periods. Lastly, *chlorosis* or the "green sickness" was a disease affecting adolescent girls, characterized by a sallow complexion, weight loss, and digestive complaints.[26] Cullen and others considered it a species of amenorrhea.

Among the diseases ascribed to the urinary tract – only about 8% of all cases in the genitourinary group – the labels "urinary complaint" and *nephritis* figure rather prominently. The latter constituted an entire genus in Cullen's nosology and was defined as "pain in the region of the kidney, often following the course of the ureter, frequent making of water either thin or colorless or very red,"[27] a group of symptoms suggestive of infection or renal colic.

In fact, passage of stones, usually bladder stones, was not an infrequent occurrence; the general term *calculus* was differentiated into "gravel" (small stones, some presumably of renal origin) and "stone" (meaning a concretion in the bladder too large to be voided). The term *dysuria* or "difficulty of urine" characterized a painful and burning sensation as the affected person voided small amounts of urine quite frequently. Popularly called "strangury," dysuria was often related to the presence of bladder stones, which caused an inflammation of the bladder, or appeared as a result of such infections.[28]

Total suppression of urine, in turn, was called *anuria* or *ischuria,* a local affection in Cullen's classification caused by disorders in the kidney or bladder or obstructions in the urethra. Physicians blamed the formation of stones on dietary indulgences, insufficient fluid intake, and a sedentary life-style, which, some practitioners believed, would produce an accumulation of "lithic acid."[29] Another factor was the excessive retention of urine in the bladder "from a false delicacy," a practice that William Buchan blamed for many deaths as well as "tedious and incurable disorders."[30]

In the opposite situation, drinking an excessive amount of fluids, especially mineral waters, was thought to dilute the blood so that it rapidly filtered through the kidneys in ever-increasing amounts, thus giving affected individuals a rare urinary ailment called *diabetes.* Popularly known as the "pissing evil" because of its unfavorable prognosis, diabetes was defined by Cullen as "a chronic profusion of urine with the smell, color, and savoury of honey."[31] It seemingly affected people "in the decline of life," especially hard drinkers and chronically fatigued workers after a lifetime of strenuous labor, although these causal relationships were greeted with skepticism by many eighteenth-century practitioners.[32] Both diabetic patients listed in the General Register were men admitted to the teaching ward for further study and treatment.

Because most genitourinary diseases were indeed venereal, an analysis of the patients' occupations and institutional destinations confirms the previous finding that more than half of them were soldiers. The proportion of patients suffering from genitourinary ailments fluctuated significantly during the three decades of this study. From a peak of 40% in 1770, the incidence dropped sharply in the next five years to 20%, remaining between 26% and 31% during the 1780s and leveling off at 24% in 1800. These changes are closely connected with the admission of patients with venereal complaints. Among the possible reasons for the decline were a reduction in the admission of soldiers, greater accuracy in diagnosis of what constituted a genuine venereal problem, and the likelihood that a fair number of unrecorded cases in the 1790s were patients affected by syphilis.

Infectious diseases

Only a few categories listed in the General Register make up the infectious disease diagnostic cluster, dominated by the very frequently employed label "fever":

Ague or intermittent fever	58	Scarlatina or scarlet fever	1
Fever	372	Smallpox	27
Hectic fever	2	Tabes	2
Measles	3	Typhus fever	6
Mumps	3		
Pertussis or whooping cough	2		

As can be seen from this list, fever alone constituted nearly 80% of all the ailments assembled under this group, followed by the ague (12.2%) and smallpox (5.6%).

Fever

"In the language of this country, the vulgar if they are hot, say that they are in a fever," wrote the prominent physician George Fordyce (1736–1802) in one of his dissertations,[33] referring to the ailment next most often (after lues venerea) recorded in the General Register. During the eighteenth century fever was a disease or group of diseases characterized by malaise and a rise of temperature, but the symptoms defining it were somewhat elusive. In Cullen's classification, fevers were placed under the first class of *pyrexiae* and defined as possessing "a frequent pulse coming after some degree of cold shivering, considerable heat, many of the functions injured, the strength of the limbs especially diminished."[34]

According to Cullen and his followers, fevers went through three distinct periods or "fits" that determined the progression of symptoms and duration of the disease. The initial "cold stage," dominated by chills and weakness, was ascribed to the impact of agents that created a debility in the nervous system and therefore spasms in arteries irrigating the surface of the body. As a reaction to the spasms, the organic system stimulated both the heart and the arteries, creating the second or "hot stage" of fever with a frequent and stronger pulse, reddish and hot skin, and other manifestations of increased nervous excitability. A third and final stage of resolution began with a lower pulse rate, profuse sweating, and greater urinary discharge, signaling a relaxation of all excretory functions and restoration of normal excitability to the brain.[35]

The explanations offered by Cullen's medical system regarding the genesis and progress of fevers dominated Edinburgh medicine for several decades, although individual authors expressed skepticism about their validity. Cullen's dictum that "almost the whole of the phenomena of fevers lead us to believe that they chiefly depend upon changes in the state of the moving powers of the animal system" revealed the significant changes occurring in medical theory at this time, which contributed to the demise of humoralism in favor of schemes based on neurophysiological models.[36]

At the infirmary men and women suffered almost equally from fever, although women, especially those listed as servants, were slightly more affected. In fact, one out of every four patients labeled in the General Register as having fever was hospitalized in the servants' ward, information that tends to confirm previously mentioned suspicions that the removal of servants from households in which they served was largely fueled by fears of contagion. Thursdays and Fridays seem to have been the most frequent days of entry, with October and December the months most likely to see febrile cases arriving at the hospital.

Admission of fever patients tended to vary significantly from year to year, fluctuating from 8% of all registrations in 1770 to 21% in 1785. Such considerable shifts are difficult to correlate with deaths from fever recorded in the General Bill of Mortality for Edinburgh and published in *Scots Magazine*. Given the imperfect methods for reporting and registering deaths in the city and the predominant social criteria dominating hospital admissions, such a lack of correspondence is not unexpected. Moreover, the infirmary received a substantial number of patients from the surrounding countryside as well as from distant army barracks and navy vessels, all reflecting independent epidemiological settings.

Again, as in the case of venereal diseases, the Edinburgh infirmary showed a remarkable degree of liberality in admitting so many fever patients, since many of them were considered contagious and once in the institution needed to be subjected to special isolation and ventilation procedures. Both managers and attending physicians were conscious of the dangers posed to other inmates by these arrivals, and of the constant threat of an epidemic breaking out within the walls of the hospital. Nevertheless, in the view of some practitioners, these fevers were so common among the poor that their admittance could not be avoided. "After more than thirty years of attentive medical observation of the situation of the lower orders in this city," wrote James Gregory, "I am fully convinced that the common continued fever is the greatest evil to which they are exposed except one: the use of distilled spirits."[37]

A number of small wards with four beds each, located in the wings of the building, were selected as ideal for managing fevers, since the rooms could be kept reasonably clean and well ventilated. In addition, special so-called fever wards were instituted in the 1780s, wards that were, in Gregory's words, "cleaner and better ventilated than most bed-chambers in Edinburgh" and that allowed patients to recover spontaneously without the employment of medicines. "I doubt whether an hospital or any number of wards in it that may be required for this purpose can in any other way be employed so much for the benefit of the public," observed Gregory,[38] expressing the conviction widely held by contemporary medical men that hospitalization could definitely be of great benefit to patients affected with fever if proper measures were taken to contain the disease within the institution.

Ague or "intermittent fever"

"Ague" was a popular term in use for centuries in the British Isles, perhaps derived from the French word *aigu,* meaning acute.[39] The name was frequently linked with fevers and employed to characterize any acute and febrile illness such as "ague smallpox" and others. By the eighteenth century, however, ague was increasingly restricted to just one type of fever, one characterized by its regular and intermittent character. Today, there is persuasive evidence to suppose that ague was indeed malaria, a debilitating disease caused by a microscopic agent called plasmodium and transmitted to humans by anophiline mosquitoes.[40]

In his nosology Cullen, on the basis of their clinical course, divided all fevers into two fundamental types: continuous and intermittent. The latter were characterized as intense febrile episodes, each separated from the next by regular intervals in which the affected individual no longer had an elevated temperature and felt more or less recovered. Cullen and most physicians employed the Latin term *quotidian* to distinguish those intermittent fevers showing daily paroxysms. The most common type was the *tertian* fever, affecting individuals every other day, with intervals of forty-eight hours between fits. A final form, the *quartan* fever, showed a seventy-two-hour intermission from one attack to the next.[41]

Medical authors were not only confused by the frequent lack of regularity displayed by the febrile episodes but also baffled by their recurrence, no matter what pattern of fits the fever adopted. As William Buchan explained, the ailment "afforded the best opportunity both of observing the nature of fever and also the effects of medicine."[42] During the fit of ague, the human organism went rapidly through the three postulated stages of fever, only to begin them anew without any obvious cause and despite numerous therapeutic measures. Most physicians, including Cullen, considered tertian fever to be the genuine type of intermittent, and many believed that continued, remittent, and quotidian fever patterns were still "imperfectly formed," settling down as a tertian intermittent fever.[43]

Most cases of ague were observed in the autumn and spring and were thought to be caused by emanations or "effluvia" arising from places where the ground was excessively wet or marshy. These hypothetical discharges presumably arising from the putrefaction of organic matter under the action of water and heat from the sun were considered by Cullen and many others to be hurtful, acting as powerful sedatives on the bodily systems. Once inhaled, these vapors or "miasma" caused enough debility in the neuromuscular system to allow the onset of spasms leading to the first cold stage of fever, clinically characterized by intense chills.[44]

"Marsh fever," as ague was frequently called, was recognized during the eighteenth century as being a serious and disabling disease endemic to certain regions of England, especially the fens of Cambridgeshire and the regions near the estuary of the Thames River in Essex and Kent.[45] In fact, many of the patients with so-called ague seeking admission to the infirmary in this period were migrant Highlanders returning from the English fens after having contracted the disease there during harvest work. The entire marsh country of southeastern England had a long history of endemic sickness and high mortality; yet it continued to beckon "unseasoned" (not acclimated through exposure) newcomers because of its agricultural opportunities, bestowing on them in return a chronic debilitating disease. Towns like Samford in Lincolnshire, Stilton in Huntingdonshire, Wisbeck in Cambridgeshire, and Woolrich in Kent appeared in the reports given to Edinburgh hospital physicians as places in which the ague or marsh fever prevailed.[46]

Little information about the prevalence of ague in eighteenth-century Scotland is presently available. In his analysis Sinclair reported that the disease had "formerly prevailed over a large proportion of Scotland," affecting farmers especially at harvest and planting time to the extent of forcing interruptions of the "various operations of husbandry."[47] From the individual parish reports it appears that only limited marshy areas in the southeast, especially in Berwickshire near the border and similar localities near the Firth of Tay and the lower course of the Tay River in Perthshire, may have suffered endemically from intermittent fevers.[48] Cullen in his clinical lectures insisted that he had not seen a single patient with ague in his twenty years of practice near Glasgow,[49] although of Edinburgh he admitted, "It is very seldom that a spring season passes in this part of Scotland without more or less of the appearance of intermittents and especially among the vulgar."[50]

In cases recorded by the clerks the sexes seem to have been almost equally represented, with a slight predominance of women in proportion to their total numbers. A significant contingent of these patients (17%) was dispatched to the teaching ward, possibly because professors thought that the intermittent fevers not only furnished good examples for studying the various stages of fever but offered great opportunities for testing therapeutic methods designed to abort febrile episodes. Another 15% of the patients were servants, and 10% soldiers, all admitted to their respective units in the hospital.

In the sample under study, hospitalization for ague or intermittent fever reached its peak between 1780 and 1785, precisely at the time when the often-quoted statistics from the Kelso Dispensary in Berwickshire showed the highest number of ague cases.[51] However, in contrast to the ambulatory institution in the Lowlands, where ague made up more than 13% of all visits between 1780 and 1785, at the Edinburgh infirmary admissions recorded under this diagnosis amounted to only about 3% of the total for the same years.

Smallpox

Smallpox was one of the most frequent and visible diseases of the eighteenth century. Contemporary writers estimated that Great Britain lost about thirty thousand persons annually to the ravages of this disease, which felled over sixty million Europeans during the eighteenth century.[52] Cullen called it *variola* and defined it as an inflammatory fever followed by the eruption of small red pimples. He recognized two basic types, the "distinct" or "discrete" form with moderate fever and only a few pustules and the "confluent" type with numerous irregular-shaped lesions in clusters and a high fever that continued unabated even after the eruption and often proved fatal. Confluent smallpox, in turn, could be of the hemorrhagic variety, with blood in pustules, urine and stool. All forms were supposedly caused by the same specific and highly feared contagion, thought to be a "ferment" assimilated into the bodily fluids, where it vigorously multiplied. The ensuing skin manifestations were believed to be one of the mechanisms whereby the infected variolous matter was "deposited" for subsequent elimination from the organism.[53]

Smallpox cases were excluded from many voluntary hospitals of the period because of well-founded fears that those affected by the disease would promptly infect other inmates and perhaps initiate an epidemic in the institution. In addition, small children ineligible for admission were frequent sufferers. However, given the prevalence of smallpox among the British population, physicians realized that such a proscription "would be a great check upon the utility of hospitals especially as in its dangerous state it requires the close attention of medical skill."[54] With reluctance and trepidation, some hospital authorities across the country occasionally admitted a few adult cases of smallpox, provided there were sufficient facilities to isolate them and prevent institutional infection.

Cullen was realistic about the advantages of hospital care in smallpox. He thought that those who contracted the disease during the cold weather were likely to suffer a more intense inflammatory reaction that could produce a confluent type of eruption attended by high mortality. Although excessive heat was blamed for turning smallpox pustules into purulent sores, Cullen believed that "warm air cannot kill," thus justifying the early admission of smallpox patients, before the full force of the inflammation and skin eruption had taken its toll. However, there was no hope of arresting the formation of the pustules, which left the ailment's characteristically disfiguring scars. Smallpox for Cullen was an ailment that "physicians cannot cure and the nurse cannot kill," but one whose symptoms the milder hospital environment, rest, and a good diet could favorably influence.[55]

As John Aikin argued in 1771, "The frequency of this disease would always give a supply of patients in most towns," and if private philanthropy wanted to achieve its objectives, smallpox needed to be treated. The best solution for this problem, and one that took into account contemporary fears of contagion, was to establish a special wing at existing infirmaries to house smallpox victims and persons wishing to be inoculated, or even to build a separate hospital "for suitable relief."[56]

At the Royal Infirmary twenty of the twenty-seven patients recorded in the General Register as afflicted with smallpox were men, half of them soldiers. Since the disease was more common in summer, half of the cases entered the institution between May and August. Because of the dangers from contagion, hospital regulations again demanded that patients be admitted to small rooms located next to the wards with only two beds in them, "the patients to be moved from time to time from one of these beds to the other if unoccupied." Ventilation, frequent changes in bedclothing, and turning of mattresses were all recommended. Vapors of warm vinegar and even the burning of tobacco leaves were used as air "correctors" to block the movement of smallpox contagion.[57]

Typhus fever

Finally, among the so-called noninflammatory or nervous fevers considered by Cullen was *typhus,* a severe febrile illness that began insidiously with malaise, severe headaches, and rising temperatures, which were followed by delirium or "typhomania." Most patients with typhus were admitted to the teaching ward for closer observation and treatment. Some ended with complications like *putrid* fevers, displaying gangrene of fingers and toes, diarrhea, and infected bedsores.[58]

In summary, then, female servants and later in the century seamen were both proportionately more affected by infectious diseases than any other occupational group. One of every three patients suffering from such an ailment was a servant ending up in the servants' ward. Another 20% of infectious cases were referred to the teaching ward because most university professors wanted their students to acquire firsthand knowledge of fevers. During the three decades under study, incidence of these diseases fluctuated significantly, reaching a peak in 1785 (31% of all admissions), only to decline ten years later to 12%.

Surgical infections

"Inflammation," admitted Benjamin Bell, "is the most frequent as it is perhaps the most important object of the surgeon's attention and a fit subject for the first article of a system of surgery."[59] The next most frequent group of ailments comprised fifty-five categories inscribed into the General Register, which can be lumped together as follows:

Abscesses	10	Sores	5
Bone caries	1	Miscellaneous ulcers	7
Fistulas	15	Suppurations	4
Miscellaneous sores	55	Swellings	16
Phlegmons	7	Ulcer on leg	23
Sore (on) arm	17	Ulcers	83
Sore (on) foot	19	White swellings	12
Sore (on) leg	73		

Ulcers and leg sores

The two most common categories in the preceding list substantially overlap: For practical purposes the terms "ulcer" and "sore" must be considered virtually synonymous, although the former was employed by medical professionals while the latter remained primarily a lay designation for the same type of lesion. Benjamin Bell defined *ulcer* as a "solution of continuity in any of the softer parts of the body."[60]

The random sample of inscriptions into the General Register for the decades 1770–1800 contains eighty-three cases simply listed as "ulcer," twenty-three additional entries called "ulcer on leg," and seven instances in which the word "ulcer" was attached to another anatomical part, including the nose, arm, finger, foot, toe and anus. The word "sore" presents problems because in a number of cases it was meant simply to convey a painful condition, such as "sore throat," "sore head," or "sore breast." Sometimes the label "sore on leg" clearly indicated an ulcerated condition, but it is difficult to judge just how many patients admitted under that category actually had open and discharging ulcers instead of pains in their legs. Perhaps a number of these cases had painful abrasions or skin conditions evolving toward ulceration and serious enough to warrant admission. One real clue was their destination. In the sample under study, less than 7% of those patients registered with sore leg went into the medical ward, a clear indication that the condition of the rest was judged a surgical problem.

Given the extraordinary frequency of leg ulcers reported in other eighteenth-century British hospitals – between 16% and 23% of all admissions at the Devon and Exeter Hospital in the period 1760–1800[61] – it would not be inappropriate to combine the diagnoses "ulcer on leg" and "sore leg" and add at least two-thirds of those patients simply entered as suffering from ulcers on the assumption that they probably also represented lesions located on the legs. Such a consolidation of diagnoses would indicate that leg ulcers represented close to 5% of all hospital admissions and thus constituted the third most common condition, behind venereal diseases and fevers.

The frequency of leg ulcers among the lower classes was occasionally pointed out by contemporary medical authors. One London surgeon, Charles Brown, estimated in 1799 that 20% of the poor suffered from this ailment and that given their numbers, many of those seeking treatment were being turned away from the hospitals.[62] Since Brown was trying to make a case for the foundation of a charitable institution devoted solely to the treatment of leg ulcers, his assessment may have been exaggerated. Nevertheless, the condition must have been quite prevalent at the time to warrant extensive medical discussions. Surgeons such as Benjamin Bell listed bruises, wounds, burns, and skin inflammations as causes of localized ulcerations.[63] Given lack of personal hygiene, dirty clothing, and the prevalence of scabies, any abrasion caused by scratching could turn into an ulcer. The same thing happened with flea and louse bites.

Whereas these events were recognized as local ailments, others seemed to be "constitutional," reflections of a systemic disease – for example, scurvy and venereal disease. So-called scorbutic ulcers not only were recognized in eighteenth-century naval personnel but frequently appeared among common people seeking entrance to the hospital. "In the Royal Infirmary sores of this kind are frequently met with," admitted Bell, "accompanied sometimes with even the most characteristic symptom of scurvy: soft, spongy gums."[64]

In other instances the ulceration was the result of a "scorbutic taint," meaning certain clinical conditions suggestive of nutritional deficiency without the specific pathognomonic signs of any disease. Bell was quite aware of the causal links between poor nutrition and the appearance of ulcers: "The foul old ulcers of poor people in every country are most frequently induced by indigence and are kept up by a real want of nourishment."[65] Treatment was therefore simple: Patients needed to receive a "well regulated nourishing diet." Contended Bell: "The practice of hospitals would probably prove more beneficial by laying the use of internal medicines almost totally aside and by employing the savings thus produced in furnishing such a diet."[66]

Among local ulcers, Bell distinguished eight classes beginning with the *simple purulent* and *simple vitiated*. The former was characterized by its low degree of inflammation and mild purulent discharge. The latter, in turn, emitted some foul-smelling matter called "sanies" if it was greenish, "ichor" if acrid and red, and "sordes" if brown like coffee grounds. The *fungous ulcer* showed spongy, unhealthy granulation tissue; the *sinuous ulcer* communicated with a cavity or structure in the form of a fistula. Most *callous ulcers,* lesions with ragged and thick edges, were associated in the eighteenth century with the nearby presence of varicose veins. Finally, Bell distinguished the so-called *carious ulcer,* a bone lesion often leading to separation of the dead fragments; *cancerous ulcer,* with hard edges and irregular growth; and *cutaneous ulcer,* including pustules, shingled, and ringworm.[67]

Lively debates about the meaning of ulcers and their management occurred during the last decade of the eighteenth century. Hitherto under the guidance of humoral theories, practitioners had viewed ulcers as convenient outlets for the discharge of harmful and unwanted matter. Therefore ulcers were generally kept open in the belief that serious illnesses would ensue if the flow were to be stopped and the purulent matter thus diverted to other internal organs. On the basis of new clinical insights, many of them obtained from military and naval medicine by physicians like James Lind and Gilbert Blane, progressive surgeons such as Benjamin and John Bell began to look for new methods to heal ulcers.[68] But all known measures were doomed by the "emaciated state of the system from want of food" displayed by hospitalized patients, a condition that Benjamin Bell considered "very prejudicial" to the healing process.[69]

More than two-thirds of all the patients affected with sore leg, ulcer on leg, or simply ulcer between 1770 and 1800 were men, and between 63% and 82% of them were admitted to the surgical wards of the infirmary. Of the rest about 15%–20% went into the soldiers' ward, 2%–8% to the servants' ward, and the remaining fraction to the teaching and medical ordinary units.

From a check of the evolution of these disease categories over the three decades of this study, it appears that the popularity of the label "sore leg" dwindled considerably after 1780, at about the time when terms such as "ulcer" and "ulcer on leg"became more frequent. In the statistical study half of the cases recorded as either "leg ulcer" or "ulcer on leg" were hospitalized during the year 1800, in part because of the influx of Russian soldiers.

Benjamin Bell agreed with Cullen's notion of inflammation as a condition in which increased tone or contraction of the arterial system induced local plethora or blood accumulation with tension, redness, and throbbing pain. If circumscribed, the swellings were often called *phlegmons* or inflamed tumors, which could simply disappear and heal by "resolution" or which might have to be "brought to suppuration" and then evacuated. Suppuration was defined as a process whereby the contents of swellings and ulcers were converted into a thick, whitish substance called pus. Contemporary surgeons felt that pus formation was the effect of "A natural exertion of the system," a local fermentation of blood serum under the impact of heat, a theory originally propounded by John Pringle in his *Treatise on the Diseases of the Army*.[70]

Abscesses were defined in the eighteenth century as cavities located in the tissues and already filled with pus. They usually exhibited all the symptoms of phlegmons in process of suppuration: local heat, redness, and pulsation, gradually moving toward the skin surface, where most of them eventually burst forth spontaneously, discharging the accumulated purulent matter. Surgeons expressed fear that exposure of newly opened large abscesses to air would aggravate the inflammation and lead to a series of systemic symptoms, including bouts of high "hectic" fever and even death. At the infirmary, as a result, they ceased to carry out extensive incisions into these lesions to aid the discharge of pus.[71]

A *fistula* was a kind of elongated and narrow channel in the connective tissue resembling a pipe with small permanent openings formed by a discharging abscess or ulcer. Benjamin Bell placed this lesion among his various categories of ulcer, calling it a "sinnuous ulcer" that opened to the skin or a neighboring natural cavity.[72] In the sample under study half of the cases were simply labeled "fistula." Four occurred in women and may have been vesicovaginal (passage between the bladder and vagina) or rectovaginal (opening between the rectum and vagina) fistulas secondary to childbirth injuries. The most commonly registered fistula was the *fistula in ano* located in the lower portion of the rectum, often the result of infected hemorrhoids or other anal infections that turned into abscesses. Another was the *fistula lachrymalis,* an abnormal communication between the lachrymal sac and the skin generally located midway between the angle of the eye and the nose. This fistula occurred following purulent eye infections that blocked and destroyed the duct normally allowing tears to flow into the nose.

Finally, there were a number of patients suffering from *white swellings,* painful enlargements of certain major joints without the usual inflammatory symptoms characteristic of acute rheumatism. Loss of motion, accumulation of fluid, and abscess formation were followed by spontaneous discharges of a thin, whitish fluid. Eighteenth-century surgeons were acutely aware of the progressive and severe systemic manifestations accompanying this joint disorder, especially weight loss, night sweats, and gradual weakness leading to death, and they blamed the condition on chronic rheumatism or consumption with scrofula. The almost predictable outcome created dilemmas for contemporary hospital surgeons, who were faced with limited options: amputation in the first stages of the disease, followed by a dangerous postoperative infection, or conservative management with gradual destruction of cartilage and bone tissue in the affected joints as the patient inexorably wasted away.[73]

In all, surgically treatable infections occurred more among men (61.3%) than among women (38.6%). Two-thirds of the patients entered the surgical ward for treatment, 13% the soldiers' ward, 12.4% the teaching unit, and 5.2% the servants' ward. The overall incidence fluctuated significantly, from 15.5% of total admissions between 1775 and 1780 to 8.6% in 1800. Within all affections considered to be surgical, the inflammatory or infectious conditions made up 42%–90% of all cases admitted to the house between 1770 and 1800.

Respiratory diseases

The following categories from the General Register were brought together under the heading "respiratory diseases":

Angina	10	Hemoptysis or spitting of blood	13
Asthma	10	Inflamed breast	1
Breast complaint	5	Pain (in) breast	5
Breast pain	1	Pain (in) side	7
Catarrh	47	Pectoral complaint	139
Cold	1	Phthisis or consumption	34
Cough	11	Pleurisy	8
Cynanche	11	Pneumonia	18
Dyspnea	5	Sore throat	14

Pectoral complaint

Over 40% of the cases grouped as respiratory were categorized by the hospital clerks simply as "pectoral complaints." This popular eighteenth-century term covered a multitude of ailments vaguely located in the chest, most of them of respiratory origin. Given the paucity of cases specifically labeled as pleurisy, pneumonia, and especially "consumption," pectoral complaint must have included almost all diseases affecting the bronchial tubes and lungs, as well as cases with detectable fluid in the chest. Cardinal symptoms were cough – the third most frequent symptom in student notebooks after pain and fever – and difficulty of breathing, called popularly "asthma" and professionally *dyspnea*. Cullen defined the latter as "a sense of fulness and infarction of the breast" and included all breathing difficulties among the spasmodic ailments caused by irregular motions of the muscular fibers lining bronchial passages.[74]

Nearly two-thirds of all patients labeled by the clerks as having pectoral complaints were men, with soldiers and servants leading the way among the occupational groups listed in the General Register. Since a fair number of those suffering from chest disorders were actually suspected of having pulmonary consumption, servants again were among those readily sent to the hospital, as masters fearing the onset of a chronic and incurable disease sought to terminate employment. Not unexpectedly, given the seasonality of most respiratory problems, the registrations show that the month of January had the highest rate of admission of this disease category.

From the distribution of this diagnosis over the three decades from 1770 to 1800, it appears that the term "pectoral complaint" gradually gained favor with hospital clerks, finally accounting for nearly 7% of all entries made in the register for the years 1790–1800. Possible reasons for reporting patients affected with respiratory ailments in this way were actual diagnostic uncertainty, expediency, and perhaps the need to disguise suspected cases of pulmonary tuberculosis considered "improper for hospitals" according to infirmary statutes. In fact, many of these so-called pectoral complaints were recorded as cases of incipient "phthisis" or "consumption" in student notebooks. As soon as warmer weather set in, they were discharged for clean "country air," considered the only useful remedy. "Patients labouring under pulmonary consumption if the disease be advanced to the second or last stage, will suffer from the air of the hospital," read one of the infirmary's directives,[75] reflecting the concerns of both managers and practitioners about the vitiated air in the wards that was clearly not conducive to the patients' recovery. Most contemporary physicians concurred with Aikin's dictum that "all diseases affecting the lungs are of that kind which can never receive benefit from even the sweetest and best contrived hospital."[76]

Why, then, were so many patients affected with pectoral complaints allowed to enter the infirmary? The reasons were simple. As in the case of venereal diseases, the hospital had contractual obligations to admit sick soldiers and servants seeking care. Perhaps more important, such complaints were common among the "vulgar." One cause for the frequency of bronchial and pulmonary afflictions, especially during winter months, was poor housing. Another factor was Edinburgh's air pollution. Rises in living standards after the 1760s prompted a greater consumption of coal for heating purposes, and black smoke began to billow from hundreds of city chimneys, gradually converting Edinburgh into the "auld reekie" (old smoky) of nineteenth-century infamy.[77]

Catarrh

The next most frequent respiratory condition was catarrh (14% of this category), a disease that Cullen defined as "an increased excretion of mucus from the membranes of the nose, fauces, and bronchia," accompanied by fever.[78] Most of the symptoms correspond to those of the common cold, often associated with hoarseness, dry cough, and occasionally pain in the chest, but in their evolution catarrhs could exhibit more cough, breathing difficulties, and considerable expectoration. Cullen did not consider the ailment dangerous except when it affected elderly persons or those already laboring under a chronic lung disease.[79]

Most cases of catarrh occurred during the winter months, when it was the "disease of the season." It apparently affected the "poorer sort of people" with the greatest frequency and violence, to the extent that they almost became "habituated to catarrh," as Daniel Rutherford explained it. "There is no disease in this climate that is more to be dreaded," he continued, noting that frequent bouts with catarrh created a dangerous chronic condition that possibly set the stage for pulmonary consumption.[80] Infirmary physicians were convinced of the favorable effects of hospitalization in this disease. Cullen and Duncan recognized that the "shelter and protection afforded by the hospital" and the "uniform temperature of this house" were key elements in the recovery or patients afflicted with catarrh,[81] protecting the sick from the frigid northeasterly winds coming off the North Sea.

Phthisis

Following closely behind catarrh in frequency was *phthisis pulmonaris,* popularly known as "consumption of the lungs" (10% of the respiratory category), in Cullen's system a species of hemoptysis characterized by a "hectic" type of fever with several daily peaks and the expectoration of fresh blood and eventually purulent matter. Before the latter symptom appeared, Cullen and other physicians talked about an "incipient phthisis," but the appearance of an opaque, yellowish matter believed to proceed from ulcerations or tubercles located in the lungs signaled the advent of a "confirmed phthisis."[82] These medical authors believed that the matter contained in lesions frequently observed at postmortem examinations was "imbued with a peculiar noxious acrimony" that caused the fever and gradual bodily decay associated with this usually fatal disease.[83]

Consumption among the poor "carries off the greatest number of persons about the middle period of life," wrote John Sinclair in his analysis of diseases prevailing in Scotland toward the end of the eighteenth century. Sinclair blamed deficient housing, light clothing, and occupational conditions for the contemporary rise in consumption. The "coldness and dampness" of dwellings, a shift in clothing from "thick and warm Scotch plaiding to the fine but thin and cold English cloth," and lack of properly heated workshops for weavers and spinners were among the reasons given for the prevalence of this disease.[84] In Edinburgh the category "consumption," with its frequent "pectoral complaints," consistently led the city's official mortality statistics in the latter part of the eighteenth century and was responsible for about 30% of all registered burials.[85]

Cullen, for his part, recognized a frequent link between pulmonary phthisis and *scrofula*, an affliction of the lymphatic glands, especially around the neck. Known for centuries in Europe as the "King's Evil," scrofula was apparently widespread in southern Scotland at that time and seen as a product of poor nutrition and damp climate. The ensuing debility manifested itself in the form of hard, painless swellings in the neck or under the chin or armpits, occasionally draining a whitish, foul fluid that brought the patients to the attention of surgeons. According to eighteenth-century authors, both phthisis and scrofula appeared in people of a "sanguineo-melancholic temperament" with "very fine skins, rosy complexion, soft flesh, and a thick upper lip."[86]

Cullen also realized that in a number of instances pulmonary phthisis occurred in stonecutters, millers, flax dressers, and others constantly exposed to dust. In general, however, the leader of the Edinburgh Medical School was skeptical about the contagious nature of phthisis, stating in his textbook that "in many hundred instances of the disease which I have seen, there has been hardly one which to me could appear to have arisen from contagion."[87] Separating the symptoms from chronic catarrh, asthma, and other bronchopulmonary conditions was always difficult, and phthisis was only seriously suspected when cough and expectoration persisted for many months and were gradually joined by frequent night sweats, fever, weight loss, and hemoptysis during the more advanced stages of the disease.

Physicians had many reservations about admitting patients clearly suffering from phthisis, but this attitude was never based on fears of contagion. Since prognosis was for the most part unfavorable, affected individuals were seen as virtually incurable and thus "improper" candidates for hospital treatment. Cases of confirmed phthisis received only advice and some palliation of their symptoms before being sent out again. However, patients assumed to be incipient cases could sometimes hope for successful treatment and perhaps even a cure, although their chances of receiving a good diet, sailing to a warmer climate in winters, and getting gentle exercise from horseback riding were practically nil. Since these measures customarily recommended to private patients were not "practicable in the lower ranks of life," brief stays in the hospital during the coldest months with rest and an appropriate diet could achieve somewhat similar results until the warmth of spring and a chance for pure country air led to their prompt dismissal.

Of the phthisis patients listed in the General Register, 61% were men. About half of the entire group was admitted to the ordinary medical ward; equal numbers (17.6%) went to the soldiers' ward, the servants' ward, and the teaching unit. A third of the total number entered the infirmary during the month of January, a finding that confirms the physicians' statements about the desirability of admitting such persons in the winter to prevent the transformation from incipient to confirmed phthisis under the stress of exposure to cold weather.

Pneumonia and pleurisy

A final comment regarding the occurrence of *pneumonia* is in order. Cullen included under this term "the whole of the inflammations affecting either the viscera of the thorax or the membrane lining the interior surface of that cavity," with two species of the disease designated *peripneumony* and *pleurisy*, respectively.[88] His reasons for lumping them together was the conviction that all inflammatory conditions of the lungs began in the pleura and then expanded into pulmonary tissue. The principal symptoms were fever, dyspnea, cough, and bloody expectoration, as well as chest discomfort or pain. Exposure to cold was believed to be the most important cause, and not surprisingly two-thirds of the cases inscribed in the General Register were admitted between November and March. In the available sample 28% of those entering the infirmary with a diagnosis of pneumonia were sent to the soldiers' ward.

Angina or cynanche

Finally, the General Register also listed a number of patients suffering from *angina* or *quinsy*, defined as an inflammation of the throat better known in Cullen's nosology as *cynanche*. Among the most common species were *cynanche tonsillaris*, an inflammation of the tonsils with pain, redness, and swelling; *cynanche trachealis*, also known as the "croup," with hoarseness, breathing difficulties, and occasional suffocation as membranes formed in the fauces and restricted the intake of air. In addition, Cullen recognized a *cynanche maligna* or putrid quinsy, with extensive ulcerations of the tonsils and fauces, and the *cynanche parotidea,* also known as "mumps," affecting the parotid and maxillary glands.[89]

To conclude, respiratory diseases accounted for nearly 11% of all cases admitted to the infirmary from 1770 to 1800. In the final decade this group represented about 17% of all ailments considered medical, and the increase may perhaps reflect greater environmental pollution and occupational hazards linked to the Industrial Revolution. Men patients (60%) predominated over women (40%), about the average ratio for all medical and surgical inscriptions. Most patients were referred to the ordinary medical wards – 62.8% – whereas 16.8% entered the servants' ward and 16.5% the soldiers' ward.

Diseases of the digestive system

The General Register contained a fair number of diagnostic categories that can be included in the group of digestive diseases:

Bilious complaint	1	Dyspepsia or stomach complaint	120
Bowel complaint	5	Enteritis	1
Cholera	1	Hepatitis	3
Colica pictonum	1	Ileus	1
Colic or spasm	12	Jaundice or icterus	11
Costiveness	1	Stomach spasm	1
Crampish pains	1	Tympanites	1
Diarrhea	18	Vomiting	5
Diseased liver	1	Worms	5
Dysentery	8		

Dyspepsia was an eighteenth-century medical term for indigestion or difficulty of digestion. This category covered a multitude of symptoms, from want of appetite or *anorexia* to heartburn or *pyrosis,* eructation, "squeamishness," vomiting, and pain in the gastric region.[90] Cullen's genus *dyspepsia* was placed in his second class of diseases, called *neuroses,* meaning disorders of the nervous system that affected sensory impressions and motions. Dyspepsia was believed to be caused by weakness in the muscular fibers of the stomach, as a reflection of systemic debility, as the result of a local injury, or as a secondary event caused by "sympathy" with other affections in the body. The consequences of such a loss of tone or "imbecility" of the stomach affected the quality of the digesting fluids secreted in that organ, causing especially the excessive acidity perceived to be responsible for some of the dyspeptic symptoms.[91]

Admission of such a large number of patients with dyspepsia raises problems of interpretation. The diagnosis was certainly applied to people suffering from heartburn, also popularly known as "waterbrash" and professionally called *pyrosis*. According to Cullen, it was frequent in Scotland, affecting "people in lower life" who were dependent on meager diets of milk and starches. Symptoms in the form of stomach cramps and belching generally occurred before eating.[92] Whether affected with genuine hunger pangs or other disorders, poor people with heartburn must have constituted an important contingent of the dyspepsia cases to actually merit description in a medical treatise.

Another group admitted under this category included persons addicted to the use of "ardent spirits." In his *First Lines of the Practice of Physic* Cullen listed frequent alcoholic intoxication among the principal causes of dyspepsia.[93] In his analysis, Sinclair argued that the substitution of distilled liquors for ale was the most hurtful change in diet experienced by the Scottish people during the eighteenth century and he mentioned stomach complaints among the disorders that had become more frequently seen as a result of alcohol abuse.[94] This was especially true among the "lower ranks" in the city of Edinburgh, whose "high jinks" (drinking bouts) were a necessary escape from the daily vicissitudes of life. So prevalent was the "vice of drunkenness" that one contemporary Edinburgh newspaper published tongue-in-cheek a scheme for preventing it: a wooden automaton capable of absorbing wine while continuing to utter toasts.[95] "Dram" (liquor) drinking or visiting the "dram shop" was often a necessity for attainment of any kind of social recognition, and those who did not indulge in the pastime were viewed as suffering from some degree of physical feebleness and "imbecility" of character instead of stomach.[96]

Psychological factors as well as such dietary causes as fasting and hard drinking were implicated in the occurrence of stomach complaints and dyspepsia. Anxiety, "uneasiness or vexation of mind," "intense study not properly alternated with cheerful conversation or exercise," "close application to business too long continued," "disorderly passions of any kind," and "an indolent and sedentary life" were some of the situations blamed for dyspeptic disorders. Hysteria and hypochondriasis were two mental affections also displaying dyspepsia, but here the stomach trouble was usually considered a secondary symptom.[97]

Tea drinking probably swelled the rank of dyspeptics, as noted by Sinclair in his examination of Scottish health conditions. "The poor stint themselves in many essential necessaries of life in order to procure this article of luxury," he wrote. Sinclair was appalled by the quality of the "very coarse kind of black tea" sold to the poor, a "miserable and unwholesome" article generally drunk very strong and hot without milk or sugar.[98] The effect on the stomach was thought to be similar to that of other so-called narcotic substances, such as alcohol.[99]

Slightly more male than female patients (although there were a larger number of the latter in the sample) were recorded in the General Register as cases of stomach complaint and dyspepsia. No occupational preference could be detected. Usage of the term "stomach complaint" predominated in the early 1770s (not a single case of dyspepsia is recorded for the year 1770), but there was a gradual change to the term "dyspepsia" in the next decades, until by the 1790s the latter was almost exclusively employed. Taken together, the two categories show only minor fluctuations between 1770 and 1800.

Instead of being solely a symptom, *diarrhea* was also considered to be a disease in its own right, a genus in Cullen's nosology under the order of spasmodic diseases. It was characterized by frequent stools without fever or any other inflammatory manifestations. Most authors distinguished six different species of diarrhea depending on the appearance and character of the stools: *feculent* (white), *bilious* (yellow), *mucous* (whitish, semitransparent), *caeliaca* (milky), *lienteria* (mixed with undigested food), and *hepatic* (containing blood).[100]

Cullen defined the *colic* or "colica" as a "pain of the belly especially twisting around the navel, vomiting, and constipation."[101] The most common species was the so-called *spasmodic colic,* a disease characterized by constipation, abdominal cramps, and frequent nausea as well as vomiting. In extreme situations the gut became totally paralyzed and intestinal contents issued from the mouth, a fatal condition called *ileus* or *iliac passion.* Most of the colics, however, especially the flatulent or "wind colic" prevailing among country people, followed the ingestion of spoiled or indigestible foodstuffs and fermenting liquors. Others ware said to occur after exposure to cold and wet weather. Finally, a *bilious colic* with acute umbilical pains and bile-tinged vomits and a *hysteric* one with severe stomach pains and vomiting were also discerned.

A special condition was *colica pictonum,* also referred to as the *colic of Poitou* or *Devonshire colic* because of similar affections reported in those places. In addition to violent abdominal cramps and constipation appearing in the early stages of the disease, sufferers complained of tingling sensations in the extremities. Weakness, numbness, and paralysis in arms and legs followed. Stupor, delirium, and death could result if the disease was allowed to take its course.[102] Eighteenth-century physicians were aware that this ailment was due to chronic lead poisoning. For many the cause of the "nervous colic" was exposure to poisonous dust and fumes prevailing among miners, smelters of lead, plumbers, and manufacturers of white lead. Frequent cider drinkers in Devon also suffered similar symptoms, since the presses made to crush the apples were leaden.[103]

The term *enteritis* was commonly applied to nonspecific inflammations of the intestines, whereas *dysentery* was reserved for a specific epidemic disease occurring in warm weather with fever, abdominal cramps, and frequent stools of a more or less putrid nature. Buchan blamed the advent of enteritis on the ingestion of unripe fruits, great quantities of nuts, and stale bottled beer or sour wine, as well as "hard windy malt liquors."[104] Dysentery seemed to be transmitted by a contagion and predominantly affected young children during the summer and early fall.

Cholera morbus or "bilious diarrhea" was distinguished from other conditions and viewed as a fulminant ailment spontaneously arising in young people during the warm weather, primarily characterized by intense vomiting and purging of bilious matter, cold sweats, and severe abdominal pain and distention. The acuteness of the disease and violence of its symptoms were viewed as extremely dangerous. "The patient sinks sometimes in 24 hours," stated one textbook, exhausted and thirsty from the great loss of fluids.[105]

Cullen recognized an acute and chronic inflammation of the liver or *hepatitis,* which was accompanied by fever, nausea, pain or fullness under the right lower ribs and radiating to the top of the shoulder, and a yellowish tint of the skin, eyes, and urine. At times gallstones or the frequent consumption of strong wines and spiritous liquors were implicated as causes for the jaundice. Cullen and others also believed that exposure to cold, violent exercise, or the passions of the mind could produce the disease. Hemmorhages, often in the form of nosebleeds, were observed toward the end of the clinical evolution.[106]

By contrast, chronic forms of hepatitis were generally discovered at postmortem dissections to be caused by large abscesses or tumors that virtually destroyed the organ. On occasion, the surface of the liver would adhere to the peritoneal lining or the diaphragm, and some of the pus would drain toward the skin or the chest cavity. A special type of liver enlargement was sometimes noted in the form of a *hydatis* or *hydatic cyst,* a bag lined with an opaque coat containing a number of smaller detached vesicles. The cysts had a tendency to burst into the abdominal cavity, quickly producing a fatal inflammation of the peritoneum.[107]

Icterus or jaundice was considered to be a separate disease, defined by its clinical manifestations: "yellowness of the skin and eyes, white feces, urine of a dark red tinging."[108] The most common species was the *icterus calculosus* produced by the presence of gallstones that obstructed the biliary ducts. Another was the *icterus infantum,* which according to Cullen occurred in infants a few days after birth.[109]

Eighteenth-century authors distinguished three types of worms: the tapeworm or *taenia,* a long roundworm or *teres,* and another short and rounded worm lodged in the rectum and named *ascarides.* Worms seem to have been very frequent, especially in children "who grind their teeth or pick their noses," and the high incidence in certain families suggests an important hereditary component that facilitated their appearance. Worms were believed to prosper in weak and relaxed stomachs, and children were especially vulnerable because they still lacked sufficient bile in their guts to prevent the generation of these parasites. Cullen, for his part, insisted that in many cases "worms are entirely innocent and of no prejudice to the system," merely bystanders or even "the effect rather than the cause of diseases such as smallpox and measles."[110] The problem, as he saw it, was that once worms had been detected before or after hospitalization, "anything and everything may be imputed to them," a perennial source of diagnostic confusion and error. Abdominal cramps and swelling, diarrhea, vertigo or swooning, and even epileptic fits were among the most commonly listed complaints, and anal itching suggested the presence of small white worms.[111]

The proportion of women affected with digestive diseases was significantly higher than average (47.5%), reflecting no doubt the frequent diagnosis of dyspepsia made in female patients, but all occupational groups identified by the hospital clerks shared about equally in the occurrence of these disorders. Between 1770 and 1800 the General Register disclosed only minor variations in the incidence of diseases belonging to the digestive system.

Musculoskeletal disorders

Over twenty-five separate diagnostic categories were used in the General Register to refer to musculoskeletal disorders. They can be summarized as follows:

Back pain	1	Rickets	1
Contracted thigh	2	Sciatica	5
Diseased ankle, arm, finger, hip, knee, leg, and toe	15	Spasm of breast	1
Ischias	1	Stiff arm and joint	2
Lumbago	7	Strained thigh	1
Pain (in) arm, knee, leg	3	Swollen wrist	1
Rheumatism	139	Tetanus	1
		Weak arm	1

More than half of all cases in the musculoskeletal group were listed simply as *rheumatism* or "rheumatic complaint." The terms were applied to a variety of joint and muscular affections associated with pain and restriction of motion. According to Sinclair, rheumatism was a relatively recent disease in Scotland but already the most prevalent complaint registered in all the parish reports of the country. It was believed that a moist and cold climate predisposed people to this affliction, but its incidence was decisively promoted by what Sinclair called the "miserable, cold, and damp huts in which the poorer classes reside." Sinclair was also well aware of the social and economic impact of rheumatism on Scottish life, crippling the working force and rendering "the decline of life a state of increasing misery." Direct relationships to poor housing, inadequate clothing, and unhealthy life-style among the poor made rheumatism a prime subject "to which the real philanthropist can direct his attention with a greater prospect of doing good."[112]

Popular eighteenth-century notions blamed rheumatism on the inability to perspire freely during the winter months, as a result of which noxious substances were trapped inside the body instead of being able to surface with the sweat and be eliminated. At the root of the problem was flannel. "Since people have ceased to wear flannel shirts, rheumatism has become much more general," observed Sinclair, since its capacity to ward off excessive cold while continuing to stimulate and absorb perspiration was superior to linen. "To adopt the use of flannel would do more to alleviate, if not extirpate, rheumatic and nervous disorders in general than the united powers of the materia medica," he concluded.[113]

In his classification, Cullen placed rheumatism under his first order of diseases, the pyrexiae or inflammatory ailments, although he publicly admitted that it was "one of these diseases which very much disturbs the order and method of our nosology."[114] He defined rheumatism as a disease with fever and pain "infesting the knees and other large joints."[115] Moreover, he tried to make a distinction between acute rheumatism – an inflammatory disease with symptoms of fever – and chronic rheumatism – a sequel of the former following the disappearance of fever and redness around the joints. As in other inflammatory conditions, Cullen postulated that cold applied to joints produced local vascular spasms followed by a systemic reaction similar to that observed in fevers. The increased "afflux of blood" to these joints then yielded pain, inflammation, and restricted motion. Resolution of the episode occurred in the third phase, characterized by a relaxation of the neuromuscular system and suspension of the shifting or "flying pains." "Sweating," Cullen told his audience in a lecture, "is the natural crisis to rheumatism."[116]

While able to fit the main clinical manifestations of acute rheumatism into his fever model, Cullen had great difficulties in explaining the chronic type of the disease, admitting to students that it was "one of the most difficult subjects of pathology." He imputed both the rigidity and the contraction encountered in several joints and surrounding musculature to protracted vascular spasm that reflected a state of atony or weakness in the nervous system. Though plausible within the framework of his neurovascular pathogenesis, Cullen's explanation was extremely vague and forced its author to concede, "I have not acquired any clear notion with regard to it myself."[117]

Hospital physicians were urged to make distinctions between acute and chronic rheumatism and admit only the former, because acute diseases were "likely to receive speedy relief from the skill and attention of the physician." The chronic, in contrast, led to protracted hospitalization but had "little hopes of a radical cure."[118] This distinction was, however, often difficult to make. Cullen remarked that "we are frequently puzzled to distinguish diseases from their sequels or antecedents when they cannot be put in the same place of our nosology."[119]

All cases recorded in the General Register were labeled simply "rheumatism," without reference to their acuteness or chronicity. From the available evidence it appears that women were proportionately more affected than men, although the overall percentages – men, 57.5; women, 42.4 – are almost identical to contemporary statistics presented by John Haygarth in his "clinical history of the acute rheumatism": men, 57.3%; women, 42.6%.[120] Haygarth tried to explain his findings by saying that the "men are more exposed to cold and rain than women."[121]

The relative predominance of women admitted to the infirmary with rheumatism was caused by an influx of female servants suffering from symptoms of the disease. Almost one out of every five patients entering the hospital under this heading was identified as a servant and sent to the appropriate ward for care. Eventually, toward the end of the century, seamen became the occupational group with the highest incidence of rheumatism. (In James Lind's statistics concerning sick sailors admitted to Haslar Hospital between 1758 and 1766, about 7% suffered from rheumatism.)[122]

An ailment considered to be a special form of rheumatism was *sciatica,* also called *ischias,* an affection of the hip joints and adjacent muscles producing a severe localized pain that could radiate down the thighs and legs. Another was *lumbago,* with pain in the loins aggravated by bending. A less frequent type of lumbago attacked the psoas muscle, with an attendant hectic type of fever and collection of pus.[123]

Two important diseases rare among infirmary admissions were *rickets* or *rachitis* and *tetanus.* The former was a genus in Cullen's nosology under diseases with swellings and affected young children between the ages of one and two. Because it often occurred in families, there was a suspicion among physicians that debilitated and malnourished mothers or wet nurses transmitted a certain "taint" capable of producing the skull, chest, and limb deformities.[124]

Buchan believed that rickets had "never appeared in Britain till manufacturers began to flourish and people, attracted by the love of gain, left the country to follow sedentary employments in great towns."[125] Lack of proper diet and exercise and confinement in small houses instead of exposure to fresh air were among the factors thought to cause the disease. Cullen postulated "a faulty state of ossification seemingly depending on that matter which should be deposited."[126]

Tetanus, also known, for its most prominent symptom, as "locked jaw," attacked mostly adults following their exposure to cold and moisture or lacerations and puncture wounds. The most dramatic symptoms were severe muscular spasms beginning with a painful rigidity of the neck and back (*opisthotonos* if the head was drawn back toward the spine and *emprosthotonos* if it was pulled forward, the chin resting on the chest). The muscles of the lower jaw contracted to close the mouth completely while the abdomen retracted until it felt "as hard as a piece of board."[127] Patients affected with tetanus periodically suffered violent contractions and excruciating pains. Mercifully, all those who displayed these symptoms succumbed to the disease in a matter of days. The one patient listed in the register was a man accepted to the teaching ward for further observation and treatment. He died in the hospital three days later.

Registration of cases affected with musculoskeletal disorders did not vary significantly between the years 1770 and 1800. As expected, the percentage of admissions recorded as rheumatism rose slightly after 1790 because of the arrival of sailors, but this increase was largely offset by a decrease in other categories. By 1800 musculoskeletal diseases afflicted about 6% of all patients who entered the hospital.

Neurological and mental diseases

The following categories used in the General Register were placed in the neurological and mental group:

Neurological		*Mental*	
Atrophy or atrophia	3	Hypochondriasis	13
Chorea	3	Hysteria or hysteric complaints	38
Concussion	1	Mania	1
Deafness	3	Melancholy	2
Epilepsy, convulsive affection, or fits	20	Nostalgia	1
Headaches or cephalgia	24	Senility	1
Head complaint	1		
Hemiplegia	3		
Lethargy	1		
Marasmus	2		
Paralysis or palsy	38		
Phrenitis	1		
Vertigo	6		

The most common disease listed among the neurological disorders was *paralysis* or *palsy*, defined by Cullen as "consisting of a loss of the power of voluntary motion" and affecting certain parts of the body.[128] Two frequent species were *hemiplegia*, in which only one side was affected, and *paraplegia*, where the body below the waist lost its motions. Of the patients listed in the register, 80% were men, almost all of them admitted to the ordinary medical ward and the teaching unit. All cases of palsy were explained by an "interrupted influx of the nervous power" resulting from a generalized affection.[129] Authors were quick to point out that the diagnosis was entirely based on the patients's inability to move voluntary muscles, whether or not it was accompanied by a loss of sensibility. Total absence of both motor and sensory power was said to happen in a condition called *apoplexy,* a vascular accident taking place in the brain.

Cullen believed that the interruption had its origins either in the brain or the nerves, the latter affected along their paths to the various muscles. It was postulated that a paroxysm of apoplexy often caused a fair amount of blood to escape the vessels, compressing one part of the brain and establishing a hemiplegia. Other palsies happened as a consequence of injuries to the larger nerves, as complications of various infectious diseases with delirium, or as a result of inhalation of poisonous fumes.

Another common ailment listed in the register was *cephalgia* or headache, a "dull pain of the head," generally of short duration. In most instances it was just a symptom of a forthcoming fever or catarrh. Some headaches, however, were chronic or "periodical," and constituted the entire complaint. People with the latter condition reported pain on one side of the skull: *hemicrania;* others had pain around the temples or forehead.[130] Two-thirds of those who entered the infirmary with headaches were women, half of them admitted to the ordinary medical ward during the 1770s.

Epilepsy or the "falling sickness" was another one of Cullen's diseases placed in the category of neuroses. It was characterized by sudden and involuntary convulsions, with the attacks usually preceded by headaches, lassitude, or the so-called *aura epileptica,* a premonitory sensation of something creeping like an insect or floating from the limbs toward the head.[131] After the aura, convulsions would begin without further warning, with the person generally falling to the ground, insensible, the tongue thrust out and frothy saliva issuing from the mouth.

According to contemporary reports, epilepsy mainly affected children and young adults, attacking more men than women. Of the twenty patients admitted to the infirmary, twelve were male and eight female. Half of them went into the ordinary medical wards and another quarter to the teaching ward because of the therapeutic challenges posed by the fits. Most cases were considered hereditary, but the traumatic source of others was clearly recognized.[132]

Vertigo or "swimming of the head" was usually just a symptom of "transient and short continued giration of objects," presumably produced by injuries, plethora, fever, debility, or digestive troubles. The sensation was explained as the effect of a temporary compression in the brain caused by pressure from the skull, vascular congestion, or humoral disorders.[133]

Atrophy or *atrophia,* meaning the "falling away of flesh," was a disease in Cullen's nosology defined as "leanness and asthenia without hectic fever." It was also called "nervous consumption" and characterized by a lack of appetite, bad digestion, and considerable weight loss, all caused by insufficient food intake during famines, diarrhea, emotional disturbance, or alcohol abuse. The term *marasmus* carried a similar meaning of bodily consumption but was usually employed to designate the final stages of such a disease.[134]

Cullen's definition of *chorea* included a clinical description that centered on its involuntary convulsions, often restricted to only one side of the body, "resembling the gesticulations of mountebanks" and affecting individuals before puberty. Also termed "St. Vitus' dance," the disease began with paralysis of one leg that characteristically forced those who were affected to drag the limb along.[135]

Finally, *phrenitis, frenzy,* and *cephalitis* were terms employed to describe an inflammation of the brain or its membranes. Among the principal symptoms were fever and severe pain, especially in the back of the head and neck, followed by incoherent speech, delirium, and intolerance to light and sound. At times phrenitis attacked the soldiers who were continuously exposed to the heat of the sun during their guard duty.[136]

Hysteria was frequently seen at the Edinburgh infirmary. Cullen distinguished this disease from other convulsive disorders and neuroses by its most characteristic set of symptoms: the *hysteric paroxysm.* Affected persons would first complain of abdominal fullness and pain and then describe a sensation similar to that of a ball ascending from the gut to the stomach and then to the throat, where it produced a sense of strangulation and suffocation. These feelings produced great anxiety and triggered a number of convulsions often restricted to one limb – the arm, for example, with the clenched fist repeatedly beating on the chest. These motions were joined by episodes of laughter and crying, screaming, or shouting, all seemingly carried out in a trancelike state. After some time, the convulsions and noise would cease, and those so affected would claim no recollection of the preceding events.[137]

Most eighteenth-century authors believed that hysteria attacked primarily women during their childbearing years. An indolent life-style, with lack of exercise or fresh air, and boredom were thought to enfeeble the body, making it susceptible to this affliction. Almost all patients listed in the General Register were women and about a fourth of them servants. Cullen tried hard to link this disease with the uterus, remarking in his textbook that hysteria appeared more readily before menstrual periods and in barren or nymphomaniac women of plethoric habit. Congestion within the genital system was connected with a state of excessive nervous irritability and hysteric fits.[138]

Hypochondriasis or "hypochondriac affection" was for many contemporary authors the male equivalent of hysteria. Cullen, however, made a distinction between them, insisting that hypochondriasis, also popularly known as "vapors" or "low spirits," was a condition without fits. Persons affected by it were of a melancholic temperament and felt an obstinate "apprehension of great evil." They were sad, fearful about the future, and, in Cullen's words, "particularly attentive to the state of their own health to every the smallest change of feeling in their bodies."[139]

Hypochondriasis usually occurred in middle-aged persons of both sexes. In the sample from the infirmary register nine of the patients were male, four female. The melancholic disposition and life-style that predisposed people to hysteria also had a hand in the appearance of hypochondriasis. In eighteenth-century Britain, according to Buchan, an increase in luxury and sedentary employments threatened to swell the registers with new cases. For him, hypochondriasis was a perennial companion of the studious individual submerged in deep thought. "To what a wretched condition are the best of men often reduced by it," he wrote, "their strength and appetite fail; a perpetual gloom hangs over their minds; they live in the constant dread of death and are continually in search of relief from medicine."[140]

Melancholy or *melancholia,* by contrast, was viewed by Cullen and others as a partial form of madness "without dyspepsia." Character traits disposing to the disease were caution and fear, timidity, and the tendency toward despondency that also marked hypochondriacs. What set melancholic patients apart, according to Cullen, was their defective judgment regarding issues other than their own health. Groundless fears, impatience, weariness of life, and "indisposition to action" were some of the mental traits reflective of melancholia.[141] For Buchan there existed a special type of so-called religious melancholy, whereby "persons of a religious turn of mind behave as if they thought it a crime to be cheerful."[142]

During the eighteenth-century mania was considered to be a higher and more universal form of true madness. "A hurry of mind" and "running from one train of thought to another" were among its most distinctive characteristics. Cullen also considered victims to be resentful, angry, or irascible, their confused perception and false judgments prompting impetuous and hurtful actions attended by the "incoherent and absurd speech we call raving." Like other observers, he was impressed by the resistance these persons displayed against "the powers of sleep, cold, and even hunger."[143]

Cullen believed that these mental symptoms reflected an "unusual excess in the excitement of the brain," probably produced by the passions of the mind. In his effort to link mind and body, he expressed the conviction that "the state of the intellectual functions depends chiefly upon the state and condition of what is termed the nervous power." Thus Cullen accepted the proposition that certain cases of insanity were due to localized affections of the brain interrupting free communications within the organ – a concept drawn from the pathological observations of Morgagni. However, he remained skeptical about the universal applicability of this hypothesis to all manic cases, proposing instead a functional theory, cerebral excitement, which could explain the reversible nature of certain mental affections, notably the delirium accompanying fevers.[144] In a clinical lecture delivered in 1788 James Gregory agreed: "Stupor, rage, and mania may arise without any organic lesion and this is an important piece of information both as to theory and practice."[145] To eighteenth-century practitioners brain lesions implied a state of irreversibility that discouraged treatment. Changes in nervous excitability instead suggested opportunities for improvement and even cure, bringing hope to the treatment of mentally ill patients.

Admissions for neurological and mental diseases experienced only minor fluctuations between 1770 and 1800, remaining around 6% of all authorized hospital entries. The high proportion of women among them was due to the frequency of hysteria and of headaches affecting women.

Traumatic conditions

Forty-two separate categories, most of them listed in the General Register as "surgical accidents," were brought together as indicated here:

Accident	9	Fracture of leg	5
Bruise or contusion	29	Injury (of) head, hip, eye, foot,	
Burn	15	leg	6
Cut leg, head, knee, throat	5	Luxation	4
Dislocation (of) ankle, arm, leg,		Mortification of feet	1
spine, thigh	8	Sprain	15
Dog bite	1	Sprain (of) ankle, hand, thigh,	
Fracture	15	wrist	4
Fracture (of) arm	6	Wound	11
Fracture (of) finger, rib, skull,		Wounded or hurt foot, head,	
thigh	9	scalp, throat	6

Most of the injuries listed in the folios of the register are self-explanatory. The most numerous were fractures (23.4%), bruises (19.4%), sprains (12.7%), and wounds (11.4%). The term *fracture* was reserved "for divisions in bones produced by external violence," and fractures were called either *simple* or *compound* depending on whether they communicated through a wound with the surface of the body. Compound or complicated fractures were often multiple and often became exposed to air. Aside from instances of old age, lues venerea, and scurvy, in all of which the bones were brittle or diseased, fractures arose through application of "unusual force" in a variety of circumstances, many of them already described in the survey of urban and rural accidents.[146]

A majority of cases inscribed by the hospital clerks simply carried the label "fracture" without specifying its anatomical location. Among those entries where the site was identified, fractures of the legs and arms seemed to predominate, followed by those affecting the thigh and skull. Bruises or *contusions,* often just slight injuries of the soft tissues, occasionally elicited enough local pain and inflammation to justify admission to the hospital, as did many sprains. Prevention of excessive swelling was important, because the aftermath of many sprains included some permanent distention of the injured parts and restriction of motion.[147]

Bell defined wounds as "every recent solution of continuity in whatever part of the body it may be, when attended with a corresponding division of the teguments."[148] He distinguished simple, *incised* wounds from *punctured* ones, the latter being much more dangerous because of their capacity to damage other underlying structures and greater risk of secondary infections, including tetanus. Instead of showing smooth straight edges, a *lacerated* wound exhibited ragged and unequal ones, as did a *contused* wound caused by a blunt object. "Mortification" – meaning *necrosis* – of the surrounding tissue, as well as secondary gangrene, was an ever-present threat.[149] If the wound was produced by an animal, especially a dog, there was danger of contracting *hydrophobia,* now better known as rabies.

"Burns," wrote Bell, "assume different appearances according to their degrees of violence and manner in which they are produced."[150] The least serious ones, caused by boiling water and other liquids, merely scalded the surface of the skin or created a number of blisters in proportion to the intensity of the contact. Direct touch with hot metals or combustible materials, however, created a "black mortified slough" accompanied by great pain. Indeed, it was the intensity of that pain and the danger of secondary infection that brought most burn victims to the hospital. Bell alerted his colleagues to the dangers of leaving gunpowder grains imbedded in the skin in burns caused by firearms.[151] Interestingly, none of the burn patients registered at the infirmary was identified as a soldier, a further indication that a majority of soldiers came to the hospital because of illnesses unconnected to action on the battlefield.

Of all trauma cases, 71% were reported in men, and nearly 80% of the fractures seen in the hospital occurred in men. Most of them were directly hospitalized in the surgical wards, with 6% going to the servants' ward and 4% to the soldiers' ward. Between 1770 and 1775 the clerks reported only a small number of traumatic cases, but this situation changed drastically in the 1780s and 1790s, when the total number of such patients increased sevenfold; perhaps the increase was a phenomenon associated with new hazards of the early Industrial Revolution.

Diseases of the skin

Thirteen separate categories employed by the clerks in the General Register were consolidated and brought together in the skin disease group:

Chilblain	1	Lepra	4
Eruption (of skin)	53	Psora or itch	13
Erysipelas or the rose	23	Scurvy or scorbutic eruption	18
Herpes	8	Tinea or white head	4
Impetigo	1		

In his nosology Cullen placed skin conditions under his order *impetigines,* diseases of so-called depraved or corrupted constitution. Over 40% of all cases were entered in the folios simply as *eruption* or *cutaneous eruption.* Such vagueness was not surprising, since the whole topic was in a state of clinical and theoretical confusion while physicians debated the nature and scope – local or general – of all diseases affecting the human skin.[152]

In eruptions coinciding with several childhood diseases, for example, most authors agreed with Buchan's view that "nature often attempts to free the bodies of children from bad humors by throwing them upon the skin."[153] To treat such lesions, therefore, was actually to risk blocking a health-restoring discharge, "driving it inwards" again, where it was bound to harm the patient elsewhere and perhaps even closer to a vital organ. In a word, skin diseases were expressions of the healing power of nature and better left alone except for soothing the most uncomfortable symptoms.

Contemporary explanations about the origin of skin disorders insisted that they were all the effects of concentrated acrid matter that in its movement toward the surface of the body was detained under the cuticle, where it exerted its damaging action. Under ordinary circumstances such humors were usually eliminated through normal perspiration, but with bodily moistures diminished during the winter months, these noxious substances accumulated near the surface. Then, as spring approached once more, normal perspiration and even sweating would take place, carrying the harmful substances to the outer layers of the skin, where they produced a number of injuries. Cullen adhered to this hypothetical pathogenesis and in fact tried to establish relationships between severe winters and the frequency of skin eruptions in the spring. Consequently, he often opposed the admission of patients already suffering from such ailments during the colder season, fearful that the warmer temperatures prevailing in hospital wards could possibly exacerbate the skin outbreaks through the promotion of more sweat.[154]

The next most frequent entity was *erysipelas* or "St. Anthony's fire" (18.4%), characterized by fever as well as redness and swelling of the face. This noncontagious rash generally spread to the scalp, eyelids, and other parts of the head, eventually changing into several blisters that contained a thin, yellowish fluid. At times the skin eruption extended downward to the legs, the fever was very high, and the patient suffered from mental confusion and delirium.[155]

Buchan considered erysipelas or "the rose," as it was also popularly called, to be a disease "very incident to the laborious," that is, to all types of lower-class workers. In his view it was caused by "sudden checks to the perspiration" when the laborers sat or slept on damp ground or wore wet clothing.[156] In the sample under study more than half of those admitted with a diagnosis of erysipelas were servants, with another quarter going into the soldiers' ward. It generally affected adults of "plethoric habit" between the ages of thirty and forty and erupted in the fall after the hot weather was over. Almost half of these infirmary patients entered the hospital between August and October.

Scurvy or *scorbutus* was included in the group of skin disorders (14.4%), since most patients hospitalized with the disease were admitted primarily because of their skin lesions and thus were registered as *scurvy skin, scorbutic eruption,* or *scorbutic blotches.* Besides prevailing in sailors on or after long voyages, the ailment was common in poor and weak people eating "unwholesome" food, especially smoke-dried or salted provisions in a partial state of decomposition. Few vegetables and fruits and a life in low damp places with confined air completed the list of factors favoring the appearance of the disease.[157]

The clinical manifestations of scurvy included loss of strength, swollen and bleeding gums, and a pale, dry skin covered with reddish-blue spots that gradually expanded into large, livid blotches. These lesions were usually present on arms, legs, and thighs and were susceptible to ulceration, giving off a thin, foul-smelling fluid while the underlying flesh sloughed off, discharging mixtures of blood and pus. Multiple and profuse bleedings from nose, gums, lungs, and intestines accentuated the already dramatic symptomatology.[158]

While the cure and prevention of scurvy seemed assured by the use of lemon juice, physicians vigorously debated the possible causes of the disease. James Lind and Thomas Trotter, with their extensive naval experience, led the way; others, including John Pringle and even William Cullen, offered their own explanations. A "peculiar state" of the blood was generally held responsible for the pathological bleedings, but authors could not agree whether this condition was due to nutritional deficiency alone or to a putrefaction operating within the bodily humors.

Half of the cases in the sample under scrutiny were admitted to the infirmary in the year 1775, despite the influx of seamen and Russian soldiers two decades later. The only plausible explanation is that the hospital predominantly received cases of "land scurvy" prevailing among the poor in the city of Edinburgh and surrounding countryside. At the infirmary this type was common, because only 20% of all patients admitted were seamen. Another 5% were soldiers, and an equal number identified themselves as servants. Most of them (77%) were men and about two-thirds were admitted during the winter months. Very few incoming sailors were thought to suffer from scorbutic complaints, perhaps because of the brief duration of sea voyages undertaken by the vessels of the North Sea Squadron and, after 1795, also because of the successful prevention program instituted by the Admiralty.[159]

Another disorder, the "itch" or *psora* (now known as scabies) was regarded as very common in eighteenth-century Scotland, especially among persons of lower rank. Cullen called it a local skin ailment with "itchy pustules and little ulcers."[160] They generally first appeared at the wrists and fingers but could quickly spread to arms, thighs, and legs. Clinicians distinguished a "dry itch," more common in adults, from a "wet itch" frequent in children, where the repeatedly scratched lesions became eczematous and exuded a clear or purulent matter.

Psora was thought to be caused by "a very small kind of animalcula of a whitish color shaped like a tortoise"[161] – a description of the invading mite. Poor children and all others "who despise cleanliness," asserted Buchan, "are almost constantly found to swarm with vermin and are generally covered with the scab, itch, and other eruptions."[162] Lack of hygiene and dirty clothing seemed to facilitate infection. Of the patients diagnosed as having the itch at the infirmary, two-thirds were entered as males. The servants' and soldiers' wards accepted 20% each; the rest were accepted for the ordinary medical units. Most cases were listed between 1780 and 1785.

Herpes was identified as a local disorder consisting of a great number of small ulcers, packed together in clusters "that creep on and spread about the skin."[163] Several species were recognized: *herpes simple,* consisting of single, dry, yellowish-white pustules that burned or itched; *herpes serpigo* or "ringworm," where the pustules sprouted "in heaps"; *herpes zoster* or "shingles," with large clusters of white and watery pustules located on neck, chest, hips, or thighs; and *herpes exedens* or redness resembling the skin manifestations of an ulcerated erysipelas. In the sample under discussion seven of the eight herpes patients were males, two of them soldiers.

The term *lepra graecorum* or *leprosy* designated a variety of chronic cutaneous affections characterized by rough and scaly skin and itchy red pimples spreading in a circular manner and briefly oozing thin fluid when scratched. Most formations first emerged in clusters of three or four pustules on arms, legs, or at the edge of hair on the forehead before spreading to other areas of the body. At times the name *impetigo* was used for similar manifestations. As with other skin ailments, leprosy was blamed on a stagnation of faulty or impure serum amassing under the body surface in situations of considerable debility.[164]

Eighteenth-century authors were aware that the name "leprosy" had originally meant a much more serious and disfiguring disease with extensive ulcerations, bone destruction, and loss of limbs. They also recognized that in warmer climates such a severe type of leprosy was still common. However, several contemporary writers reserved the term *black scurvy* for such cases, no doubt because of the color that the dying limbs assumed during their decay.[165] In cold climates, therefore, lepra graecorum was understood to be a chronic but benign skin disease. Of the four patients entered into the register, three were women and two of them servants. All four apparently recovered and were discharged cured.

As Buchan wrote, "The most obstinate of all eruptions incident to children are the *tinea capitis* or 'scabbed head.' "[166] Cullen defined it as a separate local scalp disorder, with small ulcers among the roots of hair leaking fluid that formed white, friable scabs. Bell, who called this disease *crusta lactea*, felt that is was just another species of herpes, although he recognized that peculiar "bulbous swellings" at the hair roots probably caused the symptoms.[167]

Circulatory disorders

A small number of diagnostic categories derived from what eighteenth-century physicians called a *general hydropic diathesis:*

Anasarca	11	Hemorrhoids or piles	4
Aneurysm	1	Hydrocephalus	3
Ascites	8	Hydrothorax	1
Dropsy	50	Plethora or congestion	1

Nearly 70% of all these cases admitted to the hospital were simply listed as *dropsy,* popularly known in the eighteenth century as "watery swelling" and defined by Cullen as "a preternatural collection of serous or watery fluids formed in different parts of the human body."[168] He and other authors concluded that dropsy occurred because of an imbalance between the constant discharge and absorption of fluids in the human organism. One perceived cause for the disorder was purely mechanical: resistance to the return of venous blood because of vascular obstructions in the liver and lungs or problems in the right ventricle of the heart. Such circulatory impairments were ascribed to tumors, aneurysms (localized arterial dilatations), or hardened tissue in the liver and lungs.

According to Cullen, general debility was another cause of dropsy, brought on by poor, watery diets or following long-standing illnesses such as pulmonary consumption and ague with enlargement of the spleen. "Intemperance in the use of intoxicating liquors" was also blamed. Most medical authorities speculated endlessly about the causes of these bodily fluid collections. Among the factors adduced in the production of dropsy were an excessive ingestion of fluids, insufficient urinary secretion, and deficiency of "gluten" and red globules in the blood, allowing for an excess of serum.[169]

One particular type of dropsy was *anasarca,* a watery swelling diffused throughout the whole body. It generally began with pitting edema in feet and ankles, discovered in the evenings after the person had remained the whole day in an erect posture. During the night the swelling went away initially, because the patient was lying down. At subsequent stages of the illness, however, the swellings remained and then gradually extended upward to include the legs, the thighs, and eventually the trunk of the body.

Cullen gave the name *ascites,* "dropsy of the belly," "to every collection of waters causing a general swelling and distention of the lower belly."[170] In most cases the fluid was present in the abdominal cavity "immediately washing the intestines"; in other instances, called *encysted dropsy,* it was contained in closed vesicles such as those located at the ovaries *(hydrops ovarii).* The effusion was initially noted in the pit of the stomach, causing some dyspnea, distention, a feeling of increased weight, and eventually a sensation of fluctuating fluid. In most instances ascites was viewed as a manifestation of a progressive anasarca, but it could also arise independently in cases where there was a scirrhous liver or spleen.[171]

Hydrothorax or "dropsy of the breast" was the name given to all fluid collections located in the chest cavity or the pericardium. Progressive dyspnea, especially after exertion or while lying flat in bed, was followed by dry cough, general uneasiness, and palpitations. Confirmation of the presence of hydrothorax was obtained when a fluctuation of fluid in the chest was perceived when the patient changed positions. The progressive dyspnea, irregular pulse, and strong palpitations made it a dangerous condition frequently ending in death.[172]

Hydrocephalus, "dropsy of the brain" or "water in the head," was a serious condition in which inflammation of the meninges or fluid collected between the brain and the skull – *internal hydrocephalus* – or in the scalp – *external hydrocephalus.* Most cases were of the former type, appearing in newborn infants or young children (many suffering from scrofula) with headaches, pain in the limbs, convulsions, and, if the patient survived for several months, enlargement of the cranium.[173]

Alcoholism or, as eighteenth-century physicians expressed it, "addiction to the use of spirits" was often causally linked with anasarca, ascites, and hydrothorax.[174] Sinclair in his assessment of contemporary dietary changes occurring in Scotland stressed the nefarious effects of substituting "ardent spirits" for the commonly consumed ale and the alcoholic's liability to "dropsical complaints." In their clinical lectures both Cullen and Andrew Duncan, Sr., frequently remarked about the relationship between ascites or anasarca and "paying too many visits to the dram shop."[175] Another association described by Cullen was the presence of hydatic cysts in the liver, diaphragm, and lungs in cases of hydrothorax and ascites.

The term *hemorrhoids* or *piles,* wrote Benjamin Bell, was applied to the distention, inflammation, and evacuation of blood from "veins running upon and in the neighborhood of the rectum."[176] If the veins were merely distended, the piles were called *blind;* if they discharged blood, they were *open.* Bell and other contemporaries rejected the traditional view that hemorrhoidal bleeding, like a safety valve, was a necessary and natural mechanism to rid the body of excessive or harmful humors. Bell thought that the trauma of large collections of hard stool lingering in the rectum and pressure from adjacent organs, as during pregnancy, impeded the proper blood circulation in the hemorrhoidal vessels and eventually caused the condition.[177]

Tumors and cancers

Twenty-one separate diagnostic categories, half of them considered surgical, were assembled under the heading of tumors and cancers:

Cancer	9	Scrofula	31
Cancer of breast	3	Steatoma	2
Cancer of lip	8	Steatoma of bladder	1
Exostosis	1	Tumor	6
Polyp	2	Tumor (of) back, cheek, jaw, lip, knee, testicle, thigh	7
Schirrhous or scirrhous tumor	2		
Scirrhous testicle, tonsil, uterus	3		

"Every preternatural enlargement, in whatever part of the body it is seated, may be termed a *tumor,*" wrote Benjamin Bell.[178] He divided tumors into two general classes, acute or inflammatory and chronic or indolent, using clinical criteria to describe their initial characteristics but quite aware that any tumor could evolve from one type to the other during the course of the disease. Among acute or inflammatory tumors Bell placed phlegmons, venereal buboes, sprains, and contusions, whereas the class of chronic tumors comprised a large number of miscellaneous swellings: cysts, aneurysms, hemorrhoids, anasarca, emphysema, tympanites, hernias, scrofula, and scirrhous tumors.[179]

The most common condition was scrofula (41.3%), followed by the general diagnosis cancer (12%) and a specific cancer, that of the lip (10.6%). *Scrofula,* otherwise called "scrofulous affection" or the "King's Evil," has already been briefly described. Cullen considered it a hereditary disease and in his nosology placed it among affections of the skin, since he felt that the characteristic neck tumors were a result of the corrupted humors that gave rise to cutaneous eruptions.[180] The hereditary nature of scrofula was concluded from observing the ailment in families, generally the poor, who lived in cold and damp quarters and survived on meager diets. The painless swellings appeared in sickly children between the ages of three and seven, "of soft and flaccid habits," joining or following another disease of want: rickets.[181]

Cullen observed a seasonal influence in the evolution of scrofula, blaming spring for the initial appearance and yearly exacerbation of the tumors, not only located around the neck but occasionally also emerging at elbow and ankle joints, where the symptoms and lesions took on the character of "white swellings." Gradually, the scrofulous tumors became larger and softer, developing a tendency to ulcerate and discharge a whitish substance that in Cullen's words resembled "the curd of milk."[182] Multiple openings occurred over the most prominent tumors, chronically oozing a substance quite distinct from normal pus. Some of these lesions tended to heal spontaneously over the years, leaving behind disfiguring scars, while new tumors made their appearance. In some instances the disease went away completely; in others the tumors became larger and the patient wasted away, often with symptoms of pulmonary phthisis.[183] Because of the presence of multiple and discharging ulcers a fair number of scrofula cases were directly referred for surgical treatment. In the sample of thirty-one cases listed in the General Register, 51% were referred to the medical wards, 22% to the surgical units, and 20% to the soldiers' ward. Only a small fraction of the patients, 6%, were identified as servants.

A *schirrous* or *scirrhous* tumor was defined by Cullen as "an hard tumor of some part, generally a gland, without pain and difficultly brought to suppuration."[184] According to contemporary views that went back to antiquity, the characteristic of a scirrhous was its increased consistency. Persons of all ages were susceptible to acquiring such growths, most of them viewed as consolidations of coagulated bodily fluids (as in the breast), congealed lymph (in nodes), or extravasated blood (following contusions). Many of these lesions could be perceived by touch, and they eventually dissolved on their own, were brought to suppuration, or were surgically removed.[185]

Cancer, on the other hand, was defined as "a painful tumor of a schirrous nature and degenerating into an ill conditioned ulcer."[186] Bell and other authors were convinced that the disease was originally local, caused by many of the factors responsible for a scirrhous tumor, which was believed to be the precursor of every cancerous growth. Eventually the scirrhous tumor changed into a cancer because of inflammation or the action of bodily fluids. Those located near the bodily surface would develop ulcers. Lancinating or burning pains, a dusky appearance of the skin covering the lesion, and the eventual formation of ulcers with ragged edges discharging a mixture of blood and pungent matter signaled the transformation of a scirrhous into cancer.[187]

Bell believed that the disease ceased at this point to be purely local, since surgical removal of the original tumor only caused further lesions near the original site or at a distance. A systemic *cancerous diathesis* was produced through absorption and distribution of the acrid matter first flowing at the original site.[188] This substance was responsible for so-called metastases, deposits in other parts of the body revealed by postmortem dissections. Thus cancer was generally seen as a "malignant" disease, usually fatal if allowed to spread beyond its original local boundaries and begin discharging its characteristic corrosive material.

In men cancer primarily affected the tongue, mouth, and testicles; women, especially unmarried and menopausal ones, usually suffered from cancers of the breast and uterus. Cancer of the lower lip was also frequently diagnosed following the appearance of fissures or warts. It probably also followed repeated burns caused by smoking clay pipes. These lesions needed to be distinguished from venereal sores present in the mouth and tongue.[189] All eight patients listed in the General Register between 1770 and 1800 as having lip cancer were men, seven of them servants. All breast cancers occurred in female servants. The general cancer category contained five men and four women, seven of them identified as servants.

Possibly the extraordinary proportion of servants among those hospitalized with cancer (85%) can be explained as cases of early detection by employers, who immediately referred their workers to the infirmary for treatment. By contrast, people not in domestic employment, when affected with cancer, usually consulted private surgeons, who according to Benjamin Bell "generally retain the patient under their own management if the case does not appear to be desperate or if any reputation is likely to be got from an operation."[190] Thus only unfavorable or terminal cases were sent to the infirmary from private practitioners, whereas of the twenty cancer patients labeled as servants in the General Register, only one perished in the hospital and fourteen were reported cured.

Lastly, the infirmary clerks registered two cases of *steatoma,* also popularly known as "wen," an encysted, sometimes fatty tumor originating in the sebaceous glands of the skin but also identified in other parts of the body. A *polyp* or *polypus* was a whitish and compact tumor believed to be formed by coagulations and concretions of blood. Many of them were actually blood clots obstructing blood vessels, but a few were recognized in other bodily organs, especially the nose, uterus, and rectum. *Exostosis* or *hyperostosis* was the name given to bony excrescences or tumors arising from bones following inflammatory processes, notably venereal disease.[191]

Eye problems

A few categories of diseases affecting the eyes were also recorded:

Amaurosis or blindness	10
Caligo	3
Opacity (of) cornea	3
Ophthalmia	45

The most frequently listed ailment was *ophthalmia* or inflammation of the eyes. In his nosology Cullen considered two basic kinds: an inflammation affecting only the eyelids – *ophthalmia tarsi* – and the more common *ophthalmia membranorum,* which had its seat in the various membranes enclosing the eyeball. Most infections arose in the conjunctiva and were accompanied by burning pains, tears, redness, swelling, and intolerance to light. Dust, exposure to cold winds, "night watching" – especially reading or writing by candlelight – and the application of strong light – from looking into snow for a long time, for example – all were considered important causes triggering the inflammation. At times ophthalmia preceded or followed the appearance of scrofula. Purulent complications and the spread of the infection to the cornea often led to its partial or total opacity and permanent damage to vision.[192]

Impairments of eyesight "on account of some opaque substance interposed between the objects and retina" received the name *caligo* in Cullen's nosology. *Caligo lentis,* a disease "occasioned by an opaque substance behind the pupil," was just another term for *cataract.* Besides *caligo cornea* or corneal opacity, popularly referred to as "specks in the eye," there was another variety: *caligo humorum* or *glaucoma,* considered a defect of the aqueous humor in the eye.[193]

When "the eyesight was diminished or totally abolished without any evident disease of the eye," Cullen termed the disease *amaurosis.* The main symptoms were a dilated and motionless pupil, loss of vision, and headaches, all happening in one or both eyes simultaneously. In a few instances, as in hysteria or other emotional states, the symptoms were just temporary or periodical. Unfortunately, in a majority of cases the symptoms were progressive and irreversible. Eighteenth-century writers linked different causes to the appearance of amaurosis, among them compression of the optical nerve by tumors or vascular congestion, external injuries, local debility, venereal disease, and rheumatism.[194]

Miscellaneous medical conditions

A few remaining categories from the General Register could not be included in the previous groups:

Anomalous complaint	5
Convalescent	1
Debility	5
Feigned complaints	2
Inoculation	1
Pain or pains	47

The most common condition was "pain" or "pains," a favorite entry especially employed by hospital clerks inscribing the register during the year 1775. Five other cases were simply called "debility"; a similar number, displaying a confused symptomatology, were recorded in the folios as suffering from an "anomalous ailment" or having anomalous complaints that could not be fitted into the existing classifications of disease.

The problem of "feigned complaints" or *morbus simulatus* also existed among admissions to the infirmary. The ailments of some persons trying to get into the hospital for reasons not readily explained were "liable to be imaginary," but they provided admitting physicians with a sufficient number of counterfeit symptoms to ensure their acceptance. Once in the house, however, these persons increasingly ran into trouble, because they had to maintain their ruses while under surveillance from other inmates, nurses, students, and attending physicians. Inconsistent reports, obvious lack of physical distress, and unpredictable reactions to the therapeutic regimes usually led to their discovery and ultimate expulsion. Others, admitted to the wards for legitimate complaints, actually found hospitalization to their liking, especially during winters. While on the road to recovery these patients were "frequently averse to leave and therefore to feign complaints," observed William Cullen.[195]

Although the problem appears to have been minor, according to hospital registrations, Cullen in his clinical lectures devoted a fair amount of time to a discussion of these cases. His pedagogical objective was to sharpen the diagnostic skills of the students, instilling in them a measure of skepticism regarding the reports furnished by patients during daily rounds at the infirmary. As mentioned before, Cullen used the nurses to expose simulators or threatened to apply blisters, a therapeutic trial that usually prompted impostors to ask for their dismissal. "Whenever I find a patient falsifying his ailments as they may make me appear ridiculous in practice," he explained about one patient, "I always think it is proper to dismiss them, and as I had signified something of this kind to him a day or two since, he has thought proper to walk off."[196]

One female patient was admitted in 1790 to be inoculated for smallpox. In spite of various popular methods prevalent at the time and inoculators roaming the countryside, some patients preferred to have the procedure performed under direct medical supervision. Such instances were extremely rare among lower-class people, but a student casebook contained another case of a young soldier "desirous to be inoculated" who entered the teaching ward of the infirmary for about three weeks to be subjected to the medical method.[197]

Miscellaneous surgical conditions

A number of patients inscribed in the register suffered from conditions that might have needed the services of a surgeon:

Cataract	15	Imperforated rectum	1
Harelip	1	Odontalgia or toothache	2
Hernia	9	Stricture of urethra	1
Hydrocele	7	Umbilical hernia	1

"Blindness, induced by an opaque body immediately behind the iris, forms a disease we name cataract," wrote Benjamin Bell in his eighteenth-century textbook.[198] He admitted that the real seat of such an "offuscation" was a recent discovery, and he postulated that the condition was the result of a vascular obstruction. Cataracts were said to occur more frequently in women near their menopause, but eleven out of the fifteen patients listed in the General Register were men, almost all of them admitted to the surgical ward.

The next most common problem in this group was *hernias*. Bell wrote that the term "might with propriety be applied to every swelling produced by the dislodgement of parts from those boundaries within which in a state of health they are contained."[199] Contemporary surgeons distinguished *inguinal* (groin), *scrotal* (scrotum), *femoral* (upper thigh), *umbilical* (navel), and *ventral* (belly) hernias, blaming severe bodily exertions, violent coughing, and accidental falls for their appearance. Quite in contrast to what was happening in France at the time, Bell noted their infrequent occurrence in both Edinburgh and London hospitals. He ascribed this phenomenon to a greater laxity of the tissues in Frenchmen reared on a diet rich in oil.[200]

The most dangerous situations ensued when hernias, generally of the inguinal type, became *incarcerated* or *strangulated* as a loop of intestine slipped into the hernial sac, became swollen, and was unable to return to the abdominal cavity. Trapped and deprived of circulation by the constraints of the hernial ring, the mortified gut became inflamed and eventually burst, spilling its fecal contents into the abdominal cavity with fatal consequences. Thus removal of the stricture was of the utmost urgency.[201]

Another problem was the formation of a *hydrocele,* according to Bell a "watery swelling in the scrotum or spermatic cord."[202] Although some of these tumors followed in the wake of external injuries, most of them seemed to have formed in patients suffering from generalized edema of dropsy.

Working at the infirmary, Bell was confident that surgical attempts to currect *harelip* could be successful. While most surgeons postponed the operation until the child was at least five years old and preferred to intervene when the patient was a teenager, Bell had other ideas. "After various trials," he began to perform the repair in infants during their third or fourth month of life, although he favored cases where the child was about one year old.[203]

"Toothache," Bell observed, "appears to be more unsupportable than any other kind of pain."[204] Individuals admitted with *odontalgia* generally had a number of decayed teeth that gave them enough trouble to request hospitalization and allow surgeons to remove the source of their pain. In other instances the discomfort was caused by so-called *gum-boils,* small abscesses located in the gums and formed by inflammations at the roots of the teeth. Cullen placed odontalgia as a genus of disease among his inflammatory diseases and considered certain cases secondary to rheumatism.

All cases of hernia obtained from the General Register occurred in men; in fact, 72% of all patients brought together in this group of miscellaneous conditions were male. Though the potential for surgical intervention was present in all cases, only 48% of these patients went directly into the surgical wards. The soldiers' ward received 28%, including all six patients suffering from hydrocele, and the rooms reserved for seamen got another 12%. Notably absent were servants, whose ward did not receive a single patient belonging to this group.

Surgical procedures

Finally, instead of providing a diagnosis, the General Register at times simply listed the surgical intervention to which incoming patients were subjected:

Amputation	14
Castration	1
Lithotomy	3
Trephined skull	1

By far the most common surgical procedure carried out at the infirmary between 1770 and 1800 seems to have been amputation (73.6%), defined by Benjamin Bell as "the removal of the whole or part of a limb."[205] Because the technical aspects involved were thought to be within the reach of every practitioner, Bell was more concerned about the need for and timing of an amputation than its actual execution. Such judgments "require more deliberation than perhaps any other in surgery," he wrote.[206]

In his textbook Bell listed eleven causes that "rendered amputation necessary," beginning with compounded fractures, lacerated and contused wounds, and extensive "mortification," meaning death or gangrene of the tissues. Further indications arose from partial and accidental amputations common during contemporary warfare as a result of cannonball fire, the presence of so-called white swellings in joints, and extensive destruction or growth of bone tissue – *caries* or *exostoses* – in limbs. Finally, tumors, cancers, and deformities also demanded from time to time the same surgical treatment.[207]

Bell presented a number of convincing arguments against early amputation in cases of compound fractures where the wounds had been exposed to air, claiming that the shock of the initial injury militated against successful surgery. Therefore he urged practitioners "never to operate but with the advice of some of his brethren in consultation,"[208] in order to avoid subsequent charges of unnecessary surgery. Bell estimated that in his time and during "the general run of hospital practice" the mortality for amputations was around 5%. By contrast, the death rate for the fourteen cases taken from the infirmary's register was 21%.[209] A possible reason for the fourfold increase may have been the low quality of operative surgery in the hospital that resulted from the chronic squabbles between the managers and the Royal College of Surgeons. Indeed, most of the surgeons rotating through the infirmary were said to be young and inexperienced.

Another procedure carried out in the Edinburgh infirmary was *lithotomy,* popularly known as "cutting for the stone." It consisted in the surgical removal of one or more bladder stones too large to pass through the urethra and thus be voided. Unlike other contemporary hospitals, notably the Norwich and Norfolk Infirmary, which had its own team of lithotomists, the Edinburgh institution only occasionally had a case requiring operation.[210]

After the presence of a large stone in the bladder had been convincingly ascertained, using a number of urethral probes and repeated rectal examinations, the question of its removal by surgical means came up if symptoms persisted and the pain was excruciating. Surgery offered the only real hope of a cure, given the common failure of a number of chemical compounds, called *lithontriptics,* designed to dissolve them.[211] As Bell explained, "Unless the operation is performed, the remainder of a miserable life will probably be cut short by the frequent return of pain and fever."[212]

Unlike amputations, lithotomy demanded a very precise knowledge of anatomy, especially of the structures that lay in the path of the operator's knife: the neck of the bladder, prostate, seminal vesicles, anal muscles, and the rectum itself. Most eighteenth-century procedures that gained favor with the surgeons were based on perineal incisions designed to enter the bladder from below without excessive hemorrhage and irreversible damage to the adjacent organs. Bell and many others were partial to the so-called lateral operation popularized by William Cheselden in London earlier in the century. Bell introduced a number of technical improvements designed to avoid cutting into the bladder at several points.

Bell was candid about the multiple hazards surrounding the extraction of bladder stones. Mortality rates in otherwise healthy subjects with small stones were said to be at that time around 5%, but if the stones exceeded seven or eight ounces in weight, more than 10% of the patients would die because of the extensive tissue damage caused by tearing out the offending concretions. Bell therefore recommended a four-inch incision, sufficient to allow the operator room to introduce his finger or a forceps and quickly extract the stone.[213] Once the bladder was breached, it was hoped that the flow of urine covering the entire wound would serve as a barrier to further contamination and subsequent infection. All three patients listed in the General Register as having been subjected to lithotomy were soldiers. Two of them were reported cured; the third one died.

Trephination, a procedure to relieve pressure in the brain from depressed bone fragments, blood clots, or even abscesses, was seldom employed by eighteenth-century surgeons. It consisted in cutting through the bones of the skull at carefully selected points with a special instrument called a *trepan.* Most trephinations were attempted in patients who had recently sustained skull fractures, many of them moribund, the outcome of the surgery remaining much in doubt.[214] The case listed in the General Register, however, was apparently cured.

Finally, the case labeled *castration* possibly involved an individual who had sustained an accident or had a testicular tumor; he died in the hospital.

Given the small number of cases involved, it is difficult to reach any meaningful conclusions about these surgical activities. Women apparently had more than their share of amputations (about 44% of amputations were carried out on women, who constituted only 38% of the hospital population); the other procedures all were done on men. All of the patients were directly admitted to the surgical wards.

LENGTH OF HOSPITALIZATION

In the sample of 3,047 entries obtained from the General Register of Patients for the period 1770–1800, both admission and discharge dates were listed for 2,973 cases. It is therefore possible to compute the time these patients remained in the hospital. The average total stay was 31.3 days, slightly over a month. Table 3.3 is a breakdown of this average according to the various disease categories previously considered.

As can be seen from the table, acute respiratory conditions required the least amount of time in the hospital – slightly more than three weeks – especially the mild catarrhs and pectoral complaints. The infectious diseases, mostly ordinary fevers, also went away in about three weeks. Longer than average hospitalization, however, was needed for chronic neurological and mental conditions such as protracted paralyses, epilepsy, and hysteria. Those suffering from venereal diseases continued in the infirmary for nearly six

Table 3.3. *Average length of stay in the infirmary, 1770–1800, by complaint*

Type of disease	Days
Medical	
All complaints	29.1
Genitourinary diseases	42.3
Infectious diseases	24.7
Respiratory ailments	23.7
Diseases of the digestive system	27.3
Musculoskeletal disorders	30.2
Neurological and mental problems	34.2
Diseases of the skin	31.0
Miscellaneous medical conditions	30.4
Surgical	
All complaints	40.0
Surgical infections	42.8
Traumatic conditions	32.5
Tumors and cancers	38.0
Miscellaneous surgical problems	38.2
Surgical procedures	55.1

weeks, which was considered the appropriate time for a cure based on mercurials.

Among surgical cases, persons sustaining injuries stayed the shortest time on the average – not surprising, given the abundance of bruises and simple sprains and the fact that more serious conditions such as skull fractures survived only a few days in the hospital. In contrast, surgical infections, largely chronic leg ulcers, required much longer treatment, and those undergoing surgical operations in the amphitheater remained for nearly eight weeks before being allowed to leave the institution.

An analysis of hospitalization by wards disclosed that the greatest turnover of patients occurred in the servants' ward, where many people with simple fevers and catarrhs were housed. Somewhat surprisingly, beginning in the early 1790s the seamen's ward kept its inmates the longest, presumably because of their chronic complaints centering on weakness, rheumatism, venereal disease, and scurvy. For the entire period the average length of stay, by ward, was as follows:

Teaching	31.8 days
Medical ordinary	31.7
Surgical ordinary	38.3
Soldiers'	35.5
Servants'	25.8
Seamen's	44.1

Table 3.4. *Average length of stay in the infirmary, 1770–1800, by year*

Year	No. of cases	Days
1770	300	43.6
1775	439	26.0
1780	486	31.2
1785	480	24.2
1790	456	30.1
1795	418	47.2
1800	395	24.9

Table 3.5. *Number of patients hospitalized for short stays, 1770–1800*

Average length of stay (days)	1770	1775	1780	1785	1790	1795	1800
7	47	59	109	100	69	80	64
14	43	55	50	76	67	61	78
21	31	83	49	65	54	55	40

From examination of hospitalization data between 1770 and 1800, no significant trends in lengths of stays can be discerned (see Table 3.4). In some years the number of brief, one-to-three-week stays increased about 60%–100%, allowing for faster patient turnover and thus higher admission rates (see Table 3.5). However, because of the contractual arrangements, a number of patients, usually soldiers and seamen, continued to lodge in the infirmary for longer periods of time before being officially declared "invalids" and removed from the institution. Some of these men actually resided in the wards for eight to twelve months.

Data obtained from the 808 clinical histories of patients hospitalized in the teaching ward confirm the foregoing observations while shedding additional light on gender breakdowns, occupations, length of symptoms prior to admission, the influence of treatment, and so on. The average length of stay in the teaching unit was 27.3 days, approximately four weeks. This figure is lower than that for the entire infirmary because of the sometimes precipitous discharge of numerous convalescent patients toward the end of each clinical rotation, when the ward was transferred to another professor or simply closed until the next academic term. In fact, admissions authorized during the months of October, November, and December tended to stay quite a bit longer than those who entered during the spring term (April) or summer (July).

Women remained 26 days in the teaching ward on the average, men, 31, a difference probably resulting from the frequency of mild colds and fevers among the former, especially a large contingent of maids. A smaller number of laborers with similar health problems stayed for only 23 days. In sharp contrast, both soldiers and seamen, with their prevalence of venereal complaints, rheumatism, and skin ailments, endured in the teaching ward for considerably longer periods of time: 43 and 48 days, respectively.

People with acute symptoms who had no therapy prior to admission were the first to leave the Edinburgh infirmary. Subacute and chronic cases lingered considerably longer. Relationships between the various types of therapy and the extent of hospitalization were determined by the clinical development of the diseases being attended; the only exception was mercury. Thus the application of emetics, cathartics, venesection, and cold baths coincided with routine one-to-three-week medical care programs adapted to the evolution of most ordinary fevers. No single measure, including bloodletting, seems to have lengthened hospital stays. People with venereal disease, on the other hand, remained in the house for nearly two months not because they were still suffering from the disease but to follow rules concerning the employment of mercurial remedies.

This brief overview and definition of the most common diseases seen at the Edinburgh infirmary between 1770 and 1800 provides one particular panorama of morbidity encountered in a British voluntary hospital of the period. Comparisons with similar contemporary institutions are difficult to make at this time, given the paucity of published statistics and insufficient archival research. However, an analysis of data obtained from the Newcastle Infirmary, the Manchester Infirmary, and the Bristol Royal Infirmary suggests that at Edinburgh surgical cases remained somewhat underrepresented – they constituted approximately 37% at Newcastle and 38% at Manchester in the early 1750s, with leg ulcers again prominently reported as the single most frequent ailment. Among medical cases, scrofulous tumors and respiratory illnesses, especially consumption, led over infectious diseases at both the Newcastle and Manchester infirmaries. The frequency of digestive and musculoskeletal complaints was about the same in all institutions. No single case of venereal disease was listed for any of these three English hospitals.[215]

Some of the differences between institutional admissions possibly reflect local disease conditions. Both Newcastle and Manchester had many cases of tuberculosis in the form of pulmonary consumption and scrofula of the neck. Edinburgh, at the crossroads for Scottish migrant workers, received many patients suffering from the ague. Other changes can be attributed to variations in diagnostic labeling and medical criteria for what were "proper" cases for hospital treatment. Nevertheless, the most significant factors were social and economic, the causes of the high admission rates for venereal diseases and fevers at the Edinburgh infirmary.

In the case of Margaret ("Peggy") Carmichael, her delirious febrile state brought her also into the teaching ward, where she was admitted just as her father before her had been with a diagnosis of typhus fever. The same thing happened a few days later to both her sister Mary and her brother Pat. The probable reason for such an inclusion among teaching cases was the fact that James Gregory, then in charge of the unit, was interested in showing students the clinical evolution and treatment of typhus fever. It is to therapeutics that we now turn.

4

Hospital care: state of the medical art

Not the least advantage which arises from hospital practice, is the simplicity with which remedies are prescribed, as to number and preparation, by which they do not disturb the operations and effects of each other, and their natural and genuine properties are discovered and ascertained, from which medicine receives much improvement.[1]

PRINCIPLES OF EIGHTEENTH-CENTURY THERAPEUTICS

Cullen defined therapeutics as the "doctrine of remedies," measures employed to improve or heal the sick and to restore the patient to health.[2] Therapeutics constituted the core of medical intervention, a set of healing schemes generating hope or fear, satisfaction or disappointment. During the eighteenth century a cure or return to health remained a praiseworthy but elusive goal, still based on the recognition of patterns of recovery observed for centuries at the sickbed. Each confrontation between disease and the individual was a specific struggle played out in multiple variations that could baffle even the most experienced clinician. During this conflict, natural healing powers inside the human organism attempted to resist the onslaught of disease and readjust lost humoral balances. Outlets were found to expel morbific matter formed in the body under the impact of sickness. The end result varied. The patient could "escape" the disease or it could move beyond "the reach of relief" and kill.

To promote cures, eighteenth-century Edinburgh physicians retained a fairly passive, noninterventionist posture. Students were directed to follow nature's own cues, first in the form of proper "markings" or characteristic symptoms, in order to make a proper diagnosis. Then practitioners were urged to pause and watch whether "nature is sufficient of itself to complete a cure" before considering the aid of drugs, physical methods, and diet to help the natural processes along. "When nature is useful," lectured Francis Home, "it is certainly prudent to follow her and the greatest physicians have done so."[3] Cullen, addressing a similar student audience, admitted that "the practice in this country has been cautious which amounts to timid."

The traditional Hippocratic injunction of avoiding harm to the patient remained paramount: "I have a rule in practice," observed Cullen; "I seldom push a remedy that may do harm as I would rather let a disease kill a patient than kill him by medicine."[4]

Thus most eighteenth-century healing strategies summarized under the rubric "art of medicine" were actions found to be clinically useful, tangible enough to evoke physiological responses, and above all, acceptable to and even welcomed by patients. Originally, most measures were not applications of prevailing theories of medicine. Even Cullen's neurophysiological framework was highly speculative and incapable of shedding much light on actual disease processes or mechanisms promoting healing. Practitioners were painfully aware that both physicochemical and neuropathological explanations consistently failed to clarify bedside events. Thus physicians were frequently forced to return and consider discredited humoral schemes that seemed to harmonize with clinical reality.

Hence no new scientific principles guiding their therapies were available to eighteenth-century physicians and surgeons. These men were forced to "practice under ambiguities" and continue employing traditional therapeutic procedures that over the centuries had become the backbone of medical intervention. Needless to say, this rather conservative approach stifled innovation and experiment in therapy. Physicians fell into a "certain routine or form of practice which afterwards prevents the necessary exertion of the mind to discover more powerful remedies or a better method of applying them in the cure of diseases."[5]

To be sure, most late eighteenth-century physicians received a systematic university education and knew a great deal about anatomy, chemistry, and botany. Yet this knowledge was only marginally related to their clinical activities. Visits to hospitals and dispensaries or brief apprenticeships bringing them into the homes of private patients revealed a world of pain and suffering where uncertainty ruled and caution was imperative.

To make sense of bedside events, practitioners interpreted clinical changes with the aid of hypothetical mechanisms that eventually became the source of biting criticism and ridicule by lay persons. "All physiology as far as it is hitherto known, is totally or nearly useless in explaining anything which happens in fever," wrote George Fordyce.[6] There was even confusion about the usefulness of postmortem findings. Though lesions could certainly explain the appearance of specific symptoms, few physicians were prepared to discuss their role in the evolution of the disease. Again Fordyce: "A fever is a disease which no knowledge of the structure of the human body could give the smallest ground of supposition that this disease could have ever existed."[7]

With their observational powers the sole compass to guide them through this clinical maze, practitioners developed a number of devices to bring order to bedside activities. One of them, the use of nosology or the classification of diseases, has already been discussed, and it had less of an impact on therapy than on diagnosis and prognosis. Nevertheless, the classification of a fever as either inflammatory or nervous, for example, had direct implications for treatment and was based on another tool: semiotics, the knowledge of signs that led physicians to recognize and identify the disease in the first place.

A third instrument as much applicable to therapeutics as to prognostics was the doctrine of "critical days," a belief that diseases run their courses within particular time frames, ending in crises that occurred on specific days after onset. The concept, first enunciated in Hippocratic medicine, was particularly applicable in fevers, especially those of an intermittent type with regular episodes every second or third day. Physicians like Cullen tried to infuse new life into this notion and use it as a practical and heuristic device. "We are exposed to certain causes that produce a regular diurnal revolution in our bodily system," insisted Cullen, and thus "there is a constant tendency in nature for fevers to observe regular movements."[8]

With such scant empirical guides at their disposal, eighteenth-century practitioners fashioned a general plan of treatment or *methodus medendi*.[9] Attention to age, sex, temperament, and habit were essential for assessing each person's constitution and predicting how the individual patient would sustain the effects of disease as well as therapy. "The constitutions of different patients are often different from each other and substances applied to different men have different effects," explained Fordyce.[10] Debilitated people were notorious for poorly tolerating bloodletting. How should a child with venereal disease be treated? Lecturing to students, Home emphasized the importance of seasonal factors in the administration of drugs. Sweat-inducing medicines were withheld during the inclement Edinburgh winter, to avoid secondary catarrhs and fevers.[11] Even geography played a role. Because of its climate, one writer traveling through Scotland in the 1770s reported that "medical people say that it is the worst climate in the world for the use of mercurial medicines."[12]

A third component in the therapeutic plan was an evaluation of the healing power of nature. How much could it be trusted in a particular case? Were some of the spontaneous bodily reactions actually harmful instead of beneficial? If nature did indeed refuse to "give a solution of the disease," how long should the practitioner remain passive? Did a particular disease really "admit of a cure"? All these questions were of paramount interest to physicians, who often agonized over the wisdom of therapeutic activism. "Practitioners really well informed find it often much more proper to leave diseases to go through their natural course," wrote Fordyce.[13] Yet in hospital practice a compromise was struck between such a noninterventionist, "natural" approach placing priority on the avoidance of further harm and a more active posture that promoted treatment to supplement or correct natural developments. In fact, despite early pronouncements, Cullen, Home, and other infirmary practitioners gradually adopted a more activist stance in their response to diseases seen in the hospital. This switch in therapeutic modality probably occurred in response to institutional pressures for curing hospitalized patients and better knowledge of treatments through clinical experimentation.

Those called on to treat patients were eager to review all indications and procedures that previous experience had shown to be helpful. Criteria for therapeutic usefulness or "mischief" were again purely clinical, based on visible and predictable physiological effects such as vomiting after the ingestion of an emetic or relaxation following bloodletting. During the eighteenth century this information was usually obtained from medical books and articles summarizing the limited experience of their authors. Cullen and other medical authorities urged practitioners not only to become personally acquainted with the properties of drugs they were willing to employ but to display open minds and adopt new remedies derived from folk healing, such as belladonna, cod-liver oil, and digitalis. At the same time, colleagues were exhorted to discontinue the use of ineffective or useless items still crowding the official drug registries, as well as to reject all remedies considered "secret" because of their obvious link to quackery. Among the former were the traditional cure-alls mithridate and theriac, used since antiquity.

Prominent authors preached therapeutic skepticism, especially with regard to the use of panaceas or "specifics" and the usual *post hoc ergo propter hoc* reasoning that uncritically ascribed therapeutic success to the procedure previously employed. "There is nothing more agreeable than to see the good effects of our remedies," lectured Cullen, "but we must dispute whether our remedies produced the change."[14] Cure-alls smacked of ignorance and fraud.

If therapeutic knowledge could not be "put upon proper footing" of universal scientific principles, it also resisted standardization because of its individual application. In the view of late eighteenth-century medical professionals, each patient presented a unique challenge as disease took on particular configurations when confronted by the bodily constitution. "General plans are fallacious and lead to a kind of random practice," remarked Cullen.[15] Within general guidelines treatment had to be carefully tailored to each personal case, and in the absence of comprehensive physical examinations this procedure necessitated accurate progress reports from the patient. During an extensive interview, Andrew Duncan, Sr., acknowledged making three visits daily to the infirmary to interrogate and inspect his patients and give new directions for their care.[16]

Almost all known therapeutic agents were given with the expectation that they would produce systemic changes and thus "carry off the disease" or, in certain ills, "render the crisis complete." Since all diseases were believed to take somewhat similar pathophysiological courses, eighteenth-century practitioners made few distinctions among the articles of materia medica when they ordered their treatments. The basic therapeutic intent was to place the patient "in the train," a vague phrase meaning a path that could lead to recovery.

The phenomenon of fever, with its diurnal paroxysms, served as the model for planning all treatments. Essential organic functions had to be either moderated or spurred to reverse imbalances produced by disease. If a febrile fit produced a fast pulse, hot skin, and flushed face, the physician interpreted these manifestations as reflecting a pathological arousal of all bodily systems that demanded a soothing treatment until signs of healthy balance reappeared. Conversely, if illness caused lethargy, slow pulse, and debility in the patient, these symptoms were seen as signs of a depressed organic state, often called asthenia. Here the necessary therapeutic strategy was to institute a stimulating plan of cure.

In most instances, especially in fevers, the sedative or relaxing approach was employed first until a "crisis" or critical point was reached and convalescence suspected. At that juncture, reassured by nature that the patient was on the mend, practitioners switched to methods that would excite the bodily system. Occasionally, the reverse pattern was followed. In protracted cases the two sets of procedures could be alternated "to conduct the patient through the disease," depending on the physician's perception of its natural evolution.

Closely linked to systemic sedation or excitement was routine depletion of the gastrointestinal tract. Eighteenth-century practitioners retained their forefathers' concern for emptying the *prima via* or digestive canal. Did not nature frequently show the way in fevers by spontaneously causing nausea and vomiting, abdominal discomfort and diarrhea? Were not foul-smelling stools enough evidence of an incipient internal putrefaction that could threaten other bodily systems? Within the older humoral pathology it was imperative to cleanse the digestive system lest some residual food or stool suffer transformations that could be harmful to the entire organism. Constant purgation "kept the system open" and presumably drained sufficient intestinal secretions to rob fermentation and putrefaction of its raw materials.

Within the framework of Cullen's neuropathological explanations, it was assumed that the organs of digestion, especially the stomach, were always compromised, no matter what disease affected the organism. The reason was their "sympathetic" linkage with all other bodily systems. Conditions of chronic debility and, indeed, all so-called nervous diseases seemingly impaired the muscular fibers of stomach and intestines and thus suggested an urgent need to eliminate their contents.[17]

Table 4.1. *Sedative regimen*

Type of diet	Total abstinence or low vegetable diet
Beverages	Thirst quenchers – barley water Cooling drinks – cream of tartar Antiseptic liquors – acidulated fruit juices
Physical methods	Bloodletting – phlebotomy, leeching, or cupping Cold water bath Applications of blisters Use of warm baths Application of poultices Fomentations with warm fluids Abdominal rubbing
Medications	Cathartics Diaphoretics Diuretics Emetics Expectorants Emollients Narcotics
Other measures	Bedrest Avoidance of exercise Dark room Ventilation

James Gregory admirably summarized contemporary therapeutics when he declared that "the greater part of a physician's practice consists in exciting, promoting, restraining, and sometimes irritating by art various operations of nature in the human body."[18] Tables 4.1 and 4.2 give schematic summaries of the two basic approaches to disease during the latter part of the eighteenth century.

THE CONTEXT OF HOSPITAL CARE

Treatments to restrain or stimulate the organism, as well as the traditional depletion of the digestive system, were carried out at Edinburgh in a new clinical setting and on the basis of an entirely new patient–healer relationship. As noted, the sick poor applying for admission generally approached the institution with a mixture of fear and hope. Almost all of them viewed the hospital with some apprehension as an "abode of sorrow"[19] to which they resorted because the suffering had become unbearable or had failed to respond to the usual domestic measures. Some probably did not even come voluntarily but, as in the case of soldiers, sailors, and servants, followed

Table 4.2. *Stimulant regimen*

Type of diet	Full diet containing meat
Beverages	Warm or cold water
	Wines
	Cider and beer
	Liquors – brandy or rum
Physical methods	Cold or warm baths
	Blisters – use of issues, setons
	Local heat with bricks, tiles, cloths, and plasters
	Fomentations to legs and thighs
	Electricity
	Bodily rubbing with brush, flannels, or woolen gloves
Medications	Astringents
	Bitters and tonics
	Diaphoretics
	Diuretics
	Emetics
	Expectorants
	Emmenagogues and sialogogues
Other measures	Exercise – walking, horseback riding, dancing, traveling in carriage

orders from their superiors and masters. Others sustained sudden injuries during work or leisure that required prompt intervention. A few had lost consciousness and were brought in by well-meaning friends, relatives, or even strangers. Finally, a small group of patients went to the infirmary for shelter and care because they lacked relatives or friends who could look after them.

At the bottom of their anxiety, triggered by the symptoms of sickness, the poor feared death or, almost as terrible, permanent disability with its specter of abandonment or becoming a public charge. Death might even be preferable to "lonesome decrepitude" in a workhouse. But was there still a chance for recovery? Soon they would definitely find out, as the physicians – "judges of life and death" – passed their sentences.[20] Some already felt guilty about their procrastination in seeking professional help. Given the frequency of illness, disability, and death among them, others probably were ambivalent about their choice to seek hospitalization.

Fear or loathing was an obstacle to the establishment of a good rapport with the medical profession. The first contact in the admitting room was generally frustrating and confusing, as the prospective patients tried to tell the "right" stories about their sufferings, stories that would make them "proper" objects for hospital treatment. Since the clinical history was the key criterion used for admission, diagnosis, and treatment, during its taking the sick and the medical professionals got their first chance to meet. Conflicting world views and contrasting concepts of illness, not to mention the profound social gap between them, reflected in language and manners, hampered attempts to communicate.

This situation often encouraged patients to manipulate the attending physicians and sometimes to commit outright fraud, as those anxious to gain admission framed their complaints appropriately to impress the medical personnel. The latter, in turn, expressed frustration if the symptoms enumerated by patients were not sufficient to pinpoint or "mark" the disease for diagnosis. Clues vital for medical treatment were perhaps distorted by previous medications. At other times the sick remained silent, in awe or fear, as they faced the mighty professionals who were expected to take control over their lives.[21]

The formidable social position of the professionals could be both daunting and therapeutic for those admitted to the Edinburgh infirmary. Here were a number of men with considerable power and status contractually obligated to treat lowly, poor people who could probably never have afforded their private services. University professors, attending physicians, and surgeons were all recognized by their peers as competent healers, members of local professional associations such as the Royal College of Physicians and the Incorporation of Surgeons. Many of them also had extensive private practices, personal wealth, and social contacts with aristocrats and government officials, intellectuals and bankers. Their medical authority was highly respected by colleagues and patients. In the eyes of society, these men brought to their infirmary tasks the best knowledge eighteenth-century medicine had to offer. In this sense hospital care was really a true reflection of the contemporary "state of the medical art."

Within the institutional setting, medical practitioners could use their power over patients in many ways. Greater control over clinical management in the hospital assured them of better patient compliance with the therapeutic regimen than they could exact from private patients and opportunities to follow up as well as to verify the success of treatments. New freedom to pursue the effects of drugs and other procedures fostered clinical experimentation and collection of statistical information. Even some incurable ailments were temporarily palliated. Of course, new sources of professional frustration arose when the periodic interrogation of patients and nurses yielded insufficient or false information on which therapeutic decisions had to be made. Given existing communication difficulties, hospital physicians might, like William Cullen, become almost obsessed about the reliability of patients' accounts, since practitioners would be held accountable for subsequent errors or failures in treatment based on these reports.[22]

The newly acquired medical power also promoted arrogance and condescension. There was cause for patients to fear exploitation and harassment. A satirical work ironically recommended that hospital physicians "by every stratagem in your power contrive to insult and domineer over every patient committed to your care."[23] Instances of intimidation and abuse were reported, although they were more often perpetrated by nurses and servants, perhaps because they had greater contact with patients. Not unexpectedly, several medical authors, including Thomas Percival, exhorted their colleagues to respect the feelings of their patients.[24] John Gregory, for his part, emphasized the importance of "sympathy," a human quality that allowed people to identify with each other's emotions. In his view patient and physicians needed to become friends. The advantages accruing to both parties and to the therapeutic process in general were clearly recognized.[25]

One healing ritual was the daily visit to the wards scheduled by the attending physicians, surgeons, and professors. Followed by a "train" of assistants and students, hospital practitioners made their entrance at a predetermined hour to question the patients and perhaps issue new orders. According to one account, each ward greeted the visitors in solemn silence at the appointed time, with those inmates able to leave their beds standing erect next to them in military formation.[26]

Although the patient's institutional isolation could be harmful, new sources of support and sympathy appeared in the form of fellow patients. The practice of employing ambulant and convalescent inmates to care for those still bedridden created ideal conditions for sharing concerns and experiences. "Social chats" and "harmless jest" lightened the burdens and more than made up for the temporary loss of family networks and friends. As one eyewitness wrote, "Grief attracts by stronger bonds than pleasure ever knew."[27] Moreover, a generous visiting program at the Edinburgh infirmary allowed family members daily access to the wards. Finally, ambulatory patients even received permission to leave the hospital for several hours and thus briefly return to their circles of relatives and friends.

For the opportunity of closely observing large numbers of patients and becoming more proficient in clinical skills, hospital practitioners gave up some of the freedom and power they enjoyed in private practice. At the Edinburgh infirmary they owed their appointments to lay managers who demanded an oath of allegiance and promises to follow the institution's statutes and regulations. All budgetary decisions and the authority to hire ancillary personnel were out of the physicians' hands. Fiscal constraints even affected treatment plans, including the quantity and quality of the diet, the need to prescribe in-house remedies, and limits on the use of beer and wine.

Such bureaucratic rules tended to streamline and standardize medical treatments, in direct opposition to the practitioners' desire to assert their professional prerogatives in individualized care. The resulting tensions between hospital authorities and medical staff could never be totally avoided and were the source of innumerable conflicts. At the same time, medical men were constantly subjected to close professional scrutiny by their peers, clerks, and students. Physicians were indeed "obliged" to change their medicines if no favorable results were forthcoming. "A hospital is the worst [place] for a dunce who in private practice might long have escaped detection and enjoyed undeserved riches and honour," remarked James Gregory.[28]

Peer control required new guidelines for professional behavior set down in the form of ethical codes such as Percival's, ostensibly designed to avoid conflicts among practitioners at the Manchester Infirmary. Working in the limelight demanded personal circumspection not only to protect one's own reputation but, more important, to defend the standing of the institution. Hospital practitioners indeed needed to convey to the public at large the notion that they would refrain from taking advantage of their patients. If the latter "get into their heads that more freedom is used here [by physicians] than elsewhere, it will confirm their aversion to hospitals," observed Cullen. Managers also feared that all irregular activities and improper experimentation would be quickly conveyed to other patients in the house, students, and inhabitants of the city, thus jeopardizing donations. "It is necessary to give our patients some confidence in us and a good opinion of our attention," lectured Cullen.[29]

Maintaining a good opinion of the hospital was essential to the success of the charity. As in private practice, it was often necessary for practitioners to pay attention first to the "prejudices" of hospitalized people, who together with their relatives and sponsors were often "unacquainted" with institutional routines, reacting with fear and distrust to the therapeutic orders. Beyond these people, there was an even larger constituency to impress: the donors and subscribers. Expenditures, admissions, and mortality rates in the Edinburgh infirmary were frequently compared with those of comparable voluntary hospitals, especially the ones located in London.[30] Scottish subscribers needed encouragement to continue supporting their expensive charity, and they periodically got it in the form of favorable statistics. At the same time, physicians were told that attending poor people in such charitable institutions was honorable work. It was a splendid opportunity to improve the physical and moral well-being of large numbers of sick persons who otherwise would remain without care. Yet medical care was also public business, a service seen as benefiting society at large, since it put the "deserving" poor back on their feet, thereby making them again productive members instead of public burdens.

THERAPEUTIC EFFECTS OF HOSPITALIZATION

Hospital practitioners were conscious of the therapeutic effects of the "cover of the house." Cullen welcomed the infirmary's "uniform temperature," especially during the cold months of winter.[31] It seemed to do wonders for those admitted with catarrhs or other respiratory ailments, particularly the "poorer sort of people who are exposed to frequent attacks of cold and more especially in elderly people."[32] In several instances Cullen even admitted violating hospital rules by refusing to discharge such patients, instead keeping them in the "warmth and shelter of the house in hopes of a better season."[33]

He did the same thing for a number of persons suffering from incurable ailments, where hospitalization was authorized as a palliative treatment. At times, as with patients in incipient or more advanced stages of phthisis, who really were in need of fresh air and moderate exercise, confinement and warm chambers were seen as perhaps detrimental. Cullen realized the dilemma but, if it was winter, kept the patients in the house nonetheless, "defending them against cold," because he considered the hospital stay less evil than repeated exposure to "cold and starving habitations."[34]

Of greater importance were measures designed to treat fever and prevent its in-house transmission. As mentioned earlier, voluntary hospitals like the Edinburgh infirmary adopted a number of measures designed to promote adequate ventilation and cleanliness, which were believed sufficiently therapeutic to cure many fevers without any medical aid. "I would rather undertake the cure of any number of patients with the help of cleanliness, pure cool air, and cold water without any medications," wrote James Gregory.[35] During the late eighteenth century such environmental actions seemed effective enough so that many patients resting in their hospital beds appeared to rally and recover without further therapeutic measures.

The Edinburgh infirmary was built before the tenets of a new public hygiene formulated in army barracks, in field hospitals, and on board ships became sufficiently successful to be implemented in civilian hospitals. Its windows were only twelve feet in height, and the flow of air in the ward was somewhat hindered by closets and partitions, many of which were finally removed after 1800. Curtains that could be drawn around the beds to ensure privacy were at the same time obstacles to the circulation of fresh air. Moreover, the active fireplaces located at the end of each ward were considered inadequate to draw out all the stagnant air from the center of the rooms. Reformers recommended that ventilators be placed in windows to draw greater quantities of fresh air into the wards and that stoves be installed at the opposite end from the fireplaces, with long tubes connecting them to the chimneys.[36] The ensuing drafts of air were strong enough between windows and central staircase so that they even caused a recurrence of cold symptoms in a number of convalescents.[37]

In spite of such structural deficiencies, the infirmary pursued a comprehensive program of institutional hygiene, including the instant removal of all patients' "discharges" (ideally, each patient was supposed to have a chamberpot in a small closet next to the bed, but at times there were only two in a ward of twenty to twenty-five patients). The tiled floors were supposed to be mopped daily by convalescent patients and nurses, and the walls received a periodic treatment of whitewashing with lime. One such whitewashing was reported by John Hope, in the early 1780s, following a hospital epidemic of "putrid" fever.[38] John Howard, inspecting the infirmary in the late 1770s and again a few years later, gave the institution good marks because of its "airiness and cleanliness," in spite of the perceived shortcomings.[39] James Gregory wrote that the women's fever ward was "cleaner and better ventilated than most bed-chambers in Edinburgh,"[40] a fact confirmed by another attending physician, James Hamilton.[41]

Another Edinburgh deficiency, pointed out in 1800 and subsequent years, was the lack of a clear policy regarding the personal hygiene of individuals admitted to the charity. After arriving in the wards, many of them were sent to bed with their dirty clothes on, since the hospital lacked enough clean gowns or shirts for routine issue to newcomers. Others, ordered to surrender their rags to the hospital laundry, were "obliged" to lie without shirts until the washing was done.[42]

Bathing patients was part of the medical regimen and subject to special orders from physicians, issued the day following admission, if they perceived the need. At the Edinburgh infirmary the order was executed with increasing difficulty, because the central bathing facilities were also used for washing an expanding volume of laundry. To remedy the situation, portable tubs and barrels were brought into individual wards, but the difficulties of obtaining and carrying enough water to the units, as well as lack of privacy – these arrangements were "indecent to patients" in spite of surrounding curtains – sharply curtailed their employment.[43]

Although most women appeared "clean enough," men were frequently dirty, with an "unpleasant foetor attached." In the 1790s some were infested with vermin – generally meaning lice – and therefore fumigated. According to Duncan, patients arriving in the infirmary's teaching ward were carefully examined for cleanliness and the rooms fumigated daily with muriatic acid gas. The heads of some men were promptly shaved, their skin rubbed with mercury ointment, and a few clean shirts issued. In spite of the measures, lice infestation remained, the prevailing view being that "it seems impossible to answer for the transit of a louse."[44]

If the patient's personal cleanliness was an important factor in the recovery from certain fevers, the condition of beds and bed linens was regarded as playing an equally prominent role. Iron bedsteads in use at the Edinburgh infirmary were easier to clean than wooden ones, but the straw-filled mattresses rested on an absorbent base made of rope and seemed capable of retaining "every kind of contagious mischief."[45] Under normal circumstances there was an understanding that after admission every new patient was to receive clean sheets and that these had to be changed at least every two to three weeks if not sooner because of soiling by human wastes or draining wounds.[46] Here again reality fell short of the proposed ideal, because escalating admissions at the infirmary rapidly exhausted the available clean linen supplies, while the institution's laundry facilities nearly collapsed under the additional burden.[47]

In spite of shortcomings – and these occurred mostly toward the end of the century during a period of fiscal difficulties – patients at the Edinburgh infirmary were considerably better off in the hospital than in their own dilapidated quarters. In fevers, especially the typhus variety, James Gregory detected "great and favorable changes in a few hours after they are laid in the wards of this hospital and before they get any powerful medicines or perhaps any medicines at all."[48] He judged that ventilation and cleanliness in hospital wards not only prevented the accumulation of contagious matter but safely diffused it to levels no longer dangerous to patients. Following Pringle, practitioners tried to explain the appearance of typhus fever through the spontaneous generation of poison arising in the stale air of small, windowless, and crowded rooms. Part of it was believed to be human perspiration, the rest simply vapor emanating from decaying food and plain filth. It was the gradual concentration of this contagion that finally overwhelmed people living under such conditions. Their removal to properly ventilated quarters with improved cleanliness was a necessary precondition for recovery. Hence the hospital became, according to Gregory, the "best or only hitherto known contrivance" for curing and preventing such "slow," continuous fevers.[49]

THE USE OF DRUGS

Drugs were the most frequent therapeutic articles employed in the hospital. Most of them were traditional herbal products "afforded by nature" and chemical preparations "compounded by art," all listed in official compilations called pharmacopoeias or dispensatories. In Britain these lists were approved and published by the Colleges of Physicians in London and Edinburgh.[50] The Edinburgh infirmary had its own in-house dispensatory, the *Pharmacopoeia Pauperum*, a standard reference for prescriptions by physicians and surgeons attending the hospital.[51]

During the eighteenth century knowledge about drugs was largely based on empirical evidence accumulated at the bedside, often in the form of individual case reports or textbooks on materia medica containing information about the botanical origins and chemical qualities of drugs and food articles.[52] Because most therapeutic measures only possessed a clinical rationale instead of being proposed because of experimental physiological and pharmacological reasons, treatment depended on the individual experience of a practitioner and was subjected to frequent changes on a trial-and-error basis. Ruled by the imperative to "exert" themselves, physicians "exhibited" or administered whatever promised relief. Cullen, for example, pledged to students that he would never "sit down in despair and do nothing. I commonly take up a supposition that will admit of practice."[53]

Whether the success of particular medicines was based on hearsay, biased testimonials, erroneous inferences, or insufficient experience mattered very little. Uncritical physicians were, of course, "dazzled with any surprising discovery and immediately employ it for the cure of diseases, not considering how difficult an art medicine is," complained George Fordyce.[54] Others loosely reasoned by analogy and established cure-alls or panaceas based on the faulty premise that products helpful in a limited number of conditions would also work in other problems. At the end of the spectrum were "ignorant and lazy practitioners who commonly take the medicines presented to their hands" without any effort to judge their propriety in a specific situation.[55]

The hospital setting allowed physicians to temper their therapeutic compulsions and avoid the extremes of uncritical activism or conservatism. Given new opportunities for direct patient observation and collection of reports about the clinical effects of remedies, Cullen, Home, and their colleagues at the Edinburgh infirmary encouraged the use of simple drugs. Indeed, adhering to institutional constraints, most hospital practitioners confined their prescribing to one or two formulas for each medicine and seldom administered more than one active drug at a time. "I have a rule of sticking to a single remedy," stressed Cullen, "for otherwise in the case of a single change we do not know to what it is to be imputed."[56] However, when in doubt about using a drug, it was better not to prescribe any: "In every case where medicines are not actually indicated," wrote Duncan, "their use is undoubtedly to be avoided."[57]

Clinical experimentation

To render their hospital practices "subservient to medical improvement," Edinburgh practitioners engaged in certain forms of clinical experimentation using a number of drugs whose efficacy or timing for administration were in question. Cullen, for example, conducted a number of "random trials" – meaning tests without a fixed purpose. The investigations were designed to ascertain the efficacy of new compounds or establish additional indications for items already listed in the official pharmacopoeias. Cullen's use of a hyoscyamus extract, "a remedy whose effects I was desirous to learn," fell into the first category, whereas his administration of opiates in epilepsy and corrosive mercury in leprosy were examples of the latter.[58]

From the casebooks it appears that Home and Duncan were the most active infirmary practitioners conducting tests with drugs. Home's trials with Peruvian bark in the treatment of fourteen patients suffering from intermittent fevers lasted between 1769 and 1779. The purpose of the investigation was to ascertain the most effective time for administering the drug. Home divided his sample about in half, with one group receiving bark before and the other getting it after their febrile fits. His final conclusion was that the drug was more effective when given at the end of a paroxysm.[59] Duncan, in turn, tried a number of new botanicals, some of them sent from America and grown in the university's botanical gardens.[60] Their findings generally revealed significant variations in patient response to the drugs and thus supported the need for individualized therapy.

The eagerness for "experiments" displayed by Home and Duncan came under a fair amount of criticism from James Gregory, who cautioned his colleagues not to expose patients to unnecessary dangers. "Corio humano ludere" (playing with the human hide) was his rather scornful phrase for clinical experimentation.[61] Gregory recognized the need for such trials if there was a chance that the tests would benefit the patients subjected to them. At the same time, however, he considered it a "high misdemeanor" if dangerous medicines were given just "to gratify our own curiosity or zeal for science."[62] He did not object to practitioners engaging in self-experiments, but he doubted strongly that "they have any right at all to send their patients out of the world that way, who have no ambition for that crown of martyrdom."[63]

The "natural order" of medicines

To avoid the "promiscuous" employment of drugs, eighteenth-century physicians created "assemblages" or "limited associations" of drugs based on a similarity of clinical effects.[64] Duncan considered such classifications "analogous to natural orders in botany," with every category including a number of compounds that produced the same results.[65] His "natural order of medicines" contained twenty-four separate classes of drugs, each possessing a number of orders or subgroups with distinctive secondary properties. Cullen's categories in his *Materia Medica* were less elaborate, but the two showed enough agreement to provide a number of fundamental headings employed in Edinburgh during the latter decades of the eighteenth century and useful for an analysis of drug utilization at the infirmary. The histories contained in student casebooks give the prescription frequencies indicated in Table 4.3.

Table 4.3. *Drugs used at the infirmary,*
1771–1799 (N = 808)

Drug class	Frequency	%
Cathartics	523	26.2
Anodynes or analgesics	326	16.3
Emetics	278	13.9
Diaphoretics	217	10.8
Expectorants	162	8.1
Tonics	151	7.5
Diuretics	111	5.5
Mercurials	87	4.3

Cathartics

Medicines grouped in the *cathartic* class were believed to stir the bowels and increase the evacuation of stools. Their action was somewhat stimulating to the entire system and led to the expulsion of undigested matter, intestinal secretions – in particular, mucus – and hardened feces, always suspected of causing irritation and obstructions. Such effects were usually considered beneficial since purgatives were said to remove any "morbid" matter lodged in the intestines and to help the blood circulate in the lower half of the body. More important, these medicines cleared the way for absorption of fresh nutriment in the gut, where it could contribute to the final recovery.[66]

Cathartics were commonly divided into *laxatives, purgatives,* and *drastics,* depending on the intensity of the intestinal stimulation. Those of lesser action included such products as acid fruits (tamarinds, apples, and prunes), juice from the manna tree, syrup of pale roses or violets, and infusions of chamomile. Among the popular purgatives were aloes, rhubarb, senna, jalap, and castor oil, employed in the form of powders, infusions, and tinctures. A number of salts used for the same purpose were sodium sulfate (Glauber's salts), antimony potassium tartrate (tartar emetic), sodium potassium tartrate (cream of tartar), and magnesium sulfate. One mercurial compound, calomel or mercurous chloride, was quite popular and, according to Cullen, "one of the most certain and effectual purgatives that we know of."[67] Calomel was usually prescribed in association with jalap or rhubarb and would "run off by stool," meaning that in small doses of two to five grains it would not produce the usual systemic reactions attributed to mercury.[68] to mercury.[68]

Finally, among the drastics, hospital practitioners selected the tincture of white and black hellebore, wild cucumber, the pulp of a bitter apple, colocynth, and resins from the scammony root and gamboge tree. The Edinburgh infirmary dispensatory listed some large pills or *boluses* of castor oil, jalap, and calomel, as well as the popular decoction of tamarinds with senna. A purging glyster or enema contained white soap and syrup of blackthorn.

Edinburgh professors in charge of the teaching ward prescribed cathartics for one of every four patients under their care. About a third of them were affected with febrile diseases, although proportionately the highest use was registered among patients with skin conditions (close to half of them received a cathartic). Here practitioners repeatedly tried to eliminate "morbid" matter using the normal outlet, rather than allowing its elimination through the pores of the skin in the form of rashes and eruptions.

Predictably, frequent use of purgatives was also observed in cases of venereal disease and gastrointestinal ailments in which a removal of poisons was judged essential to achieve a cure. The overall strategy in employing cathartics was summarized by John Gregory: "Keep a gentle diarrhea without impairing health or strength."[69] In at least 25% of all cases, however, patients undergoing purgation experienced abdominal cramps, excessive diarrhea, vertigo, and debility. Thus physicians were forced at times to administer enemas – a less desirable substitute – to procure or maintain "plentiful discharges." Repeated trips to ward latrines and, for recumbent patients, countless exertions on chamberpots surely took their toll, often weakening patients and prolonging their convalescence.

Such a preoccupation with cleansing the bowels evidently stemmed from the traditional view, widely shared by the laity and professionals, that "the constipated and loaded state of the intestinal canal is a common cause of bad health." Domestic measures frequently aimed at a similar purification and were employed before people sought admission to hospitals. "How to regulate the alvine (belly) evacuation constitutes much of the prophylactic part of medicine," observed James Hamilton, a notorious enthusiast of purgation and one of the physicians-in-ordinary at the infirmary.[70]

Many diseases, especially fevers, caused changes in bowel habits, with "costiveness" or diarrhea virtually becoming the rule as the disease progressed. If febrile manifestations were linked with the onset of bowel "irregularities," was it not logical to blame the abnormal accumulation of stool in part for subsequent symptoms? The feces were waste products no longer needed and already "out of the course of circulation," extraneous to the body. Was it not prudent to hasten their elimination, lest they undergo putrefaction changes or by their sheer bulk disturb and obstruct the absorption of badly needed nutrients?[71]

Anodynes or analgesics

Eighteenth-century physicians defined *anodynes* as "medicines which ease pain and produce sleep," including among them *paregorics,* true pain-killers, *hypnotics,* and *narcotics,* all employed in fighting pain and inducing sleep.[72] All of them were known to be sedative agents that diminished the sensibility and irritability of the human system. The most important drug in this category was opium, generally given in the form of anodyne drafts containing liquid laudanum or paregoric elixir. The liquid laudanum of Sydenham, also named thebaic extract or simply tincture of opium, was the most popular prescription among Edinburgh professors. Other narcotics were aconite, hemlock, belladonna, and henbane. The hospital prepared enemas with laudanum and linseed infusions, as well as an analgesic ointment made of egg whites and containing opium used for painful hemorrhoids. Laudanum eye drops were recommended in many ophthalmias.[73]

During the 1770s and 1780s Edinburgh physicians heatedly debated whether opium was a sedative or a stimulant. It was a major argument dividing the adherents of William Cullen and his disciple, John Brown.[74] Cullen stressed the sedative qualities of opium, whereas Brown and his followers considered it a stimulant. Such theoretical disputes, though important for the defense of specific medical systems and the personal credibility of their respective authors, had little impact on the clinical use of opium as the ideal pain-killer of the period. The drug worked so effectively that the physicians were elated and uninhibitedly resorted to opium preparations for the treatment of many conditions, unaware as yet of its addicting qualities. "The danger which physicians formerly apprehended from the use of this remedy seems now to have vanished," wrote one of them in 1785.[75]

At the infirmary analgesics were given more frequently to female patients in all categories of sickness, since it was widely assumed in the eighteenth century that their constitution made women more sensitive to pain. The greatest usage occurred in musculoskeletal problems for the amelioration of arthritic pains and in respiratory conditions to suppress severe coughing. In fevers opium was also frequently used, especially in slow, nervous varieties, including typhus, that lacked true inflammatory characteristics but produced considerable delirium and agitation.[76] Various types of diarrhea were significantly helped by opium, often administered in the form of enemas containing laudanum. Finally, convulsions associated with tetanus, epilepsy, and even hysteria could be temporarily controlled by opium preparations, as could an acutely inflamed toe in cases of gout. From the clinical reports one gains the impression that the management of pain with opiates constituted one of the most successful aspects of eighteenth-century therapeutics. Hospital practitioners seldom hesitated to prescribe analgesics for pain – often almost indiscriminately – and their enthusiasm clearly obscured all side effects attributable to opium.

Emetics

Most neurophysiological schemes of the eighteenth century assigned to the stomach a central place in the transmission of nervous impulses to other organ systems through a phenomenon called "sympathy." It was generally believed that fevers and other diseases displayed a lack of appetite, nausea, and even vomiting because of weakness and relaxation in the muscular fibers girding the stomach. Before such a dangerous state became diffused throughout the body, practitioners argued, it was imperative to remove all the remaining contents from the stomach.[77]

According to Duncan, *emetics* were "medicines which taken into the stomach are capable of exciting vomiting."[78] Such an effect eliminated burdensome matter "being prepared for deposit in the alimentary canal" precisely at a time when stomach and bowels were ill prepared to digest anything because they were in the throes of disease. In respiratory diseases emetics disposed of the various products of expectoration swallowed by the patients. Eighteenth-century physicians also believed that vomiting would free up the gastrointestinal circulation, assist in the secretion and discharge of bile, and thus facilitate the future absorption of new nutrients.[79]

Most contemporary pharmacopoeias listed among mild emetics the root of ipecacuanha and antimony preparations, both given in the form of wines. Others were white vitriol (zinc sulphate) and the sea onion or squill, given as a drink mixed with vinegar and honey. The most popular emetic and a favorite of Cullen was tartar emetic (antimonial potassium tartrate). Others prescribed mineral turpeth (sulphate of mercury) and blue vitriol (copper sulphate).[80] The Edinburgh infirmary prepared a number of institutional juleps or sweet drinks as well as pills containing squill.

In fevers Cullen preferred to "wash out the stomach" with tartar emetic, because its dosage could be easily standardized while the effects were quite predictable. Since the drug also showed a "tendency to run off by stool," it fulfilled the dual goals of vomiting and purging so common in the treatment of febrile illnesses.[81] Indeed, according to the information obtained from student casebooks, more than 18% of all fever patients received an emetic. Nearly as many patients suffering from respiratory diseases were treated in this way. Here the need to "unload the breast through vomiting" was often paramount and even occurred spontaneously.[82]

As in cases of catharsis, "taking a vomit" was a common course of action in both domestic and professional medicine, practiced in imitation of natural events taking place during many inflammatory conditions. Patient demand and the physician's desire to remove any obstacles standing in the way of recovery usually led to the prescription of emetics.[83] Vomiting was in fact continued until the patient no longer complained of gastric heaviness or distress. Then the recovery of appetite signaled the stomach's renewed capacity to accept food and was generally viewed as a watershed in the evolution of fevers, marking the onset of convalescence and eventual recovery.

Diaphoretics

Diaphoretics were drugs capable of modestly increasing normal perspiration; the name *sudorifics* was reserved for a group of compounds promoting copious sweat. Both actions were favorably interpreted, especially in fevers, because they seemed to happen spontaneously at the end of febrile fits and usually signaled recovery. Moreover, physicians assumed that by relaxing the skin's pores and allowing a discharge of sweat, they not only increased the superficial circulation but helped the human organism shed the residual morbid matter in the form of vapor and condensed fluid.[84]

Diaphoresis, therefore, was seen as a stimulating procedure, enhanced by the application of heat in the form of baths or fomentations. Among the more powerful sudorifics employed were volatile alkali, opium, camphor, and musk. A more gentle perspiration deemed relaxing was achieved through the usage of mild aromatics such as sage and mint, served in the form of teas. Others were tinctures of saffron and crocus, vinegar, guaiac powder, arnica, and decoctions of sarsaparilla and snakeroot.[85]

Nitrous, antimonial, and common salts in the form of drafts and juleps were popular at the Edinburgh infirmary. The hospital listed a diaphoretic bolus containing ammonia salt and powder of contrayerva, a tropical American root previously used against snakebites. The standard saline draft contained wormwood salt and lemon juice. Cullen's favorite in fevers was *julapium salinum,* made with the same ingredients but also containing mint water and syrup.[86]

From the student notebooks it appears that the most frequent use of diaphoretic drugs occurred in musculoskeletal conditions, especially in cases of acute and chronic rheumatism (24% of all cases). Here the drugs were usually supplemented with baths, fomentations, and the wearing of flannel shirts. During winters, however, profuse sweating was sparingly attempted because hospital practitioners feared that patients in the drafty wards would come down with colds. Like the measures hitherto examined, diaphoresis on the whole enjoyed broad popular and professional support and was viewed as a natural cleansing technique that could rid the body of disease-producing matter.

Expectorants

According to Cullen, the *expectorants,* also termed *pectorals,* helped to "bring up the contents of the cavity of the lungs."[87] These medicines comprised a number of so-called *attenuant* or *demulcent* drugs designed to help dissolve the thick bronchial secretions and thereby contribute to their eventual elimination. Among the most frequently prescribed products were fresh and dried garlic in syrup, squill, flowers of benjamin, decoction of licorice, and gum arabic. Another group, called *incrassants,* neutralized thin, acrid secretions and also facilitated their expectoration. Linseed tea, syrup of coltsfoot, balsam of Tolu, decoction of marshmallow, and mucilage of gum arabic were the favorites of Edinburgh practitioners.[88] Opiates were given in combination with these expectorants if the cough was excessive.

At the infirmary practitioners usually ordered a so-called pectoral bolus prepared from spermaceti, a fatty substance derived from sperm whales, an infusion of linseed, or a mucilaginous mixture containing gum arabic, Cullen's standard prescription.[89] Almost half of the expectorants dispensed in the teaching ward were indeed used for patients suffering from respiratory ailments. Their action was again explained in neurophysiological terms as being both relaxing and stimulant, depending on the physician's own clinical perceptions. If excessive cough was controlled and bronchial spasms were reduced, expectorants were said to relax the organic system. However, if the patient seemed weak and the respiratory system was unable to expel the secretions, any improvement from the medicines was ascribed to a stimulating action.[90]

Tonics

Tonics were medicines designed to increase the general tone or strength of the body. Cullen included among them the so-called *astringents,* drugs capable of local effects interpreted as increasing fiber density. Substances such as alum, iron, copper, and lead preparations were included under this class. Botanicals prescribed were cinnamon bark, logwood, pomegranate, snakeweed, and lemon juice. The infirmary prepared an astringent gargle for sore throats that contained boiled oak bark.

Another group of tonics was the *bitters,* believed to promote appetite and digestion by increasing the tone of gastric muscular fibers. Through "sympathy," this local effect was then communicated to the rest of the system and served to invigorate the entire body. The most popular preparations contained cascarilla bark, Virginia snakeroot, wild cinnamon, wormwood, cardamom seeds, chamomile, gentian root, ginger, and Angostura bark. Chemical preparations also considered tonics included nitrous and muriatic acid diluted in water, and arsenical compounds.[91]

The most popular tonic in the late eighteenth century was the *cortex peruvianus,* or Peruvian bark containing quinine, which in Cullen's words was "one of the most considerable articles of the materia medica."[92] Prepared from the bark of a Peruvian shrub called *Cinchona* and used in the form of extract, decoction, or tincture, this drug had had quite a checkered history since its introduction to European medicine more than a century earlier.[93] Its greatest utility appeared to be in the treatment of intermittent fevers, but by the 1780s the bark was also prescribed in remittent fevers, typhus, and many ordinary fevers after the initial inflammatory signs abated.[94]

In 1782 William Saunders, physician to Guy's Hospital in London, drew attention to the superior qualities of a so-called red Peruvian bark derived from older trees. His observations were quickly confirmed by other practitioners, who also claimed better results with the new preparation. Better tasting and much more potent, the red bark became an effective remedy against intermittent fevers, displacing its predecessor, the "quilled" bark.[95]

According to the student casebooks, virtually half of the tonics prescribed in the teaching ward went to fever patients. Other groups getting tonics were persons suffering from mental depression, women with "suppressed" menses, and paralytics, all needing strong stimulating measures to overcome their illnesses. Unfortunately, the Peruvian bark "sat" badly on the stomach and soon caused enough nausea and vomiting in patients taking it to force its discontinuance.

Diuretics

Drugs classified as *diuretics* were believed to promote the secretion of urine from the kidneys. Eighteenth-century physicians postulated that this action would not only diminish an excess of fluids in the body but also remove "morbid" matter.[96] Included among the diuretics were so-called *diluents,* a group of substances that diluted the blood and thereby facilitated the excretion of its serum, together with whatever "acrimonies" were believed mixed with it and threatening bodily decay. Water, especially several types of mineral water, fruit juices, and cider were most commonly used.[97]

Another category of diuretics were designated *attenuants,* since they "attenuated" or thinned the blood by chemical means. Physicians prescribed carbonated salts of sodium, antimony, and niter as well as myrrh, licorice, and syrups. The sugar products, including honey, were employed because of the belief that their ingestion promoted a significant amount of urine, as observed in cases of diabetes.[98]

Among the true diuretics ordered by infirmary practitioners were extracts of juniper berries, artichoke juice, garlic, decoctions of burdock and seneka root, squill syrup, guaiac bark, horseradish, and mercurial preparations. The in-house dispensatory registered a number of diuretic boluses, ales, pills, and drafts containing garlic, white soap, juniper, seeds of wild carrots, raisins, and sugar.[99] A new, powerful drug listed among the diuretics was digitalis, introduced in 1785 by a student of Cullen, William Withering.[100] Cullen acknowledged its usefulness in his 1789 *Materia Medica,* writing that "the powers of this plant are now ascertained by numberless experiments."[101] Unfortunately, the actions of this new medicine were poorly understood, and many eighteenth-century physicians hesitated to use it. Cullen, for one, was convinced that digitalis was not even a true diuretic, since it slowed the pulse and sometimes diminished palpitations of the heart.[102]

Diuretics were primarily prescribed in circulatory disorders accompanied by significant fluid collections: pitting edema of the legs, ascites, and generalized swelling or anasarca. In the notebooks students recorded that 25% of the patients labeled by the professors as suffering from these conditions were subjected to treatment with diuretics, with only a third of them getting any results from the drugs. Another high-user group was affected with chest ailments, notably pleural and pericardial effusions. In general, patients treated with diuretics suffered from very serious diseases, experiencing the highest mortality rate (15%) of any group being cared for in the hospital.

Mercurials

Mercury or quicksilver preparations were classified during the eighteenth century as *sialagogues,* medicines promoting the flow of saliva into the mouth. This effect was believed to be the most characteristic sign that the drugs had been absorbed into the organism and were "exerting" their action on various bodily systems. Mercury was for Cullen "one of the most universal stimulants that we know of," inducing the stomach to vomit, purging the intestines, promoting the flow of urine, and inciting perspiration.[103]

In addition to its specific action against the venereal poison, mercury was very popular in the treatment of skin and circulatory disorders and one of the favorite purgatives routinely dispensed to clear the gastrointestinal tract. Practitioners prescribed limewater solutions of corrosive sublimate (mercuric chloride) and ointments containing ammoniated mercuric chloride for herpes and other skin eruptions. So-called mercurial unctions using such an ointment or elemental mercury were primarily applied to the genital lesions of syphilis. Ulcerated buboes received the caustic mercury (mercurous nitrate) or cinnabar, a red precipitate of mercuric oxide, both designed to keep the sores open for a continuous discharge of the presumed venereal poison.[104]

For oral administration physicians relied on a number of mercurial pills containing elementary mercury, mercuric and mercurous chloride, or mercurous acetate. The infirmary usually prepared a large pill or bolus containing five to fifteen grains of calomel. Because of the drug's perceived stimulant powers and gastrointestinal irritation, patients receiving mercurials were placed on a meatless, bland diet supplemented with milk and barley water.[105]

Edinburgh physicians were well aware of the "disagreeable accidents" of mercurial therapy. "To keep the patient upon the verge of a salivation" was Duncan's professed goal in the treatment of venereal complaints.[106] He felt that excessive salivation would discharge the mercury before it had a chance to diffuse into the body's circulating fluids and reach areas tainted by the poison. Especially the mouth could be quickly "offended." The patient first experienced a kind of "copper taste" and foul breath; then the gums turned "spongy" and "teeth began to vacillate in their sockets" as the constitution became "charged" with as little as three grains of calomel or seven grains of crude mercury per day for less than a week.[107]

Such complications occurred in about half of the cases of patients receiving mercurials in the teaching ward, for once making it necessary to pay careful attention to the quantity of drug employed. Because hospital practitioners wanted to correlate dosage with optimal amounts of "active mercury circulating in the system," they monitored all evacuations and even measured the discharge of saliva by boxfuls. Calomel or mercurous chloride was "the preparation in most esteem at Edinburgh," given in small doses for about a month or until all symptoms ascribed to venereal disease vanished. Its purgative effects and lack of disagreeable taste made it even more attractive to physicians who wanted to counteract the otherwise stimulating character of mercurial treatment by keeping the patient's bowels open. The oral route had a decided advantage over the much more cumbersome and painful regimen of mercurial frictions routinely recommended by French practitioners.[108]

At the infirmary practitioners were confident about their ability to control the use of mercury and achieve complete cures in cases of venereal disease, with a minimum of side effects and complications. "I am well persuaded that in most cases, mercury properly employed will prove a very certain and effectual remedy," wrote Cullen, adding, "if practitioners will attend and patients submit to the general rules given, they will seldom fail of obtaining a certain and speedy cure of the disease."[109]

Other classes of drugs

Less frequently dispensed but included in Duncan's and Cullen's classifications were *absorbents* or *antacids* capable of neutralizing stomach acidity and distress. The infirmary recommended chalk, hartshorn, magnesium, carbonate quicklime, and Japonic earth for this purpose. Closely related were the *carminatives,* drugs capable of eliminating gas and curing the bloated feeling of gastrointestinal discomfort. Coriander, dill, sweet fennel, and caraway frequently appeared on prescriptions.[110]

Emmenagogues were medicines with the presumed power to restore menstrual periods. They were supposed to stimulate pelvic circulation and specifically increase the flow through the uterine vessels. Listed in the pharmacopoeias were iron and mercurial preparations, asafetida, tincture of castor, rue, infusion of madder root, mugwort leaves, and decoctions of savin berries.[111]

Emollients or *demulcents* relaxed bodily fibers and were applied locally in the form of gargles, poultices, or plasters. A number of such preparations appeared in the infirmary's dispensatory, including a barley decoction; a plaster made with bread, white soap, and milk; and another containing roasted onions to speed up suppuration of wounds and ulcers.[112] Mentioned in various casebooks were oats and wheat flour, carrots, turnips, and even cabbage leaves, applied to skin eruptions and ulcers and used in fevers.[113]

Antispasmodic drugs possessed the power of suppressing spasms in the involuntary muscular system.[114] These medicines were closely related to the so-called sedatives and were therefore believed to diminish sensibility and excitability in the body. Castor, rue, amber, wild valerian, sagapenum, asafetida, ether, and other volatile alkaline salts were among the most prescribed. The hospital prepared several drafts and boluses for his purpose, also distributing a special antihysteric julep containing tincture of castor, hartshorn, and amber. The use of ether preparations was frequent in hysteria and epilepsy.[115]

A final category worth mentioning is the *errhines,* a class of drugs applied topically inside the nose with the purpose of exciting sneezing and creating a nasal discharge.[116] A remnant of the older depleting strategy of "purging the head" associated with humoral pathology, errhines or sneezing powders made of hazelwort and thyme survived well into the eighteenth century, and even Cullen and Duncan used them in trying to cure headaches,[117] earaches, and eye infections.[118]

Placebos

In its eighteenth-century meaning, a *placebo* was a drug given more to please the patient than to affect the bodily systems. Placebos were frequently used when practitioners were still confused about the true nature of a disease and wanted to gain time, or in hopeless cases where palliation was the sole course of action left. "Where the only intention of prescription is to satisfy a patient," wrote Duncan, "it is easy to order something which, although it may be found in a list of materia medica, does not deserve to be esteemed a medicine."[119] Instead of prescribing inert or ineffective products of the pharmacopoeia, Cullen and James Gregory employed regular drugs as placebos, although at lower doses. Said Cullen: "I make it a rule even in employing placebos to give what would have a tendency to be of use to the patient."[120] All practitioners of course realized that their mere contact with patients could trigger favorable therapeutic results.

Dispensing drugs

Prescriptions ordered by hospital practitioners were not always properly prepared by the hospital apothecary. Occasionally his shop sent out the wrong powder, an insufficient dose, or a drug prescribed for another patient.[121] At the same time, there were occasional problems with administering medicines to the sick because of nurses' neglect or patients' refusal to ingest what everybody agreed were mostly bad-tasting drafts. From a "little grousing" to outright rejection, the clinical histories contain a number of commentaries about how medicines "loaded" or "sat upon" the patients' stomachs.[122] Special problems arose in the case of small children; their mothers were usually employed to coax them to swallow unpalatable compounds.[123]

Finally, female patients frequently refused to take medicines or even be bled if their menstrual periods began in the hospital. While Cullen and other physicians ascribed this behavior to "popular prejudice" and complained that "we pay more regard to their presence [meaning the menses] than is necessary," they nevertheless seemed to have respected it, admitting that "we must comply in some measure with their opinion." In fact, by agreeing that the menstrual flow occurred under conditions of increased systemic irritability, practitioners established their own rationale concerning the harmfulness of drug usage during menstruation.[124]

PHYSICAL METHODS

In conjunction with the administration of drugs, infirmary patients were subjected to a variety of physical procedures designed to support the basic sedative or stimulating character of each therapeutic regimen. For these purposes the hospital possessed baths, an electrical machine, and devices for exercise. Availability of surgical personnel ensured the performance of bleedings and blistering. Nurses aided with fomentations, frictions, sponging, and bathing.

An analysis of the student casebooks (Table 4.4) reveals a number of practices prescribed by university professors in the teaching ward.

Bloodletting

The withdrawal of blood from the sick was the most frequent physical method of therapy employed in patients hospitalized in the teaching ward. Traditionally considered the mainstay of the medical regimen, bloodletting had a long history in Western therapeutics that could be traced at least to ancient Greece. Over the centuries it retained its prominence within the framework of humoral pathology.[125] The traditional explanation given for the removal of blood was correction of humoral excesses of "plethora" causing harmful congestion, especially in inflammatory conditions.

Under the influence of new mechanical and neuropathological theories, physicians during the late eighteenth century explained bloodletting as a key

Table 4.4. *Physical methods used at the infirmary,*
1771–1799 (N = 808)

	Frequency	%
Bloodletting (303 cases, 25% of total)		
Venesection	172	14.20
Leeches	85	7.00
Cupping	46	3.70
Blistering	285	23.50
Issue	11	0.90
Seton	7	0.50
Head shaving	25	2.00
Bathing (138 cases, 11.3% of total)		
Cold bath	26	2.10
Warm bath	65	5.30
Half bath	3	0.20
Sitz bath	2	0.10
Foot bath	30	1.00
Vapor bath	12	1.00
Fomentation	201	16.50
Friction	81	6.60
Sweat box	2	0.10
Poultices and plasters	60	4.90
Electricity	62	5.10
Abdominal paracentesis	5	0.40
Foot puncture	1	0.08
Eye scarification	18	1.40
Arterial compression	1	0.08
Catheterization	11	0.90
Total	1,211	

measure designed to lessen the tension and spasms prevailing in the human organism. "Nothing is more evident," wrote Cullen, "than that bloodletting is one of the most powerful means of diminishing the activity of the whole body, especially of the sanguiferous system."[126]

Such a view of bloodletting as an antiphlogistic remedy was based, to a great extent, on careful clinical observations. Indeed, sudden removal of four to eight ounces of blood temporarily improved several cardinal symptoms evident in fevers. The pulse rate fell, body temperature declined, pain sensations lessened, and the usual skin congestion disappeared. Following bleeding, a feeling of relaxation and faintness took over, often followed by slumber and sweating. Such physiological responses, albeit temporary, were impressive enough to make bloodletting the principal measure in all ailments considered to be inflammatory. For practitioners the effects of bleeding simulated the usual spontaneous recovery phase observed in fevers and held the promise of accomplishing a permanent recuperation. If the response to bloodletting coincided with a spontaneous improvement of the patient, the method was nevertheless credited with the cure; if the benefit was only short-lived or failed to materialize, practitioners reasoned that perhaps further withdrawals were in order.

In general, eighteenth-century practitioners resisted suggestions that bloodletting could be harmful, especially if small amounts were withdrawn. They were impressed by the swiftness of the circulatory changes and unable to obtain similar prompt effects from their arsenal of drugs. Yet caution was in order. Excessive bleeding was debilitating and not only delayed convalescence but could also predispose patients to new diseases. "The weakly state that we leave convalescents in consequence of large venesections makes them more liable to be affected by cold," warned Cullen in 1772.[127]

To make matters worse, bloodletting was poorly tolerated by most paents admitted to the Edinburgh infirmary with a diagnosis of typhus fever. Most of them were already malnourished and feeble, products of an urban society in which physical vigor was rapidly sapped by long fasting and hard labor.[128] In such circumstances physicians were in a real quandary, tempted to act quickly to remove symptoms suggestive of an inflammatory state but aware that the original debility would be exacerbated. At best, bleeding promised a protracted period of recovery while threatening to precipitate a fatal crisis. "I have sometimes been led to employ it from the apparent urgency of those symptoms but had often occasion to regret it afterwards," admitted James Gregory.[129] Gregory especially favored a proscription of bloodletting in typhus fever, seeing this step as a "complete revolution" in the traditional treatment of fevers.

Physicians and surgeons used several traditional methods of withdrawing blood. One of the most popular was venesection or phlebotomy, guaranteed to produce quick and general effects by opening a superficial vein in the neck, arm, hand, leg, or foot.[130] A less common procedure – arteriotomy – was to puncture an artery, perhaps the temporal arteries at the level of the temples or the digital arteries running at the sides of fingers. If local bleeding was preferred, scarifications were made by a lancet or scarificator instrument and small amounts of blood obtained through the use of suction cups. Similar results could be achieved through the topical application of leeches, which bit through the skin and ingested a small amount of blood.

Venesection

The actual execution of prescribed venesections was left in the hands of surgeons attending the infirmary, who in turn delegated such chores to their clerks and dressers, prompting Benjamin Bell to observe, "I have seldom seen bloodletting with the lancet correctly done."[131] Preferred sites for obtaining blood were the superficial veins at the elbow, but failing to obtain it there, the operators went to vessels located in the back of the hand, legs, or feet. In the case of severe headaches, eye infections, or even epileptic fits, phlebotomy was carried out closer to the presumed sites of trouble: the jugular veins in the neck.[132] Large bleedings were carried out "after the patient is laid in bed."[133]

With optimal lighting – day- or candlelight – the operator seated himself next to the patient and placed a moderately tight ligature around the arm or leg above the area to be lanced. Once the veins were properly swollen and visible, the surgeon employed a lancet or small knife to make an incision in the skin and the vein located immediately below. Most lancets possessed a spring mechanism that allowed the blade to hit the predetermined area with considerable force, but there was danger of injuring or completely perforating the vessel with this device.

Plunging the spear-pointed knife into a vein through an oblique incision created an orifice of about an eighth of an inch, generally sufficient to allow the flow of blood to gush out because of the ligature. Yet operators often "failed in the blooding," either because a viable vein could not be found or because the flow stopped as the patient fainted. "Our operator could not find a vein in her arm," complained Cullen, who persuaded the surgeon to search for other vessels in the hand.[134] These sites, however, usually yielded considerably smaller amounts of blood and thus forced the clerks to repeat the procedure.[135]

When blood flowed very slowly out of the incision or stopped altogether, physicians became worried because the dribble suggested systemic debility in which bloodletting was usually harmful.[136] One of the adverse effects of bloodletting was fainting, the most common effect for patients who did not "bear the bleeding well." Some of them became pale and threatened to black out at the first sight of blood, whereas others did so after various encounters with the lancet.[137] Fresh air, wine, and rest were employed to overcome the sensations. Posture was an obvious factor. Before two ounces had been taken away one patient fainted "from her being raised up," related Cullen about a case of inflammatory fever.[138] In a few cases the sight of blood flowing down the arm even triggered hysterical fits.[139]

After the prescribed amount of blood had been evacuated, operators released the ligature and manually compressed the site of incision until no further discharges occurred. The wound was washed and an adhesive plaster bandage applied in hopes that the cut would heal without infection.[140] Some patients experienced further blood loss because the edges of the wound had not been properly lined up.[141] Repeated venesections were not uncommon. They were monitored through pulse frequency: A faster pulse usually suggested further bleeding.

At the infirmary the venous blood was successively collected into three tin platters and allowed to clot. These filled bowls were kept in the wards until the next day for inspection by the attending physicians, although there were instances in which careless nurses just threw the contents out before the visit.[142] This traditional method of collection was designed to detect the presence of "sizy" blood, usually more noticeable in the second and third platter. The term described the semisolid or jellylike surface of clotted blood deposited in the container, approaching the consistency of size. If conspicuous, such a layer was also called a "buffy coat" because of its light buff or yellowish color and greater density. It usually covered the compact parts of the clot, called the *crassamentum,* formed by red globules. In most cases, the first blood samples generally coagulated quickly, leaving behind a firm clot, but if the withdrawal of blood continued, there was a greater proportion of serum and thus an increase in the yellow crust.[143]

In humoral pathology increased "siziness" of the blood was equated with systemic inflammation. Physicians believed that the buffy substance was an undesirable product of faulty bodily processes and directly responsible for the febrile symptoms. Its discovery in bleeding bowls generally confirmed the clinical suspicions and furnished a persuasive evidence for removing more blood believed tainted with noxious substances. Eighteenth-century practitioners retained faith in such relationships between inflammation and blood siziness, although all blood and circulatory disorders associated with an inflamed state were ostensibly subsumed under Cullen's neurophysiological mechanisms. Other causes believed to cause sizy blood were indigestion, excessive intake of strong liquors, too much meat in the diet, inactivity, and plethora.[144]

Contemporary physicians and surgeons were aware that blood rapidly coagulated in the platters if it only trickled down the arm or if the room in which the procedure was carried out remained warm. Colder air in well-ventilated wards affected the separation of serum and red globules, with changes in the consistency of the buffy coat.[145] Pewter receptacles were said to delay the separation. Finally, repeated or larger bleedings apparently increased the amount of serum while changing the usual "florid" color of the clot to the point at which blood could "issue almost white from a vein."[146]

In response to a 1772 query, "Is the sizy covering which is often seen upon the blood of any use in directing the method of cure?" William Heberden responded in the negative.[147] Gradually other medical authorities also expressed reservations, since the behavior of extravasated blood was indeed dependent on factors that were not operative within the living body. "I seldom can venture upon a conclusion," responded William Cullen, who ascribed the absence of a buffy coat to changes in body gluten, a substance included in blood serum.[148] The result was that practitioners increasingly made their decisions about bloodletting regardless of appearances in the collecting platters.[149]

Table 4.5. *Venesections at the infirmary, 1771–1779*

Casebook	No. of cases bled	Cases bled as a % of all cases recorded	Average amount bled (oz.)[a]
John Gregory, 1771–1772	20	40	11.8
William Cullen, 1772–1773	28	53	14.8
William Cullen, 1773–1774	12	36	15.4
James Gregory, 1779–1780	12	14	9.8
Francis Home, 1780–1781	23	41	14.1
John Hope, 1781	10	30	13.5
James Gregory, 1781–1782	16	15	15.2
James Gregory, 1785–1786	7	12	22.0
Francis Home, 1786–1787	14	26	15.3
Andrew Duncan, 1795	2	3	18.0
James Gregory, 1795–1796	11	17	25.8
Thomas C. Hope, 1796–1797	6	9	14.3
Daniel Rutherford, 1799	6	6	10.6
	Total: 167	Ave.: 23.2	Ave.: 15.4

[a]These measures are probably actual weights, rather than fluid measures.

According to student casebooks, professors in charge of the teaching ward, especially Francis Home and James Gregory, bled more female than male patients. One in every five people suffering from respiratory diseases was subjected to at least one phlebotomy while in the house, with cases of rheumatism and amenorrhea the next most frequent indications for bleeding. From the available information, more than half of Cullen's fever cases between 1771 and 1773 were bled (about 15 ounces each); the highest average amount of blood withdrawn belonged to persons hospitalized under the care of James Gregory in 1795–1796 (25.8 ounces) and 1785–1786 (22 ounces). In one case diagnosed as pneumonia in 1795, Gregory extracted a total of 68 ounces of blood over a period of five days, the greatest in the entire sample. Another of his female patients, affected with chronic rheumatism, lost 62 ounces in the same amount of time. Less aggressive venesections were ordered by Daniel Rutherford in 1799 (an average of 10 ounces) and Thomas C. Hope in 1796–1797 (an average of 14 ounces) (see Table 4.5).

All practitioners reported excellent results with venesection in at least half of their cases and were certainly convinced of its utility. Lay persons agreed with the professionals and were sometimes "desirous to be bled" after admission.[150] In the eighteenth century bloodletting was still a lingering folk practice in Scotland, both as a prophylactic cleansing rite in the spring and as a curative measure in fevers, and several patients had blood removed before seeking admission to the Edinburgh infirmary. "When a person feels sick," wrote John Sinclair, "he first bleeds and then consults his physician."[151]

Given the frequency of bloodletting, complications following the performance of venesection were common enough to demand a flawless technique and cautious follow-up.[152] Puncture of nerves in the arm and injury to the biceps tendon were not uncommon.[153] Another serious but rare problem was the puncture of an artery, resulting in arteriovenous fistulas or aneurysms.[154] Because of dirty lancets, a patient frequently experienced a local infection at the site of the phlebotomy, which in some instances developed into an abscess.[155] A more serious and potentially lethal complication was thrombophlebitis, still imperfectly understood in the late eighteenth century. John Hunter described one such inflammation, usually discovered at postmortem examinations in the form of intravascular clots and a string of abscesses following the course of the vein upward.[156] One patient under the care of William Brown, surgeon to the infirmary, died suddenly two weeks following a venesection in the elbow in 1803. The autopsy disclosed a local abscess near the original orifice followed by extensive suppuration around the vein and numerous blood clots reaching at least to the axilla, indications that death may have been due to a massive pulmonary embolism.[157]

Leeches

A popular procedure for removing blood locally was the application of leeches, small aquatic worms capable of biting through the skin and sucking blood into their stomachs. These creatures – the species commonly used in Edinburgh was *Hirudo medicinalis,* the Swedish leech easily found in northern European streams – were employed in domestic and professional medicine for centuries as an adjunct to or substitute for phlebotomy.[158] Usually each worm was capable of absorbing about one ounce of blood, but the effects of its bite – it injected an anticoagulant substance into the skin – prolonged the bleeding after the parasite had completed its feeding and dropped off.

The usual procedure was to collect the leeches in bottles containing water, adding a little sugar to keep them alive but hungry for a blood meal. To apply the leeches the operator transferred them from the original jar to a small empty glass that was placed upside down over the selected site. This area was previously wetted with warm water to cause more local congestion and frequently sprinkled with milk or syrup drops to lure the leeches.

Edinburgh physicians ordered leeches primarily in venereal diseases (15% of the cases) and musculoskeletal disorders (11%), especially acute and chronic rheumatism, to treat local pain, buboes, and inflammation. Four to eight, and sometimes even twelve, animals "fixed" themselves onto the skin over wrists and ankles.[159] Severe headaches in fevers prompted their application to both temples. Another popular indication was ophthalmia or inflammation of the eye, when leeches were placed around the eye or on the eyelids.[160]

After the leeches completed their meal and dropped off, the bleeding usually continued for a number of hours, deliberately aided by the application of a warm cloth previously dipped in hot water. This method usually yielded another two to three ounces of blood per leech, but on occasion the oozing became uncontrollable and had to be finally stopped with styptic powders or pressure bandages.[161] Considering these complications and periodic shortages of leeches during the winter months, their use at the Edinburgh infirmary remained restricted. A few decades later, European practitioners would employ more than 250 leeches in relays of 50 or 60 at any one time for several days as their only bloodletting method. The procedure had advantages over cupping because of the leeches' capacity to attach themselves to bodily cavities such as the mouth, anus, urethra, and vagina. Just as in cupping, however, leeching produced secondary skin infections at the site of the bites, which occasionally evolved into dangerous abscesses.

Cupping

The application of cupping glasses was closely related to the use of leeches and constituted another form of local bloodletting. Also a treatment of great antiquity, cupping meant attaching certain vessels, from horns to glass cups, to the skin, where they remained because of the partial vacuum produced inside them. The purpose was to draw blood containing "morbid" matter toward selected places of the skin for removal away from vital organs. At times the withdrawal was intended to diminish local pain, congestion, and infection.[162]

For centuries, practitioners used a method of "dry" cupping in which the glasses were simply fastened to certain areas of the body until local redness and pain appeared. All cases at the Edinburgh infirmary, however, were subjected to a "wet" cupping procedure. The sites selected for this operation were previously scarified with a lancet or mechanical device activated by a spring. On applying the cups, these areas "brought off" a variable amount of blood, depending on the number of incisions, their depth, and the degree of vacuum present in the vessel. In most instances practitioners were able to collect between two and four ounces of blood in each cup.[163]

The clinical data supplied in the casebooks reveal that cupping was not frequently employed at the infirmary's teaching ward during the last decades of the eighteenth century. "I have not been able to obtain the execution of it properly," admitted Cullen, presumably owing to deficiencies in the action of the small airpumps that replaced the older method of putting small platforms with lighted candles over the scarifications to create the necessary vacuum in the cups.[164] In many cases of recurrent headaches and delirium, cups were placed on both temples.[165] People suffering from depression or respiratory ailments also received them, with these two groups accounting for more than half of all the cuppings performed in the ward.

Blisters, issues, and setons

The traditional practice of selectively producing running sores on several areas of the body was also originally explained within the tenets of humoralism. The sores supposedly removed harmful substances considered responsible for disease, especially fevers. In the second half of the eighteenth century, although the practice persisted, its rationale had changed. As with other therapies, neurophysiological concepts provided an updated explanation for the traditional curing efforts. Thus, for most Edinburgh physicians, the reason for creating a blister was to stimulate the bodily system.[166]

To establish a blister, hospital practitioners applied to the skin an adhesive plaster or dressing with sticky edges covered with very irritating substances called *vesicants* or *caustics*. The most commonly employed product was an ointment or powder made of Spanish flies or *cantharides,* a type of Mediterranean beetle in use since Roman times.[167] Other drugs with similar action were mustard, onion, and leek. Blister dressings ware generally placed on the shaved crown of the head, on the nape of the neck, between the shoulder blades, on the sternum, and on the back, after the skin had been cleansed with a vinegar solution. The selected site usually "answered" within twelve to twenty-four hours by "rising" and forming a vesicle that was then pierced without removing its cuticle. This opening allowed the discharge of a clear fluid, and the blister was accordingly "dressed" every day with new bandages.

Blisters ordinarily dried up within two or three days unless practitioners reapplied irritating plasters to promote more discharge. Such successive administrations were part of an elaborate "blistering schedule" popularized by Boerhaave earlier in the eighteenth century. In Edinburgh, Cullen and others promoted the continuous application of mustard flour, garlic, and sulphuric acid to prolong the irritating effects for a week or longer.[168]

To obtain more drainage, many blisters were eventually converted into *issues,* larger sores kept open by placement of a foreign object like a pea or kidney bean or a caustic paste. Finally, hospital surgeons were occasionally called on to transform the blister into a *seton* by piercing the skin adjacent to the sore and placing cords of silk or cotton into the wound to stimulate more drainage. Like blisters, issues or setons were also "dressed" daily, with new bandages replacing the soiled ones that covered the lesions.[169]

According to Cullen's student Thomas Fowler, "Blistering plasters certainly constitute one of the most efficacious remedies we have to boast in the practice of physic."[170] In the course of treatment almost one out of every four patients admitted to the teaching ward received a blister. The highest percentage was among people suffering from respiratory problems (39%), since in catarrhs and so-called pectoral complaints blisters were said to alleviate pain and cough while promoting expectoration.[171]

Moreover, infirmary physicians also used blisters in intractable cases of chronic rheumatism and paralysis (25%), hoping to improve the symptoms. Another major indication for blistering was fever, especially of the typhus variety, where strong stimulation was recommended. The serous discharge was expected to remove corrupted matter from the body.[172]

Because of pain and the danger of secondary infection, most patients seem to have dreaded blisters and issues, often refusing them outright and at times pretending that the symptoms prompting physicians to order such measures had suddenly vanished. Excessive or repeated use of cantharides powder produced severe bladder irritation with painful micturation and even blood in the urine. As previously described, Cullen used the threat of applying blisters effectively to rid himself of unwanted hospital patients feigning illness. If they were ambulatory, patients confronting a prolonged blistering schedule simply packed their belongings and left the infirmary.[173]

Bathing

The student casebooks reveal that more than 10% of the patients hospitalized in the teaching ward received a bath as part of their treatment. After 1770 at the latest, the Edinburgh infirmary had in use a set of cold and hot baths for patients only, located on the ground floor and completely separated from the luxurious public bagnio.[174] Toward the end of the century, the growing demands for clean laundry unfortunately displaced the patients from these facilities, and they were forced to bathe in portable barrels and tubs placed in the wards.

To reach the baths, patients wrapped themselves in their blankets and used the drafty central stairway to the lower floor. For this and other reasons, physicians preferred to order a half bath or *semicupium*, in which the person was submerged up to the navel in a vat, or simpler yet, a footbath or *pediluvium* requiring a minimum of staff assistance. In both instances practitioners hoped that the beneficial effects of warm water would be propagated to the rest of the body.[175]

A warm bath lasting between fifteen and twenty minutes was believed to have relaxing effects in a variety of spasmodic affections, including chronic rheumatism and postparalytic muscular contractions. At the same time, baths were said to exert a tonic effect on the nervous system because of the stimulation of peripheral blood vessels. For that reason hospital physicians ordered immersion baths in intermittent fevers to prevent paroxysms, or in convalescent cases of typhus fever to restore bodily strength.[176] For similar conditions of debility or hysteric fits, a complete or partial bath such as a sitz bath or *cluniluvium* was recommended. Menstrual suppression and hemorrhoidal inflammation also prompted orders for hot sitz baths, designed to enhance pelvic congestion and, it was hoped, promote the discharge of blood.[177]

Because of their alleged power to attract internal acrimonies to the skin and thus facilitate their eventual discharge, warm baths were also frequently prescribed in the treatment of skin diseases, including the latter stages of smallpox, when there was a need to remove the scabs. More than a third of all those patients in the teaching ward who were suffering from skin disorders and venereal diseases with cutaneous manifestations received some form of warm bath during the course of their hospitalization.[178]

Physicians tried to stimulate sweating by ordering their patients, after warm baths, to wear flannel shirts and cover themselves with extra blankets. Others had their legs placed in so-called sweat boxes, small heated cases, for several hours or their feet kept warm with boiled bricks or hot water bottles.[179] Cullen and other medical authorities were impressed with the usefulness of vapor baths, which could deliver a greater amount of heat and "continuously support pretty constant sweat." Cullen believed that warmth and moisture were the only effective ingredients in the famous mineral baths of Europe, "not the particular impregnations which carry people a thousand miles to obtain it."[180]

More limited steam applications were employed when patients had difficulties with expectoration. Some patients were obliged to breathe through the spout of a funnel that covered a bowl of boiling water. Later in the century James Gregory used a "vaporizing machine" for the treatment of pneumonia and typhus fever.[181]

"Cold applied to the body can be astringent, strengthening and stimulant," taught Cullen, although the initial effect was mostly sedative and designed to ameliorate the inflammatory symptoms in fevers.[182] In cases of typhus fever and especially if delirium was present, physicians ordered sponges of cold water placed on the head and trunk of the patient. At other times hospital practitioners favored "cold air baths," exposing the partly clad bodies of their patients to cold air.[183]

Fomentations and frictions

Given the inconveniences of carrying large quantities of water to the wards and keeping it properly heated, hospital patients usually received a substitute for a warm bath: fomentations, carried out for about half an hour by nurses or convalescent patients. Two flannel cloths dipped in hot water were alternatively placed on the skin and left there until the warming effect wore off. The water temperature was about 100°F, and the entire operation was repeated two or three times daily, especially at bedtime.[184]

One of the major indications for fomentations was fever, especially typhus, when patients were restless, delirious, or experiencing chills. In the teaching ward nearly 20% of all such cases received fomentations. Edinburgh physicians claimed that the procedure had a relaxing and soothing effect, and clinical reports contained a number of entries claiming that the patient in question "was laid asleep by the fomentations." Cullen explained the success of fomentations by claiming a "sympathy" between the skin and the rest of the organism.[185] Fomentations were employed in circulatory disorders, namely, anasarca, ascites, and edema of the legs. One out of every four patients affected with these diseases was fomented, many of them repeatedly, in the hope that their swellings would decrease. Fomentations were also applied in cases of chronic rheumatism and paralysis, using either hot water or, as *embrocations,* volatile ingredients such as camphorated oil specifically directed to the affected joints. Decoctions of chamomile flowers were employed in the fomentation of bruises and ulcers.[186]

Closely related were a number of rubbing activities designed to relax or stimulate specific areas of the body. Gentle massage "with a warm hand," employing camphorated oil, created "moderate and frequently repeated oscillations in the whole of the fibres," helping to overcome muscular contractures and painful joints in chronic rheumatism. When ordered by physicians, the "grateful warmth" was repeated daily for a week to ten days.[187]

In recalcitrant cases more stimulating frictions were attempted, using rough clothes, woolen gloves, or pieces of flannel impregnated with benzoin or turpentine.[188] They were designed to promote perspiration and, it was hoped, to lead to a termination of bothersome symptoms.

Cullen believed that a flesh brush was more convenient than flannel cloth in achieving proper tissue oscillations, though he objected that contemporary manufacturers had made brushes too stiff and hard. In cases of hemiplegia he ordered the paralyzed side rubbed with a brush for about half an hour every morning.[189] Although the effects were sometimes encouraging, Cullen admitted that it was inconvenient to demand the procedure from unskilled nurses, particularly in the teaching ward, where rapid patient turnover was essential for the fulfillment of educational objectives.[190]

Electricity

Soon after the principles of electricity became sufficiently known in the early eighteenth century, experimenters directed their attention to possible medical applications. The first physician to deal specifically with electricity was Johann G. Krueger (1715–1759), professor of medicine at the University of Halle and successor to Friedrich Hoffmann. In a series of lectures delivered in 1743 Krueger expressed his conviction that electricity was a new and promising form of therapy, especially useful in restoring motion to paralyzed limbs. Krueger and his student Christian G. Kratzenstein set out to collect further clinical data; Kratzenstein experimented with electricity on himself, studying its effects on pulse rate, circulation, and perspiration.[191]

Kratzenstein's essays, first published in 1744, went through additional editions in 1745 and 1746 and helped to generate considerable interest in the subject among German physicians. Unfortunately, these writings conveyed an uncritical picture of the favorable effects observed in all electrical treatments, summarized by Kratzenstein's dictum, "I do not exaggerate when I introduce electrification as a panacea."[192]

French authors, notably the physicist Abbé Nollet, pursued medical uses of electricity further by installing in 1746 an electric machine in the Hôtel des Invalides in Paris, a famous military hospital. The results subsequently obtained with paralytic patients were ambiguous, but success reported in 1748 by a colleague of Nollet's, Jean L. Jallabert, professor of physics at the University of Geneva, vindicated the Parisian studies. Further clinical trials at Montpellier, under the direction of the professor of medicine, François B. de Sauvages, seemed promising. His student, Jean E. Deshais, even attempted in his 1749 dissertation to explain the effects of electricity in the body by postulating that it increased pressure of the nervous fluid and therefore could overcome a series of obstructions responsible for paralysis.[193] sis.[193]

On the Continent the fortunes of medical electricity suffered a severe blow because of the activities of several quacks in Venice and Turin who used medicated electrical globes and tubes. Physicians, however, continued to conduct clinical experiments designed to ascertain the proper indications for this therapy and the best methods of applying the electrical fluid. Publication of Anton de Haen's *Ratio Medendi* in 1758 revealed that the Austrian physician had extensively employed electricity in cases of partial paralysis and St. Vitus' dance. In the same year Benjamin Franklin, in a letter to John Pringle, communicated his experiences with electricity in the treatment of amenorrhea.[194]

These reports and others from France persuaded some members of the medical profession to drop their reservations about the use of electricity, and the publication in 1759 of John Wesley's *Desideratum, or Electricity Made Plain and Useful,* led to its widespread popular use by laypersons. In a few years the work of the founder of Methodism went through several editions and spurred the design of numerous portable electrical machines, as well as the emergence of "medical electricians" who administered such treatments in London and several provincial towns.[195] Yet in spite of several valuable publications by medical authorities in Britain and abroad, the use of electricity retained a certain aura of quackery among many respectable professional healers. William Cullen, for example, stated that "in this country it is very doubtfully spoken of."[196]

Scotland, despite Cullen's disclaimer, proved to be quite receptive to the potential benefits of electricity. According to the records, the Edinburgh infirmary received its first electrical apparatus from John Rutherford, professor of the practice of medicine at the university, in April 1750. The static electrical machine was placed in a corner of the consulting room, and the surgical clerk was entrusted with the treatments. From the early regulations it appears that electricity was not only administered to inpatients but on occasion applied to persons sent expressly for this purpose to the hospital.[197] This installation preceded by almost two decades the reported placement of a similar machine at the Middlesex Hospital in London.

As early as 1757, a case was communicated to Edinburgh physicians and read at a meeting of the Philosophical Society of Edinburgh. It dealt with the cure of a paralysis through the employment of sparks from an electrical machine.[198] A set of examples selected from the practice of James Saunders, a physician in Banff, was discussed by William Cullen at another meeting of the same society, presumably during the 1760s. Saunders exchanged clinical information with Andrew St. Clair, professor of medical theory, about the latter's experience in the infirmary and published his own cases gathered from private practice between 1752 and 1761 in Andrew Duncan, Sr.'s, *Medical and Philosophical Commentaries* for the year 1774.[199]

In Cullen's neurophysiological framework, electricity was considered to be a powerful stimulus capable of exciting the nervous power inherent in muscular fibers. Such tonic qualities were revealed through the increased circulation, pulse frequency, and perspiration that followed even the most mild electrification. While temporary, the stimulation was believed to dissipate localized pain and restore a measure of flexibility to contracted muscles and rigid joints. Obvious warmth and exhilaration following certain electrical treatments were interpreted as corrections of general debility, which was often blamed for hysteria and menstrual suppressions.[200] In spite of certain reservations and an awareness that the effects were usually transient, Edinburgh professors continued to order electrical treatments for their infirmary patients. In 1771 a petition by William Cullen in the name of both ordinary and university physicians requested the purchase of an additional "small electrical apparatus which could be carried to a patient's bedside." As the necessary funds seem to have been available, the device was probably procured.[201] Reports about the Edinburgh infirmary submitted to a German medical journal in 1781 indicated that the hospital had put aside a room to house its electrical machine; at specially scheduled hours the surgical clerk carried out the various treatments prescribed by physicians.[202]

In those years three principal methods of supplying static electricity were in vogue. The first, *simple electrification,* also termed *positive* or *negative bath,* allowed the patient to sit on an insulated stool or chair and be connected to the positive or negative terminal of the machine while it was being activated. The small amount of electricity thus perfusing the body created an agreeable sensation of warmth and animation, revealed by faster pulse and increase in perspiration. According to Tiberius Cavallo, a contemporary Italian authority on medical electricity, the degree of electrification was to be regulated by how the patient reacted to treatment.[203] These "baths" generally lasted for about half an hour and were repeated once or twice a day for several days to remove weakness, improve appetite, or decrease swelling in cases of dropsy.

The second method of "drawing sparks" from the patient was through contact with the electrified patient using wooden or metal points attached to chain conductors. The conductor touched bare skin, interposed pieces of tinfoil, or simply the patient's clothing. A popular version, "sparks drawn across the flannel," lasted between ten and fifteen minutes and again was performed once or twice daily. Unlike the "baths," these treatments could be directed to specific areas of the body, such as nerves, muscles, and joints. In cases of amenorrhea, "gentle" sparks were administered to the pelvic area for two to three minutes, generally through clothing to avoid "shocking the delicacy of tender females."[204] In intermittent fevers treatments were administered before onset of the next fit in hopes that sweating would abort the ensuing paroxysm.[205]

Finally, physicians ordered the "electric fluid thrown" in the form of strong shocks through contact with electrodes connected to a Leyden jar that had stored sufficient electricity. Again the electrodes had wooden or metal points allowing delivery to selected parts of the body. If intense, shocks could be quite painful, especially when the jolts were applied with the help of metal surfaces and from large jars. By the 1780s such treatments had largely fallen into disuse, not only because they terrified the patients but also because the sparks could prove fatal if applied to the head in cases of suspected stroke or the chest in agues.[206] "I have seen instances where upon the application of it in such cases, the patients were as certainly killed as if a bullet had been shot through the heart," commented Cullen in 1772.[207]

Toward the end of the eighteenth century most electrical shocks administered to patients were of moderate intensity, the sparks measuring between a tenth and a twentieth of an inch and discharged from a one-gallon Leyden jar only about half charged. Ten to fifteen separate shocks were usually administered to the patient within a period of two to five minutes, the sessions perhaps repeated daily for about a week. Most conditions originally slated for treatment with electrical sparks also qualified for shock therapy if advanced, chronic, and unresponsive to other treatments. In cases of amenorrhea, the shocks sent through the pelvis usually caused a considerable vaginal discharge.

Orders for electrical treatment appeared from time to time in the student casebooks, but their overall frequency remained low: 5% of all cases receiving some form of physical treatment and 7% of patients admitted to the teaching ward. Not surprisingly, the largest contingent of infirmary inmates electrified by orders of the attending professors suffered from either paralysis of their limbs or the effects of rheumatism, especially in its chronic form. In such instances repeated sparks were drawn or more intense shocks administered in the hope that some form of motion could be restored. In those persons believed to be hysteric, the sparks were actually drawn from the throat to remove the sensation of globus. One blind person labeled as suffering from amaurosis told her physicians that "she thought she saw sparks passing before her while she was electrified."[208] In retrospect, it seems that the infirmary physicians took advantage of the electrical technology available to them but remained selective in its use, seeing it principally as a supplement to other forms of treatment.

Paracentesis and other punctures

In cases of ascites when patients had large accumulations of fluids in their bellies, orders for paracenteses or abdominal evacuations were issued by infirmary physicians. Armed with a lancet, the surgeon made a small skin incision, preferably near the navel, and then pushed a trocar through the underlying tissues until it pierced the peritoneal membrane and reached the fluid. The operation was fraught with considerable danger since the unguided instrument penetrated into a vastly distended cavity and could perforate the intestines or spleen.[209]

The fluid was drawn off through a canula while the surgeon carefully monitored the removal to avoid syncope or sections of bowel drawn into the orifice. After the spontaneous discharge had ended, the operator used his hands, rollers, or a waistcoat to extract additional amounts. Among patients subjected to this procedure at the infirmary, withdrawals of 150–480 ounces were not uncommon.[210] Most candidates were apparently afraid of this measure and had to be strongly persuaded to submit to it. Complications were frequent, especially infection around the incision and, always fatal, peritonitis or inflammation of the intra-abdominal lining following the insertion of presumably unclean instruments.[211]

Physicians were also interested in reducing localized swellings, especially in the legs when edema became very pronounced and threatened to burst the skin, through multiple punctures. Similar scarifications were recommended in scrotal swellings. "Two punctures to be made in feet with the point of a lancet," read one of the prescriptions; another ordered surgeons to "make two punctures on the inside of each thigh, a little above the knee."[212] Cullen was reluctant to order such scarifications because of his fear of secondary infection, possibly progressing to gangrene and death. Such a complication seemed a high price to pay for "removing a present uneasiness without touching the cause of the disease." Instead, he paradoxically recommended larger and deeper gashes in the limbs, which would "draw off water with less danger."[213]

Eye scarifications

In severe cases of ophthalmia, hospital physicians not only prescribed local bloodletting in the form of leeches and wet cupping but also called in the surgeons to scarify the inflamed vessels of the cornea and conjunctiva. To avoid injuring the eyelids, Benjamin Bell even designed a special knife. With two assistants, one standing behind to support the head of the patient and the other at the side holding the hands and body, the surgeon would sit and face the patient. Exposing the eyeball as much as possible, the surgeon would cut into all visible engorged vessels.[214] To promote an increased flow of blood, the eye was subsequently washed with warm water or milk using an eyecup, and the procedure repeated "as may seem proper and admissible."[215]

Infirmary practitioners seemed pleased with the effects of such scarifications, Bell even writing that a "plentiful discharge gives more relief in the pain arising from ophthalmia than any other remedy we employ."[216] The procedure, however, was by no means popular among patients. In half of the cases recorded in notebooks, there are entries stating that those scheduled to undergo the procedure simply refused to submit to it.[217]

Miscellaneous procedures

The following procedures were all carried out by the attending surgeons or their clerks, called in consultation by medical professors running the teaching ward. Such referrals were common and covered a broad range of conditions from suspected abscesses, spoiled teeth, and hernias to a variety of ulcers including gangrenous bedsores and bladder stones. To ensure better care, many of these patients were directly transferred to the surgical ward.[218]

In two cases of amenorrhea infirmary physicians sought to create greater pelvic congestion by the use of arterial pressure. Using a tourniquet, the surgeons compressed both femoral arteries for a period of forty minutes without much success but with substantial side effects in the form of impaired leg circulation and abdominal pain. A similar procedure was employed by Cullen on a patient suffering from epilepsy who reported tingling sensations in one arm before his fits. With each aura, Cullen had a ligature applied around the arm in an effort to block these sensations from reaching the head and thus to prevent a full seizure.[219]

Catheters were employed in acute cases of "suppressed urine." Surgeons were summoned to insert a hard instrument made of silver before the bladder could burst. The most common condition requiring catheterization was obstruction at the neck of the bladder. Surgeons were reluctant to leave catheters in place for any prolonged period of time, presumably because they feared urinary tract infections. If the problem persisted, tubes made of resin were selected and kept in the bladder for one or two weeks.[220] Ordinarily, however, physicians ordered repeated insertions of the hard catheter – at least every twelve hours – in cases where the patient had a chronically distended bladder and diminished sensitivity about its fullness. The insertion was accompanied by a "pretty strong push" of the lower abdomen to empty the contents of the bladder.[221]

Practitioners also ordered special bandages in a variety of ailments. The casebooks recorded the use of tight bindings around the waist and lower chest for cases of hydrothorax with considerable pain in the side.[222] Flannel bandages to encircle the abdomen in ascites and suspensory ones in testicular swellings were common.[223] Lastly, the clinical histories recorded the case of a delirious female suffering from typhus who had to be restrained "by means of a strict waistcoat."[224]

EXERCISE

Physical exercise was an important companion of many prescribed cures. Whereas the initial antiphlogistic approach in fevers demanded strict bed rest and minimal physical as well as mental exertions, convalescence usually allowed a resumption of normal activities. Unfortunately, the three traditional forms of prescribed exercise, namely, horseback riding, traveling in carriages, and sailing, were upper- and middle-class pursuits seldom available to the poor.[225] Moreover, confinement in the hospital further restricted opportunities for therapeutic exercise. One activity frequently encouraged was participation in hospital routines. "Patients shall work as the matron or clerks shall desire them," proclaimed one infirmary regulation.[226] Some of this work consisted in "scraping and drawing cotton" (making lint) for bandages and dressings; other inmates simply assisted with housekeeping chores and the feeding of patients.[227]

Because exercise gave strength to muscular fibers and promoted circulation, convalescing patients with musculoskeletal conditions were encouraged to take walks outdoors, weather permitting, either behind the hospital or through the city. Others were "to use dumb bells for exercising the hands" or to mount a "wooden horse" – presumably a rocking one, to achieve the results of horseback riding.[228] The infirmary also had a "swinging chair" used for periods of fifteen to thirty minutes daily by persons recovering from pectoral complaints. Through "sympathy," such exertions could fortify the entire system and especially the stomach – a theory that prompted women labeled hysteric or dyspeptic to spend a fair amount of their hospitalization exercising on a wooden bench with a spring mechanism variously dubbed the "exercise machine" or "spring deal."[229] These workouts were considered powerful stimulants, also capable of restoring suppressed menstrual periods. "I have known women who rubbed the floor of a room for half an hour," commented James Gregory, but the activity proved fruitless, at least as far as a return of the menses was concerned.[230]

DIETETICS

In his lectures Cullen indicated that he considered dietary prescriptions the first order of therapeutics, and he also acknowledged that this part of medicine had been somewhat neglected.[231] Before the end of the eighteenth century, however, several physicians had established a detailed classification of foodstuffs as well as a plausible physiology of digestion based on both humoral and neuropathological principles.[232] Being firmly in control of their patients within the hospital, practitioners had reasonable assurances that their orders were going to be carried out. Accordingly, they set out to establish specific indications for the administration of various foods, confident that subsequent observations would prove or disprove the usefulness of their dietary formulas.

Thus, when physicians and surgeons made their rounds and decided on a therapeutic regimen, instructions concerning food usually accompanied orders for drugs and physical procedures. Like other voluntary hospitals of the period, the Edinburgh infirmary established a number of diets that were officially incorporated into the regulations of the institution.[233] Perhaps publishing these diets was designed to protect patients from arbitrary changes instituted by a thrifty or dishonest administration. More important, however, printing the diets was a calculated public relations effort, telling potential benefactors and the Edinburgh citizenry at large how well the hospital provided for its inmates.[234]

Indeed, infirmary officials regularly reassured the public that the meals provided were "proper and suitable," though they added the qualifying phrase "keeping in view the ordinary food of the poor in Scotland."[235] Such periodic pronouncements were apparently needed to refute a host of protests and criticisms concerning the quality and quantity of food distributed to patients. Among the most common complainers were soldiers and supernumerary patients, who paid for their own hospitalization and therefore felt less inhibited than others about commenting on perceived shortcomings.[236] Other disgruntled customers were the clerks and nurses who lived in the infirmary and received somewhat similar meals as part of their compensation.

A more visible attack on the hospital's management and diet occurred in 1782, when a printed pamphlet appeared in Edinburgh addressed to John Hope, then one of the attending physicians. Simply signed "Veri Amicus" (friend of the truth), the publication opened with the premise that "common sense dictates that the first duty of a physician is to prescribe as much wholesome food for the patient as his stomach is able to bear."[237] The author then went on to claim that most infirmary patients were placed on debilitating diets that "would hardly support the vital vigour of a kitten."[238] Comparing the Edinburgh diet to that served at St. George's Hospital in London, the anonymous critic focused on the breakfast porridge – "sometimes boiled into water gruel" – the dinner and supper broths – "better qualified to operate as an emetic" – and finally the beer – "not always tolerable even to the palate of an alehouse scullion."[239] Accordingly, during visiting hours, suitable provisions were smuggled into the house by compassionate relatives and friends.

Part of the criticism stemmed from misunderstandings and disagreements among lay people and medical personnel about the role of diet in the management of sickness. Since food in general was considered a stimulus to the human system, physicians tried to reduce its ingestion to a minimum during the early phase of their antiphlogistic or sedative regimen. The result was either total abstinence or the prescription of a "low," "fever" diet lacking all "animal food" products – primarily meaning meat. Physicians believed that they were strictly following nature: "Loss of appetite is one of the most constant symptoms of fever," lectured Cullen, "and the return of appetite is one of the most certain symptoms of the solution."[240]

Thus the Edinburgh infirmary's low diet was usually prescribed in all conditions deemed to be inflammatory. Starving a fever meant that patients were offered bread and milk, porridge made of oats and barley, or a panada, bread boiled to a pulp with sugar and nutmeg. Actually, a breakfast of this sort was typical for most poorer-class Scots.[241] At times the traditional oatmeal pottage was eschewed by English patients, who claimed that "nothing but horses, hogs, and Scotsmen can digest oats," an assertion that gave Cullen pause enough to admit the nutritional superiority of wheat.[242]

Both dinner at noon and supper in the evening featured similar items, with the addition of boiled rice with milk or barley cooked with currants. For drinks, physicians ordered plenty of water or milk, water gruel acidulated with vinegar, and barley or rice water. Certain patients from the countryside requested and received "sowans" for supper, a typical Scottish dish consisting of a light pudding prepared with flour extracted from oat husks.[243]

According to Duncan, the Edinburgh infirmary had a very good supply of fresh milk, and in favorable financial times the porridge was excellent, with each patient receiving a "mutchkin" – about three-quarters of a pint – per day. The quality of the bread also remained high throughout the period; bread allowances varied from twelve to sixteen ounces a day during good times. During crises, however, these quantities were reduced and the porridge turned thinner "than a Scotch stomach is used to."[244]

For patients convalescing from febrile ailments or those suffering from chronic, nondigestive complaints, Edinburgh physicians ordered a "full," "regular" diet. The breakfast remained essentially unchanged, except for additional allowances of light beer, but this meal plan introduced a certain amount of meat in the form of beef tea, a thicker beef broth, and boiled or roasted beef, mutton, and chicken for both dinner and supper. Meat was considered a powerful stimulant and served only on medical orders when the patients' appetites appeared to return. Beef tea was on occasion used with opium as a nourishing enema if the oral route could not be employed.

At Edinburgh the popular hospital broth was prepared in a sixty-gallon copper boiler according to a recipe that called for 24 pounds of meat, 14 of barley, and 3½ of oats, together with 2 pecks of potatoes and some turnips.[245] At times, attending physicians and clerks nevertheless found the broth "defective in nutritious matter," with too much water, insufficient barley, and meat represented only by chunks of bone, fat, and skin.[246]

Before the end of the century, ordinary households in Edinbrugh had difficulty obtaining fresh meat during the winter months and relied instead on salted beef.[247] Not surprisingly, the infirmary also reduced its daily allowances of 1½ ounces per patient from time to time. Items such as "cowhead and calfsfoot jelly" were prescribed instead of steaks. The meat was often said to be tough, with too much fat and gristle. If supplies were plentiful, however, the nurses would bring the raw, "undressed" meat into the wards on a board and place it near a window. The steaks were roasted, presumably in the fireplaces, and distributed hot and in small bits to patients confined to their beds. Ambulatory convalescents were "indulged with more" and ate at a dressing table. At least in the infirmary's teaching ward, they could on occasion cook their own meat if extra allowances were ordered by the professor in charge.[248] All food was served in wooden "cogues" or "cogs" (cups) of different sizes – no plates – and the hospital seldom if ever furnished spoons, knives, and forks. If used, these items were usually brought in by the patients themselves or their visitors, though an occasional horn or pewter spoon could be obtained from the nurses for a small gratuity.

To supplement the regular diet, hospital authorities relied on an ample supply of fresh vegetables and fruits available throughout the year in the city of Edinburgh.[249] Infirmary regulations called for the distribution of "various fruits in their respective seasons," including cherries, gooseberries, pears, and strawberries. Potatoes were gradually incorporated and after 1800 prepared in the form of a nourishing soup. Student casebooks reveal special prescriptions for turnips and strawberries, oranges and apples. In one case of diabetes physicians even ordered two eggs for breakfast in a futile attempt to stop the bodily wasting.[250]

Finally, the Edinburgh infirmary had an official "middle" diet containing the same items as the full diet but dispensing only half the amount of food. Except for patients still starving their fevers and those well fed because they were expected to recover from diseases of debility, the middle diet was perhaps the most frequently employed meal plan in the hospital. Special diets such as one based primarily on milk were ordered in cases of phthisis. When the patient labored under a dropsy, physicians prescribed a so-called dry diet consisting of generous portions of meat, butter, and cheese but a limit on fluids of about one pint per day. A liquid "salivating" diet was administered to patients receiving doses of mercury sufficiently large to cause a flow of saliva. It featured milk, various broths, and an allowance of warm beer.

In general, hospital physicians were cautious about giving too much food, especially since most patients did not display a great appetite while treated with emetics and other nauseating drugs. For others already suffering from digestive complaints, including severe malnutrition, regular amounts of food proved an additional burden. Confinement and the lack of exercise also hindered a return of appetite. Moreover, physicians were in constant fear that febrile illnesses could turn into "putrid" fevers, the criteria for putrefaction being foul breath and sweat, gastrointestinal fermentation, and offensive-smelling stools. To preclude such an eventuality, physicians enforced virtually meat-free meals and prescribed great quantities of diluted, acid fruit drinks believed to possess antiseptic qualities.[251]

Besides the medical reasons in its favor, the middle diet also appealed to budget-conscious hospital administrators constantly struggling to avoid deficits. While leaving the actual prescribing of diets in the hands of the "medical establishment," the managers played a key role in allocating sufficient funds for food. At the same time, they successfully insulated themselves from complaints about the quality and quantity of foodstuffs by insisting on formal, written protests conveyed through proper channels, a procedure seldom if ever employed. Blocked by formalities, physicians and surgeons complained directly to the matron in charge, who politely listened, promised improvements, and continued to act within the constraints imposed on her by the budget. It is no wonder that in the last decades of the eighteenth century and beyond, matrons on the average lasted only about four years in their positions.

Beer, wine, and spirits

Although at Edinburgh alcoholic beverages were most often considered medicines and had to be specifically prescribed by the attending physicians and surgeons, their inclusion among the usual articles of drink made them part of the dietary prescriptions. All of them were viewed as stimulants to be administered in clinical situations reflecting systemic debility, that is, in cases of certain fevers, especially typhus, and in all convalescent states where recovery depended on proper sustenance.

A "small" or "house" beer of low alcoholic content (1.2%) was usually available in quantities of about a quart per day or prescribed without restrictions. Brewed near the infirmary and generally unadulterated, this quite nourishing beer was served during breakfast and supper. A dark, stronger beer called porter (6.8% alcohol) was given in amounts of two to four pints per day to patients requiring a greater tonic effect, as well as to people who disliked drinking wine.[252]

Wine, according to one contemporary practitioner, was "within limits, undoubtedly one of those real blessings with which a kind of Providence had favoured us."[253] Its employment, justified as a tonic, diuretic, and antiseptic, certainly raised the pulse, warmed the stomach, and promoted urinary discharge and gentle sweating, restoring well-being and constitutional strength. Nevertheless, Cullen was quite aware of the secondary narcotic qualities of wine and found it difficult to decide whether the stimulation would outlast the sedative side effects.[254] Many infirmary physicians ordered claret, a light red wine generally imported from France and served diluted with 30% water or milk. Other stronger white or full-bodied red wines and a sweet port were also employed. Practitioners considered the white wines, usually from the Rhine, to be diuretics and gentle stimulants and allowed patients to drink two to three pints daily. Red wines were judged to be astringents and more powerful tonics; port, sherry, and Madeira wines were true cordials with the highest nutritional and stimulating value, ideal for slowly convalescent patients. All could be served warm mixed with sugar or panada. Daily allowances of red wine fluctuated between half a pint and one and a half pints, sometimes given between meals in amounts of two to three ounces every hour, morning and afternoon.[255] The standard mixture consisted of eight ounces of red wine and four ounces of water, served three or four times daily. Two ounces of port wine diluted in one ounce of water was usually administered every four hours in serious cases.

More than 60% of all the wine prescribed at the infirmary's teaching ward was given to patients suffering from typhus fever. The clinical histories in casebooks contain a number of remarks such as "the patient relishes the wine very much" or "has very little complaints but from want of wine."[256] In truth, once their appetites returned, some patients took advantage of their situation and demanded generous allowances of alcoholic beverages capable of "making glad the heart of man."[257] One patient under the care of Francis Home received port wine without restrictions and managed to consume more than a quart in a twenty-four-hour period.

Finally, some hospital inmates received one to two pints of diluted "spirits" – mostly brandy or rum in the form of punch – for stronger stimulation or prevention of gastrointestinal putrefaction. Of the gin punch served in the infirmary's teaching ward, 80% went to patients with circulatory disorders, but from progress notes it apparently had no favorable effects in two-thirds of the cases. People suffering from other diseases of debility, such as nervous fevers, also received liquor. In one such fever case Cullen ordered a spoonful of brandy together with four spoonfuls of water, the mixture to be taken with meals.[258]

Given the cost of these items to the hospital, the use of alcoholic beverages remained under strict professional control. In fact, increased consumption of port wine forced the infirmary in 1790 to tighten its procedures for prescribing all alcohol-containing drinks. Thereafter, attending physicians had to reorder wine and liquor each day on their rounds and send a written note to the apothecary.[259] Later, in 1795, these procedures were also extended to the consumption of porter beer.[260]

At the bottom of the restrictions was an increasingly negative attitude about alcohol as medicine, given the evils surrounding its chronic use and abuse so eloquently portrayed by advocates of temperance.[261] In Edinburgh some fears were raised in the early 1780s because of the popularity of John Brown's system of medicine among the medical students. Brownianism considered almost all diseases to be the results or systemic debility asthenia and vigorously advocated the use of alcoholic products in therapeutics.[262] In London similar sentiments against the use of alcohol emerged. John Fothergill, before dying in 1780, was quoted as saying that he felt guilty about his previous wine prescriptions because they could have fostered or encouraged alcoholism in his patients. John Lettsom suspected that patients demanding beer or wine at dispensaries or hospitals were "at the brink of destruction."[263] Although the gin epidemic had somewhat subsided, the substitution of "ardent spirits" for ale among the common people of Scotland was believed to be widespread and was already blamed for many ills, among them insanity and dropsy.

EFFECTS OF TREATMENT

In their clinical lectures, university professors in charge of the teaching ward frequently commented on the success or failure of their treatments. These judgments were based on personal observations at the bedside and a number of oral reports furnished by clerks, nurses, and the patients themselves. Some physicians, including Cullen, exposed their errors freely and discussed results with the medical students during subsequent clinical lectures. Together with discharge categories, such professional conclusions furnish the best clues about how eighteenth-century practitioners interpreted their own activities and defined the contemporary success of medical intervention.

Clinical progress was measured to some extent by paying attention to the patients' new "circumstances," sometimes distorted by flawed accounts. "Recovery was the progress of nature" or "the patient continues easy" were among the remarks entered into ward journals and ledgers after busy, daily round. Frequently employed in individual clinical histories were the terms "good," "fair," and "none" to evaluate the overall results of hospital treatment, and such pronouncements have been collected and analyzed. On the basis of 808 complete records, the results of medical therapy in the teaching ward were judged as follows:

Good	328 cases	40.5%
Fair	281 cases	34.7%
None	147 cases	18.1%
Unknown	52 cases	6.4%

Of those for whom good outcomes were reported, 62% were women and a large number were listed as servants. The patients with favorable results were on the average younger than others (twenty-six years old). About two-thirds suffered from acute diseases, meaning those of recent onset, especially fevers, sore throats, catarrhs, and gastrointestinal upsets; indeed, 61% of them were listed as suffering from infectious diseases. They received emetics and purgatives, diaphoretics and expectorants, gargles and vapor inhalations, fomentations and bloodletting. The fact that the patients were young and resilient, and the diseases mostly self-limited, undoubtedly contributed to the favorable outcomes.

The category of fair results represented a degree of temporary improvement achieved after the use of medicines that it was hoped would evolve toward permanent cures. Men and women were equally represented in this group, and their average age was thirty years. Included here were 83% of all cases suffering from venereal disease and half of those with skin disorders and gynecological complaints. The ambiguous finding reflects the dilemma of contemporary physicians, who in protracted clinical situations had trouble judging the extent and permanence of their cures.

The third medical determination, no effect, applied to more men than women. The average age of patients in this group was thirty-two; they came to the infirmary with well-established, chronic problems, notably circulatory disorders (anasarca and ascites), neurological deficits (paralysis of limbs), urinary difficulties (kidney and bladder ailments), and cancers. A high proportion of seamen – nearly 40% of them – were among those affected by these long-standing diseases. Consequently, use of diuretics, gin punch, catheterization, and paracentesis, although ordered to alleviate the manifestations of sickness, proved largely ineffective.

COMPLICATIONS

Patient histories occasionally reported clinical complications, phenomena that were either part of the evolution of disease or consequences of medical treatment, an almost impossible distinction for eighteenth-century practitioners to make. Of the 808 cases contained in student notebooks, almost 20% listed complications. The most common problems were these:

Sore mouth	23 cases
Skin rash	15
Generalized weakness	14
Bedsores	13
Diarrhea	10
Pus formation	10
Respiratory symptoms	10

Sore mouth and inflamed gums were typical manifestations of mercurial therapy instituted in the treatment of several diseases, notably venereal complaints. Both were among the few symptoms physicians could ascribe directly to the administration of a remedy. A third of the affected patients were servants; more women than men were troubled, a distinction that led to the contemporary supposition that females showed a greater sensitivity to the effects of mercury.

Skin problems, more in men than women, followed in the wake of numerous fevers and were often attributed to the efforts of natural forces trying to rid the body of impurities. Some were simply cases of "itch" or scabies reaching the period of maximum sensitization. General weakness, in turn, was predominantly reported in severe cases of typhus fever, as well as in obstinate circulatory disorders with generalized swelling. Bedsores happened in more protracted cases of typhus, chronic rheumatism, and paralysis, "from rubbing of bedclothes and urinary incontinence."[264]

More dangerous were instances referred to as "frequent calls to go to stool." Some of the diarrhea was possibly caused by the frequent use of purgatives; other cases were part of several inflammatory and circulatory

Table 4.6. *General Register of Patients: discharges, 1770–1800 (% of all discharges)*

Category	1770	1775	1780	1785	1790	1795	1800
Cured	74.9	85.1	68.7	70.4	70.8	65.4	60.5
Relieved	12.3	4.8	9.7	11.2	15.0	14.2	6.3
By desire	6.8	1.7	10.4	4.5	5.8	4.7	4.5
Dead	1.9	4.2	3.4	4.7	2.8	5.4	5.4
Improper	—	0.2	5.5	5.2	1.7	5.9	7.2
By advice	—	—	—	2.9	3.4	0.7	3.4
Irregular	1.3	0.6	1.6	0.8	0.2	2.6	2.0
Incurable	0.3	0.4	0.2	—	—	—	—
No entry	2.2	2.6	0.2	0	0	0.9	10.2

Note: Dashes indicate that the category in question does not appear for that year.

disorders. Pus formation or suppuration was an infrequent event in a variety of tumors and swellings, some of them clearly labeled cancers. Lastly, symptoms such as dyspnea, cough, and expectoration appeared in the course of many colds and sore throats already under treatment.

DISCHARGE FROM THE HOSPITAL

After hospital patients seemingly recovered from their ailments or all means believed to aid the sick were exhausted, it was time for them to go home. Discharge orders were issued daily by attending physicians, surgeons, and university professors, using a number of categories in accordance with institutional regulations. In the years under study the Edinburgh infirmary adopted a number of official labels such as "cured," "relieved," "by desire," "dead," "improper," "for irregularities," "incurable," and "by advice" to characterize the dismissals. Under these headings clerks inscribed all departures into the ward journals, ledgers, and General Register of Patients. They were tabulated monthly and again at the end of the year, since discharges represented the core of the infirmary's published statistics (see Table 4.6).

Establishing and employing these categories therefore served more administrative than strictly medical purposes. Most contemporary hospitals in Britain published their admission and discharge statistics as part of annual reports to subscribers and tried to present them in the most favorable light. Institutional success was indeed equated with high cure and low mortality rates, which allowed managers to justify expenditures and launch new fundraising drives. Inevitably, the desire for favorable statistics exerted a great deal of pressure on hospital practitioners ordering the discharge of the patients. There is sufficient evidence to show that Edinburgh physicians were sensitive to the administrative needs and in many instances deliberately embellished the discharge status to improve the infirmary's statistics.

The official statutes acknowledged that "it is not always an easy matter for a physician to judge with precision when a patient ought to be discharged from the hospital."[265] Proper timing was important, taking into account factors such as the season, the weather, the distance to the patient's home, and the demand for beds in the various wards. Cold weather certainly delayed for days and even weeks the discharge of many persons from the "warmth and shelter of the house," until conditions improved sufficiently for a safe journey back home.[266] Many were dismissed "for the benefit of country air" or "obliged to go into the country" when spring arrived, since it was widely assumed that pure air and free exercise were effective measures in the cure of incipient tuberculosis and other ailments, including chronic rheumatism and paralysis.[267] Some patients dying in the hospital requested to be discharged and brought back to their own homes.[268]

In a few instances dismissal from the infirmary had to be delayed on account of bad weather or because patients living outside Edinburgh lacked the means to finance their transportation back home. Although the managers usually insisted on deposits to defray such costs before admitting patients, many acute and emergency cases gained entrance simply with pledges of future payment that failed to materialize. In certain instances the hospital went ahead and paid for the return trip out of its "public burdens" fund. Servants sometimes remained in the hospital on orders of their employers: "Perfectly well but it being inconvenient for him to go home to his master's house where there are a number of young children, he is to be allowed to stay there till called for – his master paying 6d per night."[269]

Some persons were reluctant to leave the infirmary because they had lost their jobs, were destitute, and had no place to go.[270] Others had adjusted to the hospital routines and were quite comfortable, "not very willing to return to their former labours."[271] Under those circumstances, it was common for patients "to loiter in the house" and "amuse the physician with fictitious feelings."[272] Cullen alerted his students: "When our patients are in a way of recovery I find them frequently averse to leave us and therefore to feign complaints."[273] A battle of wits pitting "sly and cunning" patients against the hospital practitioners was played out in unending variations. "I wish that in such cases you could keep your countenance as well as I can," Cullen confided to his students.[274] If caught, those falsifying symptoms were summarily dismissed from the institution.[275]

On the basis of the sample of 3,047 cases obtained from the General Register, the following discharge categories appeared in the folios:

Status	No. of cases	%
Cured	2,155	70.7
Relieved	319	10.4
By desire	169	5.5
Dead	125	4.1
Improper	118	3.8
By advice	48	1.5
Irregular	40	1.3
Incurable	4	0.1
No entry	69	2.2

For the 808 complete clinical histories obtained from student casebooks, representing the discharges from the teaching ward between 1771 and 1799, university professors employed the following categories:

Status	No. of cases	%
Cured	452	55.9
Relieved	136	16.8
By desire	79	9.7
Dead	63	7.8
Improper	10	1.2
Irregular	5	0.6
Incurable	2	0.2
By advice	1	0.1
No entry	60	7.4

As can be seen, the Edinburgh teaching ward had a lower cure rate than the one reported for the entire hospital. In part, the difference reflected the fact that university professors invariably selected more complicated and serious cases for the teaching unit, a situation also apparent in its higher mortality rate (almost double the official total) and its greater proportion of dissatisfied patients who demanded or "desired" to be released.

"Cured" and "relieved" patients

British hospital physicians applied the term "cured" with great liberality to any patient who appeared to be on the mend, even if the recovery was partial or temporary. To be sure, the professional judgment that a cure had taken place was justified in most self-limited diseases showing definite signs of recovery. Logically, it was also applied to 97% of the patients whose treatments were evaluated by Edinbrugh hospital practitioners as causing "good" effects. Yet only 70% of all persons labeled "cured" were among those who experienced good effects; about a third were clearly listed as cured for statistical reasons without proper symptomatic improvement. This label was applied to patients with generalized edema and symptoms of pulmonary congestion who merely lost some fluid after prolonged bedrest, and to paralytic persons whose limbs failed to regain the slightest motion.[276] In another typical case, a male patient admitted with a severe eye infection was dismissed five weeks later by John Hope, "cured of ophthalmia but has lost the light of his eye."[277]

From the notebooks it appears that Francis Home, periodically in charge of the Edinburgh teaching ward during the 1780s, was especially generous with the label "cured," bestowing it on most of his patients. "Of those dismissed cured, I could name some who directly relapsed into their old complaints on the very day they left the Royal Infirmary," wrote the anonymous critic in 1782.[278] Indeed, the notebooks contain a number of cases where so-called cured people were readmitted within days of their discharge for complaints similar to those that had prompted the first hospitalization.

One anecdote, recounted by a German visitor in 1781, involved a patient of Home's who apparently was not improving in spite of the treatments prescribed by the professor. Having one day expressed his wish to be discharged, the man was relieved when Home granted the request. Turning to his clerk, the professor dictated "dismissed cured" for inscription into the ward journal, whereupon the patient is said to have angrily replied, "That is a damned lie, I am worse than ever."[279]

A study of the Edinburgh cases inscribed into the General Register reveals a decrease in the proportion of "cured" cases during the decade 1790–1800, from 70% to about 60%, but the significance of this decline remains unclear because it coincided with clerical omissions and recording gaps that reached as high as 10% in 1800. Undoubtedly, there was a perceptible increase in the number of seriously ill patients admitted to the house in the last decade of the century. This situation was reflected in part by slightly higher mortality rates and a profusion of "improper" cases found unsuitable for further hospital treatment. Yet given the institutional penchant for recording cures even in cases where the results of treatment were barely judged to be fair, it is difficult to reach firm conclusions.

Women had slightly higher cure rates than men (71% to 69%). A check of individual wards reveals that the best ratings were achieved in the soldiers' ward, where most cases of venereal disease were hospitalized. The percentage of patients discharged as cured by ward is as follows:

Soldiers' ward	81
Servants' ward	79
Surgical ordinary	71
Medical ordinary	65
Teaching ward	63
Seamen's ward	60

Not surprisingly, more than 90% of all patients with infectious and 84% of those with genitourinary diseases were released as cured. Surgical conditions such as trauma and infections were closely behind. The lowest cure rate was claimed for tumors and cancers: 30%.

Analysis of the 808 discharges from the Edinburgh teaching ward also reveals a higher rate of women (59%) than of men dismissed as cured. On the average, cured patients were younger (twenty-seven years of age) than others, and more than half of them suffered from acute ailments. People identified as servants and soldiers had the highest rates of cures: 73% and 71% respectively; laborers and seamen had the lowest: 48% and 41%. Finally, persons dismissed as cured from the teaching ward remained an average of only twenty-four days in the hospital.

Virtually all those in the infirmary who were not cured or did not die there were dismissed as "relieved," unless they chose to depart on their own accord or were officially expelled. Thus statistics from the General Register show considerable fluctuation in this discharge category, primarily related to higher or lower cure rates. The teaching ward had the highest percentage of so-called relieved patients (15). More than half of them had presented themselves with chronic health problems, and they were, as a group, somewhat older than those listed as cured: thirty-one years of age. Most suffered from stubborn gastrointestinal and urinary problems, gynecological as well as neurological diseases that stretched the average hospitalization to thirty-six days.

At the Edinburgh teaching ward the discharge label "relieved" was assigned equally to people of both sexes whose treatments were judged by the professors to yield fair (83%) or no results (12%). For the latter group, those in charge of the ward tried hard to find some measure of symptomatic relief that would justify sending the patients away as having been helped. In truth, there was no alternative. Ever sensitive of its public image, Edinburgh's charitable institution simply did not provide a category such as "unchanged" or "not improved." This would have been contrary to the infirmary notion that all suitable or "proper" patients, except for those who died, benefited from their sojourns in the hospital.

"By desire"

According to the infirmary's statutes, hospitalized patients had the option of requesting their own dismissal. Some of them suffering from mild catarrhs or fevers recovered quickly and "felt so easy" that they were anxious to leave. Others "went out on their own accord," impatient or dissatisfied with the results of treatment. In certain instances relatives or friends asked permission to take home incurable or dying patients, and the notebooks include remarks that some of them died hours or days later.[280]

Notebooks recorded a number of departures as unauthorized "withdrawals" or simply made the observation that the patient had "run away." A laborer suffering from ascites was "carried away by his wife" after eight days of ineffective therapy; one eleven-year-old epileptic slipped out of the house unseen following nine days of electrical shock treatments. Others walked out of the hospital simply to avoid taking the prescribed diet and medicines.[281]

Whether hospital physicians readily consented to their patients' wishes to leave the Edinburgh infirmary depended on a number of factors. These included the physical condition of the individual, assessment of the usefulness shown by medical treatment, the potential for disciplinary problems if the patient was kept any longer, and in the teaching ward, the educational value of the case. In general, each person listed in ward journals as leaving "by desire" expressed dissatisfaction or rejected further medical help. Therefore, with the exception of moribund patients, infirmary practitioners tried to avoid listing patients in this category, again sensitive to the image of the hospital as a very effective institution in the fight against disease.

In effect, many of the patients who left without permission were recorded as cured under the assumption that it was their impending recovery that had prompted the voluntary departure. In one instance a patient of Cullen's who was suffering from severe sciatic pain grew tired and impatient in the face of ineffective treatment and quietly left the ward. Commenting on his "elopement," Cullen openly suggested to his students that the man "would not have run away had he not found himself in a better condition." Consequently the case was entered into the registers as "relieved."[282] Similar cases exist in the notebooks.

Information obtained from the General Register demonstrates a gradual decrease in the number of infirmary patients dismissed by desire after 1780 (see Table 4.7). Males predominated (54%–58%), the average age was thirty-two years, and more than half presented chronic health problems. Nearly one out of four people affected by venereal disease was among them, having perhaps grown tired of mercurial treatments; urinary disorders and leg ulcers were also represented. A third of all seamen admitted to the Edinburgh infirmary were discharged in this category.

Most important, both the General Register and the notebooks reveal that authorized departures were closely related to longer hospital stays – over thirty days – and ineffectual treatments – in more than half of the cases practitioners admitted having no success with their therapies.

Dead

Mortality rates were the most sensitive indicators of eighteenth-century hospital performance. In Edinburgh the figures were constantly employed

Table 4.7. *General Register of Patients: patients dismissed "by desire,"*
1770–1800

	1770	1780	1790	1800	Total	% of all dismissals by desire
Gender breakdown						
Men	41	94	72	42	249	58.5
Women	37	84	25	30	176	41.4
Total	78	178[a]	97	72[b]	425	99.9
Wards						
Med. ord.	55	82	51	41	229	53.8
Surg. ord.	11	41	14	10	76	17.8
Clinical	5	8	15	8	36	8.4
Soldiers'	4	17	8	7	36	8.4
Servants'	3	27	8	3	41	9.6
High	0	1	1	0	2	0.4

[a] Ward breakdown does not include two patients considered invalids.
[b] Ward breakdown does not include three hospitalized Russian sailors.

in fund-raising efforts and compared with those from other British hospitals to demonstrate the superiority of the Edinburgh institution.[283] Because a number of very sick patients left or were removed before death, the statistics were certainly lower than they should have been. Still, it seems clear that not many people admitted to voluntary hospitals died in them, since the admissions process favored the entrance of young persons with acute, self-limited ailments. Those affected by more serious acute and chronic conditions generally left on their own accord or were discharged "relieved" before a fatal outcome could mar the record. Discharging moribund patients was not only a scheme to improve hospital statistics but a response to demands by relatives and patients themselves to die in their own homes surrounded by familiar faces.

Data from the General Register reveal a slight rise in mortality at the infirmary during the last decade of the eighteenth century (from an average of 4.1% to 5.4%; see Table 4.8). These figures are perhaps more significant given the fact that over 10% of the discharge entries were omitted for that decade. If mortality numbers reported from the 1810s (6.4%) are correct, one could indeed postulate a very gradual but steady increase, although the causes for the rise are still far from clear. In any case, entries of "dead" for the decades 1770–1800 show a higher incidence for medical afflictions (4.4%), especially fevers, phthisis, and dropsy, than for surgical problems (3.3%).

The teaching ward had the highest mortality rate in the infirmary – between 7.6% and 8% – nearly double the average for the entire hospital,

Table 4.8. *General Register of Patients: patients listed as dead,*
1770–1800

	1770	1780	1790	1800	Total	% of all in-house deaths	Average relative mortality rate (%)
Gender breakdown							
Men	33	44	36	79	192	68	3.6
Women	14	23	24	29	90	32	2.7
Total	47	67	60	108	282	100	
Wards							
Med. ord.	20	30	27	33	110	39.0	4.3
Surg. ord.	7	12	14	15	48	17.0	3.5
Clinical	8	4	8	15	35	12.4	7.6
Servants'	1	7	7	4	19	6.7	3.0
Soldiers'	11	14	4	8	37	13.1	2.7
Seamen's	[a]	[a]	[a]	2	2	0.7	6.0

[a] This ward did not exist until after 1790.

whereas the lowest came from the soldiers' ward. This finding confirms the importance of patient selection on mortality, since the teaching unit received its inmates from the general pool of applicants gathered in the admissions room. Professors obviously took the sicker people, because they presented challenges that made for better instruction. From the notebooks, it appears that men housed in the teaching ward died in greater numbers than women; their average age was thirty-two years. Because many of the patients were seriously ill and perished within a few days following admission, the average stay was relatively brief: twenty days. As expected, 98% of those who died were reported as not responding to the therapeutic regimen ordered for them. Only about half of the dead underwent postmortem examinations.

"Incurable" and "improper"

In the 1770s infirmary physicians used the category "incurable" to label all patient discharges where medical treatments had failed. "We are never to hold it as a rule to admit that any disease is uncurable till remedies have been tried to no purpose," lectured Cullen, adding that efforts to cure such diseases were to proceed "as long as they can be with any probability of safety."[284] The number of patients reported as incurable remained very small,

Table 4.9. *General Register of Patients: patients dismissed as* *"improper," 1770–1800*

	1780	1790	1800	Total	% of all dismissals as improper
Gender breakdown					
Men	74	38	70	182	65
Women	46	15	36	97	35
Total	120	53	106[a]	279	100
Wards					
Med. ord.	61	27	46	134	48.0
Surg. ord.	11	15	17	43	15.0
Clinical	3	3	4	10	3.5
Soldiers'	30	6	16	52	18.6
Seamen's	[b]	[b]	21	21	7.5
Servants'	14	2	0	16	5.7
High	1	0	0	1	0.3

[a] Ward breakdown is unavailable for two of these patients.
[b] This ward did not exist until after 1790.

and the category was eliminated in the 1780s. Henceforth, most cases beyond medical help were apparently not admitted, and others were probably dismissed as "relieved." Here again, Edinburgh hospital practitioners wjre aware of the public impact created by sending substantial numbers of incurable patients out of the house.

Incurable patients listed in the General Register were mostly men enduring medical ailments such as blindness, cancer, epilepsy, and mental retardation. Not all were hopeless cases: John Gregory warned his students that many patients "have been dismissed from hospitals as incurables who afterwards recovered, sometimes by the efforts of unassisted nature, sometimes by very simple remedies, and now and then by the random prescriptions of an ignorant quack."[285]

A new class, "improper," made its first appearance in the folios of the General Register during 1776, to replace the old "incurable" category. The term "improper" sought to indicate that the patient being discharged had been found to be unsuitable for hospital treatment, largely because the condition had become incurable. The register indicates that such a professional determination was increasingly made at the Edinburgh infirmary during the decade 1790–1800 (see Table 4.9), until in the latter year the designation was used for more than 7% of all discharges. Twice as many men as women were placed in this category. Among the people deemed improper were many seamen, and medical conditions more than double the number of surgical conditions. In general, males with chronic conditions tended to predominate, especially those afflicted with the various manifestations of tuberculosis. Other improper inmates had mental problems or seemingly feigned their complaints.

In the Edinburgh teaching ward most improper discharges dealt with stubborn gynecological problems and rheumatic conditions resistant to electricity. Before being finally dismissed, these patients endured a barrage of treatments that stretched their average hospitalization to sixty-four days. In sharp contrast, data from the General Register indicate that the average stay for improper patients was only twenty days, another reflection of the fundamental differences in the planning and execution of treatments created by the demands of clinical teaching.

"For irregularities" and "by advice"

Finally, patients who disobeyed medical orders or violated other hospital rules were immediately discharged "for irregularities." A typical example from the notebooks was a man suffering from hypochondriasis who refused to take a prescribed purgative from the nurse. "I was therefore not displeased to have the opportunity of dismissing him for irregularity," observed Duncan in 1795.[286] Others were caught feigning illness, quarreling with nurses, smuggling food, or through their behavior creating disturbances in the wards.[287]

Information from the register and notebooks reveals a considerable increase in "irregular" discharges at the infirmary during the 1790s, nearly triple the average number reported for previous decades (see Table 4.10). Perhaps the main reason was the growing influx of seamen, whose ward dismissed nearly 7% of its men for disciplinary problems. A majority suffered from venereal diseases, leg ulcers, and rheumatism.

An equally small number of persons left the Edinburgh infirmary "by advice" and occasionally with some medicines to continue treatment at home. This category was first established in 1785 to distinguish patients with protracted or nearly incurable conditions who no longer benefited from hospital treatment but still had a chance to recover in other environments. Among them were again many cases of tuberculosis, chronic "pectoral complaints," leg ulcers, and tumors. Twice as many men as women were assigned to this category (see Table 4.11).

The practice of discharging patients with a supply of drugs was common for all categories. Boxes of ointments and pills, phials of lotion and tinctures – all were ordered by hospital physicians at the time of dismissal and quickly filled by the house apothecary before the patient departed.[288]

Table 4.10. *General Register of Patients: patients dismissed* *"for irregularities," 1770–1800*

	1770	1780	1790	1800	Total	% of all dismissals for irregularities
Gender breakdown						
Men	4	14	3	29	50	52
Women	14	15	4	14	47	48
Total	18	29	7	43	97	100
Wards						
Clinical	2	1	1	1	5	5.1
Med. ord.	15	7	6	19	47	48.0
Surg. ord.	1	7	0	8	16	6.4
Soldiers'	0	8	0	14	22	22.0
Seamen's	[a]	[a]	[a]	1	1	1.0
Servants'	0	3	0	0	3	3.0
High	0	3	0	0	3	3.0

[a] This ward did not exist until after 1790.

Table 4.11. *General Register of Patients: patients dismissed* *"by advice," 1770–1800*

	1790	1800	Total	% of all dismissals by advice
Gender breakdown				
Men	38	19	57	64
Women	17	15	32	36
Total	55	34	89	100
Wards				
Clinical	1	2	3	3.3
Med. ord.	19	16	35	39.3
Surg. ord.	29	9	38	42.6
Servants'	1	1	2	2.2
Soldiers'	5	6	11	12.3

CONCLUSION

When called upon to treat patients, Edinburgh hospital physicians followed carefully laid-out plans ostensibly based on the neuropathological schemes articulated by William Cullen and his followers. In truth, however, both the sedative and the stimulating program merely paid lip service to a medical theory that predicated the central importance of the nervous system in health and disease. The apparent harmony between medical theory and practice concealed the profound differences between them in the clinical setting.

Indeed, in eighteenth-century Edinburgh the Cullenian physiopathology only provided a new set of explanations for the traditional healing approaches associated originally with humoralism and more recently with iatromechanism. Medical theories reflected new scientific discoveries and interpretations while therapeutics remained essentially unchanged, its sole and vague criterion the manifest improvement of the sick. Thus medical practice in Edinburgh, like that in other countries of Europe and America, continued to be based on time-honored measures designed to assist the natural healing powers operating within each patient. Actions taken at the bedside were generally prescribed on empirical grounds only, using drugs and other methods previously shown to have beneficial effects. Practitioners explained these effects, however, and the reasons for employing traditional procedures, within the new theoretical framework, thereby conferring a measure of rationality and modernity on the old practices.

A final word about the use of drugs in the infirmary: Many of the preparations employed by the physicians were listed in the sixth edition of the *Edinburgh Pharmacopoeia,* assembled by William Cullen and Joseph Black for the local College of Physicians and published in 1774. Like its London counterpart, this collection was widely respected and its remedies frequently prescribed in Britain and abroad. In addition, the Edinburgh infirmary published its own *Pharmacopoeia Pauperum,* containing a number of simplified formulas and preparations. Originally published in 1752, this formulary went through a number of editions, reprints, and translations, also appearing in such popular works as William Lewis's *Pharmacopoeia* (1748) and Richard Brookes's *General Dispensatory* (1753). The most important items were incorporated into a popular compendium entitled *The Practice of the British and French Hospitals* (1775), which also featured entries from British naval hospitals and Parisian institutions such as the Hôtel-Dieu and La Charité.[289] In sum, medical therapy administered at the Edinburgh infirmary was quite representative of eighteenth-century healing methods in general. Thanks to the popularity of its own in-house pharmacopoeia, the infirmary became widely known at home and abroad, its formulas frequently copied and dispensed at other hospitals.

5

Clinical instruction

The Infirmary of Edinburgh is much superior to any similar institution in Britain for the purpose of medical education. The cases of patients are all regularly registered, and an account of their situation is daily given by the attending physician.[1]

This statement, appearing in a 1792 guide for prospective medical students that is usually attributed to Alexander Hamilton, professor of midwifery, underlines the prominence of the Royal Infirmary of Edinburgh as an educational institution. Since its inception the hospital had been an important training ground for future physicians and surgeons. In 1771, nearly two decades earlier, the Edinburgh graduate John Aikin had already observed that "no school of medicine can flourish without possessing the advantage of being situated where a large hospital will at all times furnish a sufficient number of patients for lessons of real practice to the students." Aikin and others indeed concluded that Edinburgh's fame as a center for medical studies was due in great part to the clinical training offered at the infirmary.[2]

By the 1770s the role of hospitals in medical education seemed assured. "These charitable institutions amply repay the expense which the public bestows on them by promoting the study and practice of medicine," claimed Francis Home, explaining that "under one roof are collected a great variety of morbid cases to which students have an easy access, and where a wide field is opened to physicians for the improvement of their science."[3]

Thanks to its official relationships with the University of Edinburgh, the hospital established in 1756 an orderly rotation of professors responsible for patient care in its teaching ward and a systematic course of clinical lectures designed, in the words of William Cullen, to "teach the practice of physic by examples."[4] Students were allowed access to the wards during certain hours of the day, either to talk to and inspect individual patients or to make rounds in the company of clerks, attending physicians or surgeons, and university professors. Moreover, they routinely watched student dressers perform their chores and were from time to time especially summoned to the hospital to observe the management of emergency admissions, surgical operations, and autopsies.

Essential for the success of clinical instruction at Edinburgh was the integration of such training into the Medical School curriculum. The previously quoted student guide emphatically warned its readers not to attend hospital rounds until they had at least acquired a theoretical knowledge of the most frequent diseases and become familiar with the general principles of medical practice. Without such a background they would flounder, concluded the manual, and "certainly derive little profit from their labor."[5] Because the professors teaching medical theory and practice at the university were also in charge of the teaching ward and gave clinical lectures, medical training at the hospital was widely regarded by contemporaries as among the best in late eighteenth-century Europe. Edinburgh students did not randomly "walk the wards," as they did in London hospitals, frequently changing institutions and instructors while getting lost among the large retinues that followed attending practitioners. Some institutions even lacked house staff and had no fixed days for consultants willing to make their rounds.[6]

BACKGROUND

Clinical instruction in hospitals has a long tradition in medical education. In 1539 Giovanni B. da Monte (1498–1561), then professor of medicine at the University of Padua, brought his students to the Hospital of San Francesco and showed them cases of illnesses on which he was lecturing.[7] Weekend discussions with staff physicians and pupils became essential components of the medical curriculum at Padua, and the practice was brought to Holland by a number of Flemish disciples. In the seventeenth century clinical teaching reached new heights at the University of Leyden under the guidance of Otto van Heurne (1577–1652) and Franciscus de le Boe Sylvius (1616–1672), culminating in the early 1700s with the system of instruction organized by Herman Boerhaave (1668–1738).[8] His bedside teaching at the Caecilia Hospital in Leyden, where twelve beds had been set aside for such educational purposes, set new standards in medical training.[9]

Although the Leyden model was strongly favored by Alexander Monro primus when he returned from Holland to Scotland, the teaching functions of the Royal Infirmary resulted instead from local needs and a resolution of professional conflicts between Edinburgh's traditional Incorporation of Surgeons and the more recent College of Physicians.[10] Indeed, early in the eighteenth century the prosperous incorporation had already sought to expand the training facilities of its apprentices with the erection of a small hospital. At the same time surgeons elsewhere in Britain, especially in London, played leadership roles in the evolution of bedside instruction.[11]

Almost everywhere, surgeons and apothecaries considered the teaching of practical skills an essential part of their training, whereas physicians only slowly recognized the importance of acquiring clinical experience before graduation.[12] In Edinburgh, from the very beginnings of the infirmary in the small house located in Robertson's Close, students were freely allowed to observe the activities of attending surgeons and physicians. In fact, their growing numbers periodically resulted in complaints from both patients and managers, followed by efforts to restrict access.

As noted before, one effective way to regulate the flow of pupils was to issue admission tickets. As early as 1738, two years after receiving its royal charter, the infirmary's managers issued a hundred student passes at the price of two guineas each.[13] Each student was required to present his card to the porter on entering the institution, and the permit was subject to cancellation if displayed by someone other than the legitimate holder. Managers established an elaborate procedure whereby the total number of cards to be issued was determined in advance. The tickets were then printed, numbered, individually signed by one of the managers, and delivered to the treasurer, who disbursed them and kept a special account concerning their sale. Unused or canceled vouchers were returned to the managers, listed in the official minutes, and subsequently burned.

Students could request free tickets from the managers if they could prove financial hardship. Some also demanded refunds for unused portions of their vouchers, but the managers were reluctant to comply very often with these requests. Following the opening of the new building in 1741, with student attendance steadily rising, the hospital authorities sensed the economic implications of increased clinical instruction and therefore, in 1756, began issuing so-called perpetual tickets. These passes cost surgical apprentices five guineas and medical students seven and a half guineas and admitted them to the hospital for a year instead of the average three-month term of clinical lectures.[14]

Unquestionably, the sale of admission tickets generated hard cash that managers needed for the support of hospital activities, and thus it became an integral part of the yearly revenues.[15] "Clinical lectures always have added considerably to the funds of the house," noted James Gregory, adding that "many students take tickets for the Infirmary purely on account of the clinical lectures."[16] Consequently, in the last decades of the century the infirmary more than doubled its receipts from student tickets, which became the single largest item of revenue received by the managers.[17]

ORGANIZATION AND ENROLLMENT

In 1748 John Rutherford (1695–1779), then professor of the practice of medicine at the university, applied to the managers of the infirmary to organize a formal course of clinical lectures. To allow the attendance of a greater number of students, these classes were to be given in the hospital's amphitheater, primarily utilized for surgical operations. The managers immediately accepted the proposal as "of very great service to the students and likewise the house" and insisted that the course begin at once, in spite of the fact that only half of the academic winter session remained and no special tickets for attendance to the course could be issued at such short notice.[18]

Rutherford's proposal was designed to supplement the ongoing, less formal clinical instruction already given at the bedside. The necessarily limited discussion in the wards was to be expanded through the new lectures. "I shall examine every patient appearing before you that no circumstance may escape you," explained Rutherford, adding, "I shall give you the history of the disease, enquire into the cause of it, give you my opinion as to how it will terminate, lay down the indications of cure which will arise, or if any new symptoms happen, acquaint you of them that you may see how I vary my prescriptions."[19]

Rutherford's successful lectures[20] prompted the managers in 1750 to outfit a special teaching ward "not to exceed ten beds," which was to be kept open during the six months of the academic year. The idea was that the professor could now select his own patients and discuss their management in greater detail during the lectures. The expense, according to the managers, "will be much more than made up to the house by the additional number of tickets which will be taken out merely on account of these lectures." In fact, in 1749 alone, the income from ticket sales had virtually doubled, from £95 11s. to £172 4s.[21]

Not surprisingly, the excellent registration system already in place played an important role in the new clinical teaching. James Gregory pointed out that "every student attending the clinical lectures has access to the clinical books and may transcribe from them whatever he pleases."[22] In 1750 the hospital managers expanded the opportunity for this copying to two days a week, "Wednesday from 5 to 8 at night and Saturday afternoon," under the supervision of the physician's clerk.[23] Students were urged to copy cases housed in the teaching ward and presented by the professors in class. A few also took notes during their daily visits to other wards and from clinical lectures. The information, whether in short- or longhand, was generally kept as a permanent record for future reference. "I regard my clinical report book as the most valuable book in my library," concluded James Gregory.[24]

In 1756 three university professors, Alexander Monro secundus, William Cullen, and Robert Whytt, came to the aid of John Rutherford, who alone was giving clinical lectures. They contacted the hospital authorities and volunteered their services, proposing to teach jointly. Henceforth each professor was to lecture twice a week for five weeks, and the entire clinical course was expanded to last six months. The teaching ward was accordingly enlarged to a total of twenty beds in two separate rooms for an equal number of male and female patients.[25] The clinical ward was further expanded soon thereafter to twenty-nine beds, and a decade later to about fifty. On May 23, 1790, the managers announced that since "the clinical lectures continue to be of much service to the house, they thought it proper to continue the number of fixed patients as sometime ago, increased to one hundred during the time of these lectures."[26]

After the death of Robert Whytt in 1766, the retirement of John Rutherford, and the departure of Alexander Monro secundus, who assumed his father's teaching duties in anatomy, Cullen in the late 1760s divided the teaching duties with John Gregory. The latter withdrew in February 1772 because of ill health, and Cullen then taught alone for three years, imposing on himself a grueling schedule, given the numerous other obligations he had as Edinburgh's most distinguished physician. A careful perusal of a complete set of his clinical lectures, delivered during the academic year 1772–1773, sheds considerable light on the nature and methods of his instruction.[27]

Between November 12, 1772, and April 23, 1773, Cullen usually lectured twice a week at the infirmary, generally on Tuesday and Friday evenings. Forced to cancel some classes because of other urgent obligations, he scrupulously made them up in subsequent weeks, conscious of his obligations to the ticket-paying students. Before lecturing, Cullen was in the habit of making extensive notes about each clinical case he was going to discuss in class with the aid of the ward journal. Discussions of the most salient symptoms, diagnosis, and therapeutic indications were included.[28]

The time-consuming nature of these lectures was noted by Cullen's successor, James Gregory, who assumed responsibility for them in 1776: "The plain truth is that they are so severe in labour, both in point of attention and time, that all of us feel them very irksome even though our time of attendance is but three months." The result, disclosed Gregory, was that "as clinical lectures cannot be prepared beforehand, the incessant drudgery of preparing them from day to day, and the consequent interruption of all other study . . . is often inconvenient and sometimes quite intolerble."[29]

Yet it was precisely the extensive commitment of such experienced clinicians as Cullen and the Gregories that ensured the success of clinical instruction at the infirmary. Its favorable development was not ignored by the University of Edinburgh authorities. When the Senatus Academicus established on February 7, 1767, its first comprehensive regulations for conferring the M.D. degree, the statutes, while remaining vague about required courses, already indicated that all candidates were to be interrogated about practical medical matters.[30] Ten years later the university specifically included clinical lectures in the official curriculum, and from the matricu-

Table 5.1. *Enrollment for clinical lectures at the infirmary, 1770–1800*

Year	No. enrolled for clin. lects.	Total no. registrants	% enrolled for clin. lects.
1770	55	262	20
1775	55	312	17
1780	54	345	15
1785	95	420	22
1790	95	406	23
1795	122	359	33
1800	127	420	30

Source: Matriculation records, MSS Collection, University of Edinburgh. The entries counted were those inscribed in ink, since they were the only ones specifying the courses for which the student did matriculate that year. The clinical course was variously listed as Clin. lect., Clin. Praelect., Praelect. Clin., and Clin. lect., Infirm.

lation records for that period it appears that about 50–55 students per year (15%–20% of all registrants) enrolled in this course at the infirmary.[31]

Given the growing popularity of medical studies reflected in the higher enrollments, the university Senate published a new set of statutes in December 1783. Included was a requirement whereby doctoral candidates were to respond in writing to questions about the clinical management of two patients. Moreover, the university now explicitly insisted that "no person is admitted as a candidate for a degree in medicine unless he has attended these clinical lectures." The document, printed in Scottish and English newspapers, went on to publicize that "students have likewise an opportunity of attending the ordinary physicians of the Royal Infirmary" and reminded prospective newcomers that the detailed hospital journals were open to their perusal.[32]

The effects of the new statutes on clinical instruction were, however, gradual. In 1784 at least 90 matriculating students selected the infirmary course as part of their curriculum choices for that year. In 1790 95 students took the course, but the greatest increases began after the year 1795, when 122 registrants were listed. Following a decision by the managers, university professors in 1791 were authorized to conduct both a summer and a winter course of clinical lectures, which would allow students to see a variety of diseases prevalent in different seasons of the year.[33] Statistics for the year 1797, for example, indicate that 111 students registered for the summer session and 139 for the winter,[34] making the clinical lecture course one of the most popular offerings of the medical curriculum (see Tables 5.1 and 5.2).

Table 5.2. *Enrollment for clinical lectures at the infirmary, 1794–1800*

Year	Term	No. enrolled
1794		82
1795		136
1796		157
1797	Summer	111
	Winter	139
	Both terms	250
1798	Summer	83
	Winter	146
	Both terms	229
1799	Summer	101
	Winter	126
	Both terms	227
1800	Summer	74
	Winter	129
	Both terms	203

Source: Medical Matriculations, vol. 2, 1791–1795, vol. 3, 1796–1800, MSS Collection, University of Edinburgh.

STUDENTS AND CLINICAL TEACHING

Having paid for their admission tickets to the infirmary wards and for the lectures of the professors teaching the clinical course, both medical students and surgical apprentices jealously defended their hospital privileges. In January 1758, for example, after the so-called perpetual passes had already been issued, some students complained to the managers about a surgical operation for a strangulated hernia that had apparently been carried out in private, without the customary advance notification to the entire student body.[35] Similar objections about unscheduled autopsies were likewise brought to the attention of hospital authorities and vigorously voiced.[36]

Close contacts with sick patients and the dead carried considerable risks. Students were repeatedly warned by their teachers not to expose themselves unnecessarily to the effluvia believed to emanate from patients with contagious diseases. One of those who "survived the testing experience of an attack of typhus contracted on the wards of the Edinburgh Infirmary" was Peter M. Roget of *Thesaurus* fame.[37] James Gregory reported one instance when apparently eight medical students caught a febrile illness from a patient hospitalized in the teaching ward; two of them eventually died. Gregory thought that the students were partially to blame for their misfortune, since they displayed an ignorance and obstinacy regarding proper ventilation similar to that of nurses and patients.[38] During Andrew Duncan's rotation in the spring of 1793, "upwards of twenty students were infected with fever though many other precautions for preventing contagion were at that time employed."[39] This experience was promptly communicated to a committee of the House of Commons studying the effects of nitrous fumigation.

Student contact with patients was, however, strictly regulated for other reasons. Infirmary rules published in the year 1778 enjoined students to display at all times "a composed and decent carriage."[40] The danger apparently was that levity, "almost the inseparable characteristic of youth in any profession," would prevent students "from paying compassionate attention" to the patients. "I must assert with regret," wrote one contemporary, "that at present the majority of young gentlemen who walk our different hospitals are little under the dominion of the humane power of sympathy."[41] Senior attending physicians and teachers were therefore urged to "recommend by precept and enforce by example the humane attention here recommended," because "humanity will always stamp a dignity on the profession."[42] In Edinburgh a section of the hospital rules for students dealt with behavior in the operating theater, where their comings and goings were potentially disturbing to surgeons and especially patients. John Bell, a prominent surgeon attending the infirmary, also complained about too many "idle and curious" students crowding the surgical wards.[43]

Thus student visits to the infirmary increasingly began to conflict with the performance of hospital routines. On June 15, 1785, the managers saw fit to issue a series of new regulations because "much abuse and disorder has been introduced into the house by the students being admitted into the wards at irregular hours."[44] Henceforth access to the hospital was to be restricted to only two hours a day, the first from noon to one o'clock, when the ordinary physicians and clinical professors made their daily rounds. Admission to the evening lectures and a further visitation to the wards was allowed only between seven and eight o'clock in the company of the attending physicians and clerks. Surgical dressers were to conduct their tasks between four and five in the afternoon without student participation. Moreover, students were now expressly forbidden from talking directly with hospital patients; they had to present their questions to the medical staff. Lastly, copying from the ward journals and ledgers was henceforth confined to the waiting room and allowed only between eleven o'clock and noon and six and seven in the evening.[45]

Medical students quickly responded to the hospital authorities through their own organization, the Royal Medical Society. Under the chairmanship of one of its presidents, Thomas Beddoes, they formed a group called the "associated students" that vehemently protested the new rules. In a letter written to the managers of the hospital and dated June 25, 1785, the students first objected to the reasons given for the regulations, since their reputation would suffer if the public perceived them as a group of disorderly and irresponsible people. Next, they argued that the restrictions imposed on their visits to the hospital would jeopardize all direct contact with the patients. "The great object of a student's attendance at an infirmary is to examine the phenomena of diseases for himself and to see the method of treating the sick," wrote the protest committee, concluding that "these regulations have a direct tendency to prevent this. They are calculated to divert the student's attention from the patient to the physicians and clerks of the Infirmary."[46] An additional complaint voiced by students in response to actions by the hospital managers was the loss of experience in dressing wounds, applying electricity, and witnessing emergency admissions as well as occasional autopsies. Ninety-three members of the Royal Medical Society, including Beddoes, signed the letter.

In their response to the students the managers of the infirmary firmly held their ground, ostensibly making no concessions but indicating that the operating room was not off limits to ticket holders called to witness surgical operations and autopsies whenever these were scheduled. As usual, proper announcements would be posted in the waiting room. Such intransigence further angered the students, who immediately drafted a sharp reply threatening to boycott all future purchases of hospital admission tickets and promising to air their grievances in local newspapers. Finally, the students printed two thousand copies of a pamphlet for distribution to the entire student body, further detailing their objections and highlighting the callous attitude displayed by the infirmary's managers.[47]

On August 18, 1785, the hospital authorities restated their previous position but did make some concessions. The evening visit by students was expanded to a full two hours, from six to eight, and they were also allowed to be present at five in the afternoon during the activities of the dressers. Access to the institution was guaranteed whenever emergency cases were admitted and cared for.

Not entirely satisfied, the "associate students" of the Royal Medical Society now directed their protests to the medical faculty at the University of Edinburgh. Reiterating their previous contention "that little benefit can be derived from an attendance on the house unless the doors be opened to them at least from nine o'clock in the morning till eight in the night and the liberty of examining patients,"[48] the students requested that professors rescind their decision to make attendance at clinical lectures a requirement for graduation. Moreover, the protesters promised to publicize their plight further and inform potential incoming students of the restrictive policies imposed by the Edinburgh infirmary.

In a letter dated August 30, 1785, and signed by Dr. James Gregory on behalf of the professors of medicine, who were fully aware of the damaging effects that student dissatisfaction could have on actual enrollment and the international reputation of the Medical School, the faculty sought to mediate the conflict. Their proposals designed to calm the irate students included a further hour of access to patients, from eleven in the morning till noon, an addition that was planned to limit the disturbances to which patients were subjected, since house staff and the attending faculty made their rounds an hour later. Most important, the faculty conceded that "at these visits the students have the liberty of examining the patients directly and not through the intervention of a clerk."[49]

A further concession to the students was the university's proposal that "the journals of the physicians' and surgeons' practice be open to the students at all hours from nine in the morning till 8 at night," a tacit recognition of the great importance assigned to the study and copying of clinical records. As expected, the professors did not react kindly to the students' request to drop the clinical training as a requirement for graduation. Stressing the importance of this educational opportunity, "fully confirmed by many years of experience in this university" and "universally acknowledged," faculty members argued that a cancellation would only bring discredit to the institution, themselves, and ultimately the entire student body that had previously endorsed the course.[50]

Although the students persisted in characterizing the infirmary's responses to their demands as "intolerable indignities," they nevertheless accepted the terms laid out by the medical faculty and authorized the professors to discuss the proposals with hospital managers. On September 5, 1785, the infirmary accepted the compromise proposals, and the conflict seemingly ended.[51] The new regulations remained in effect until 1792, when hospital authorities again issued revisions. Noteworthy among the new directives were less liberal hours for making copies of clinical cases and special procedures to check them out from the apothecary for in-house use. Furthermore, students were now explicitly barred from the hospital's waiting room during times set aside for the admission of patients. Student reaction to the new restrictions, if any, went unregistered.[52]

CLINICAL TEACHING AND THE PATIENTS

Admission to the hospital was often a privilege of being acquainted with private subscribers. In return for free medical care, which they could hardly afford to pay for, the "deserving" poor became in a sense "clinical material," especially in institutions, like the Edinburgh infirmary, that were prominently involved in teaching. By virtue of their various ailments, hospital patients were welcome examples of a complex medical nosology as well as potential subjects for testing new treatments.

In the absence of surviving documentation it is difficult to assess tensions that existed between the needs of infirmary patients for assistence and the pedagogical demands of clinical training. James Gregory's statement that "whatever is best for the patients, is best for the students to learn" must be intended as an ideal, particularly since it was immediately followed by a warning that knowledge acquired through "unnecessary suffering, danger and harm is injustice and cruelty."[53]

Managers running the infirmary, although conscious of the economic and educational advantages of admitting students to the hospital, sought to protect their patients from excessive contact with the student body. Restrictions imposed on daily rounds, fixed hours of access, and warnings to the students not "to stroll about in the wards" were designed to protect regular hospital routines from unnecessary student intrusion. In taking these steps the administrators were motivated by fears that patients would publicly complain about invasions if they saw them as detrimental to their recovery. Such objections could easily reach present subscribers and potential donors, thereby lessening charitable gifts essential to sustain hospital activities. The 1785 conflict with the Royal Medical Society was based in a perception by hospital authorities that the comings and goings of students had got out of hand and would eventually jeopardize the charitable goals of the institution.

Throughout the entire controversy, the managers in fact justified their new rules as "consistent with the safety and proper treatment of patients for whose relief this charitable institution was established."[54] In their mediation efforts even university professors tried to temper the students' demands, rejecting all regulations "inconsistent with the welfare of the patients" and expressing the concept that "if the accommodation of the professors and the instruction of the students should ever be found, in any respect, incompatible with the immediate interess of humanity, there can be no doubt which must be preferred."[55]

Speaking more as a hospital manager (he occupied such a position for several years) than as an attending professor, James Gregory sought to reaffirm a similar concept when he emphasized in his printed memorial of 1803 that the Royal Infirmary of Edinburgh was primarily instituted for "the relief of the sick poor, not for the general interests of science." He went on to say that the latter "no doubt *must* eventually be promoted by a well-managed hospital, but this eventual benefit *must* result as a secondary object from the faithful accomplishment of the first and chief purpose of such a charitable institution."[56]

Clearly then, the managers themselves believed and the infirmary subscribers expected that the charitable goals of the hospital would receive the highest priority. Medical interests, whether investigative or educational, although they were often not incompatible with these aims, nonetheless had to take a back seat. In fact, John Bell, a hospital surgeon feuding with the clinicians around 1800, even went so far as to propose that the teaching ward be discreetly "shrouded from public view." "A clinical hospital, erected with the avowed design of receiving desperate and forlorn cases, of practicing experiments, of teaching the profession to young physicians, of proving the hypotheses of medicine and trying, by experience, the efficacy of drugs, will never pass upon the world for a mere charity," Bell wrote. He concluded his controversial sketch by remarking that "those who entered by sad necessity into such a hospital would believe themselves every way lost."[57]

In response, Gregory argued that the teaching ward could not possibly be "shrouded from public view on account of the extraordinary number of students who frequent it."[58] The best protection from potentially harmful practices directed at patients was professional scrutiny and peer pressure. Gregory was keenly aware that those responsible for patient care in the teaching unit, more so than in any other ward, operated in a true fishbowl atmosphere. They were all prominent professors of medicine with reputations to maintain, constantly forced to justify and explain their actions to colleagues, clerks, and students. "It would be for the benefit of all patients, in hospitals and not in hospitals, if their physicians were obliged to read clinical lectures on their cases," stressed Gregory. He could not conceive of any "human contrivance that can more effectually and irresistibly oblige the physician to study carefully the case of his patient." Finding himself "under the necessity of giving a minute account of everything that he has done in a very public manner, and before a number of competent judges," was a challenge that spurred the physician to do his very best.[59]

In Gregory's view the accountability of those operating in the teaching ward did not stop with the more than one hundred students frequenting the infirmary each year. Every prescription and procedure "indirectly but very speedily may be known to all their acquaintances, to every medical student at the University, and to many hundreds or thousands of the inhabitants of this city." Consequently, Gregory concluded that "any extraordinary, and especially any dangerous experiment certainly would be thus generally known and would become a subject of general animadversion."[60]

To avoid patient opposition to admission into the teaching ward, the public had to be amply reassured that medical care in that unit was at least comparable to if not better than that offered in other parts of the hospital. Gregory therefore argued in print that the teaching ward was in fact the most dangerous place to perform experiments, a word he considered misleading and an unfair label for the cautious trial-and-error approach he and others believed they were engaged in.

According to Gregory, no trials of medicines were to be conducted in the hospital before they had already been tested in private practice.[61] At least on paper, he insisted that only well-tried and universally successful remedies were to be prescribed and that theoretical schemes espoused by university professors would never affect their therapeutics. Wrote Gregory: "Supposing a professor so mad or so unprincipled as to attempt for the amusement of his pupils, to practice according to the various theories of medicine, nineteen in twenty of which he *must* know to be false; the result of his practice *must* not only be destruction to his patients but ipso facto a refutation of those theories."[62]

Gregory's remarks should be interpreted as a calculated public defense of clinical teaching, made necessary in part by the accusations of several surgeons, including John and Benjamin Bell, as well as by the writings of Francis Home. Gregory not only objected to the title *Clinical Experiments* Home had selected for his book[63] but also sought to ameliorate the overall impact of the professor's candid remarks about the utility of therapeutic trials conducted in the hospital. Home, in fact, had already written that "conclusions from experiments made in the teaching ward must meet with more credit than those derived from private practice as they are performed before so many spectators."[64]

Finally, there were also raised at the Edinburgh infirmary questions of medical etiquette characteristic of a teaching setting. Because the success of clinical instruction was partly based on bedside discussions of each case by attending physicians, university professors, clerks, and students, the patients were bound to hear at least portions of such deliberations even when carried out at some distance from the beds. In one of his works James Gregory considered the impropriety of carrying on these conferences and the "cruelty of speaking freely of the nature and danger of the diseases," a behavior necessarily bound to heighten the anxiety of the sick. In Gregory's opinion such discussions were more proper during the clinical lectures delivered away from the wards in a special room of the hospital.[65] Yet everyone in the infirmary recognized that a fair amount of discussion in the halls was inevitable, and Gregory, for one, suggested that some of the conversations, especially diagnoses and prescriptions, be uttered solely in Latin as a "matter of delicacy and kindness."[66]

Patient selection

To illustrate their lectures, professors sharing the clinical rotation admitted the necessary number of patients to the teaching ward at the start of their individual terms. The usual procedure was for the teacher and a hospital clerk to visit the infirmary's waiting room and interrogate prospective patients. Criteria for selection varied somewhat among faculty members. James Gregory, for example, explained, "My rule of choosing patients for the clinical wards, and I presume the other professors have followed nearly the same, has always been to take acute cases (fevers, inflammations) in preference to chronic cases (palsies, dropsies, convulsions, etc), and of the chronic cases to take always the *worst* and mosturgently dangerous."[67]

In fact, Gregory worried that some of his admissions could turn out to be incurable and thus according to the infirmary statutes "improper" for hospitalization. The result of his selection was a higher mortality rate among patients admitted to the teaching ward. His statement can be statistically validated. For Gregory's rotation from November 1, 1795, to January 30, 1796, sixty-four patients were admitted to the clinical ward. Their cure rate was only 46%, with a total mortality of 9.3%, while the official hospital statistics for 1795 and 1796 revealed cure rates of 70% and mortalities of 5.3% and 4.6%, respectively.[68]

Cullen was also inclined to admit and present to the students acute or subacute cases "such as will admit of frequent trials in practice," rather than protracted and chronic conditions with uncertain evolution and outcome. Whenever possible, rare clinical conditions were similarly omitted from admission and presentation, because Cullen felt that diseases of "a more ordinary appearance" were of greater didactic value to students.[69] Francis Home seemed somewhat more resigned to getting subacute and chronic cases. "The practice in hospitals is different in many respects from the private exertions of the art," he lectured to his students, adding, "As people do not come to hospitals but in obstinate cases and where a variety of medicines have been tried, hence diseases of long standing must be sent there."[70]

In addition to patients directly selected in the admissions room, professors also received a number of people whose original warrants were signed by the ordinary physicians. "Sometimes when patients having uncommon diseases are received by the ordinary physicians, they are reclaimed by the clinical professors, the rightful lords of the manor," wryly observed John Bell. Since no similar arrangement existed for surgery, Bell was jealous of the power given to the faculty members for filling up their ward with interesting cases: "They walk in among these patients, look at them, hand their nosological labels and tallies round their necks."[71]

Transfers to and from the teaching ward were often initiated by the professors a few days after admission or after the patient had reached a convalescent state.[72] Duncan insisted that the latter be sent to an ordinary ward, "that I might have a variety of cases to lecture on."[73] However, relocations could only happen with the express consent of the ordinary physicians and, more important, "if the patient himself was willing."[74] Interested in the effects of an hyoscyamus extract on a person with chronic rheumatism, Cullen "took this patient into our ward" in December 1772 to conduct further clinical tests with the drug.[75] Other people were admitted to the teaching unit simply because there was a scarcity of "interesting" patients.

During Cullen's six-month rotation in 1772–1773 he presented seventy-nine patients in class, some in more detail than others, illustrating about twenty-four clinical conditions.[76] Gregory's regular three-month rotation in 1779–1780 allowed him to present thirty-five patients afflicted with about nineteen clinical conditions.[77] Cullen's and Gregory's selection of cases each provided a cross section of the pathology most commonly seen in the infirmary. As expected, over half of the clinical sessions were devoted to discussions of fevers, catarrhs, and rheumatic ailments. Because of their seasonal incidence, both professors devoted several weeks in January to an extensive discussion of fevers, their various types, possible causes, and treatment. An examination of Andrew Duncan's lectures during his three-month rotation in 1795 discloses that patients were discussed under thirty-three different categories of disease, almost double the number presented by Cullen and Gregory.[78] Whenever possible, the instructors collected patients afflicted with similar illnesses to discuss their resemblances and point out the features that distinguished one case from another.

A foreign observer who spent two months visiting Edinburgh in 1789 had harsh criticism for the clinical instruction then given by James Gregory and Francis Home. According to this source, students were not clearly told what to observe in the patients during daily rounds, pulse taking was sloppy, and physical signs (including respiratory frequency; the condition of skin, tongue, and eyes; and palpation of the abdomen) were pretty well ignored. Professors allegedly dictated prescriptions for new medicines to the accompanying clerk without taking the trouble to explain the rationale for their employment to students. Even more serious was the charge that in those two months only four cases from the teaching ward were fully presented during clinical lectures; the other patients were considered only once each, with a perfunctory reading of symptoms and discussion of underlying pathology.[79]

From the reconstruction of the clinical courses, including those of Francis Home and John Gregory, it seems clear that the foreign source vastly exaggerated the deficiencies of Edinburgh's teaching system. Professors were always willing to discuss individual cases in greater detail and to include them in several lectures. Likewise, infirmary teachers did not just stage specific illustrations of particular diseases. Rather, they spoke about the clinical features and treatment of individual patients following admission, during hospitalization, and after discharge. From the particular clinical manifestations and reactions, the Edinburgh instructors then moved to a consideration of the disease species they seemed to embody and mode of treatment. In the discussions professors always mentioned the patient's name before considering a nosological label, although many student notebooks, for didactic reasons, often carried as title of a case the disease entity.

Cullen's 1772–1773 clinical lectures also reveal the difficulties confronting instructors in maintaining a representative number of good teaching cases. "I wish they [patients] were of a better kind but I found it difficult to select twelve patients that could be the subject of our practice," Cullen told the audience during his second lecture; "but that will mend, I hope, daily."[80] Having presented a number of simple fevers, mild skin eruptions, and rheumatic conditions, the professor found that his fortunes failed to improve. Another patient, admitted with a simple catarrh, turned out to be a malingerer. "She was one of my first patients owing to the scarcity of good patients in the house," lamented Cullen, "and she has afforded very little grounds for remarks."[81] In the ensuing weeks, Cullen continued to grumble during his lectures about being forced to discuss "insignificant" or "trifle" patients. Yet later in the course, talking about a mild respiratory ailment affecting one of the patients, he reassured his listeners that while "this was a slight case, I propose to speak of every patient upon my list and there are very few cases that will not give occasion to remarks that may be useful."[82]

At times patients were deliberately kept in the teaching ward beyond the usual discharge time. Revealing in this contest is a statement made by Cullen to his students while discussing a patient suffering from pulmonary tuberculosis. Although the routine procedure was to dismiss such cases promptly for fresh "country air" after they showed symptomatic improvement, Cullen retained this patient "to give you an opportunity of observing the progress of such a disease."[83]

As each professor's rotation came to an end, new cases ceased to be admitted to the teaching ward and every conceivable convalescent was discharged. The intent of the faculty members was to empty the unit in order to allow the incoming instructor to select his own patients. For the professor lecturing in late spring in the years before 1791, it meant closing the ward altogether until the following November, when instruction resumed at the university. Those remaining were all transferred to the care of the ordinary physician on the last day of the semester. "Good thing that poor people do not have the sensibilities of the rich," commented John Bell, in referring to this arbitrary emptying out of the clinical ward.[84] For the entire faculty this was also an excellent opportunity to eliminate from their charges what Cullen called "stick fast" patients suffering from difficult or intractable chronic conditions that were not amenable to medical treatment, persons who, as James Gregory sarcastically put it, "are so uncivil that they will neither die nor recover."[85]

Diseases in the teaching ward, 1771–1799

Information on 808 cases, which may be broken down as indicated in Table 5.3, was inscribed in casebooks between 1771 and 1799. The percentages included in Table 5.3, though they simply reflect the contents of thirteen

Table 5.3. *Cases from the teaching ward, 1771–1799*

Infectious diseases: 203 cases, 25.12% of total

Ague	31	Rubeola	5
Breast infection	1	Slow fever	2
Cynanche parotidea (mumps)	1	Smallpox	16
Fever	66	Synochus	13
Leg inflammation	1	Typhus	60
Measles	2	Ulcer of face and nose	2
Nose infection	1	Whooping cough	1
Puerperal fever	1		

Respiratory diseases: 127 cases, 15.71% of total

Asthma	3	Hemoptysis	5
Catarrh	31	Pectoral complaint	21
Cynanche tonsillaris	12	Phthisis	24
Dyspnea	3	Pleurisy	3
Epistaxis	2	Pneumonia	23

Diseases of the digestive system: 89 cases, 11.01% of total

Cholera accidentalis	1	Enteritis	2
Colic	4	Hematemesis	3
Colica pictonum	8	Hepatitis	2
Diarrhea	19	Icterus	8
Dysentery	2	Ileus	3
Dyspepsia	29	Worms	8

Neurological and mental diseases: 82 cases, 10.14% of total

Neurological		Mental	
Anesthesia	1	Apoplexia mentalis	1
Apoplexy	1	Hypochondriasis	3
Atrophy	1	Hysteria	17
Cephalgia	5	Melancholia	4
Convulsions	1		
Chorea St. Vitii	4		
Epilepsy	8		
Hemiplegia	11		
Paralysis	24		
Tinnitus	1		

Musculoskeletal disorders: 78 cases, 9.65% of total

Contraction of toe	1	Rheumatism, acute	33
Gout	2	Rheumatism, chronic	27
Rheumatism	13	Sciatica	2

Circulatory disorders: 73 cases, 9.03% of total

Anasarca	28	Hydrocephalus	3
Ascites	17	Hydrothorax	12
Dropsy	9	Palpitation	1
Hemorrhoids	3		

Table 5.3. *(cont.)*

Genitourinary diseases: 66 cases, 8.16% of total			
Amenorrhea	14	Hysteritis	1
Calculus or stone	1	Ischuria	3
Catarrh vesica (bladder)	2	Leucorrhea	8
Diabetes	5	Lues venerea	14
Dysuria	2	Menorrhagia	7
Enuresis calculosa	1	Nephritis	2
Gonorrhea	2	Phymosis	1
Hematuria	1	Sibbens	2

Eye problems: 43 cases, 5.32% of total			
Amaurosis	10	Ophthalmia	32
Caligo	1		

Diseases of the skin: 34 cases, 4.20% of total			
Erysipelas	12	Lepra	9
Erythema	1	Skin eruption	3
Herpes	7	Tinea capitis	2

Tumors and cancers: 8 cases, 0.99% of total			
Cancer of the nose	1	Scrofula	2
Hydrops ovarii	1	Tumor	3
Scirrhous mamma	1		

Miscellaneous: 5 cases, 0.61% of total			
Anomalous complaint	3	Smallpox inoculation	1
Debilitas senilis	1		

student casebooks, nevertheless confirm statements made by the clinical professors regarding patient selection. It seems clear that the teaching ward, accounting for about 10% of all hospital admissions, received a representative sample of patients suffering from medical ailments. In each category, however, the faculty tried to manage the most acute diseases, including typhus, smallpox, ophthalmia, and rheumatism, and challenging instances of such severe chronic problems as phthisis, colica pictonum, hysteria, rheumatism, anasarca, ascites, diabetes, and amenorrhea. Not unexpectedly, mortality rates for these patients were at least twice as high as in the other hospital wards.

INSTRUCTIONAL OBJECTIVES

"Clinical lectures are to the practice of medicine what dissection is to anatomy – it is demonstration," attested another contemporary student guide; "by clinical lectures disease is, as it were, embodied and brought before the student, as a subject for his leisure examination."[86] Essential for such a demonstration was breadth of scope in the health problems that could be brought before the eyes and minds of the assembled student body. Most medical educators agreed that hospital training in the late eighteenth century undoubtedly had the advantage of furnishing a larger number of cases and greater diversity of clinical situations than provided by practical apprenticeships where students just followed masters on their visits to private patients. One daily hour of rounds in the infirmary easily provided more observation and discussion than days or even weeks of individual house calls. "These advantages belong still in a higher degree to the clinical ward of the Royal Infirmary of Edinburgh," wrote Francis Home, "as the best marked diseases, the most singular in nature and the greatest variety of acute as well as chronic, are chosen for it."[87]

Just as important was continuity in the observation of patients and daily access to them. Making daily visits by themselves and in company of attending physicians and faculty members allowed for close follow-up of clinical developments and observation of the dietary and medicinal adjustments instituted in response to perceived changes. Open access to hospital patients at all times of day and night would have been ideal for the students, but such conditions would have implied a complete disregard for patient privacy and were not tolerated in Edinburgh. Yet in spite of restrictions, medical and surgical students training at the hospital during the last decades of that century could visit patient by themselves daily for one hour in the morning and then make rounds with attending staff, clerks, apothecary, or rotating faculty. In the afternoon there was one additional hour spent with surgical dressers, and finally there were at times evening rounds with the ordinary physicians.

This schedule brought students into frequent contact with patients. Consequently, a behavioral objective of clinical instruction was to sensitize the students to the plight of poor people and help them develop empathy for the sick. "In our profession," wrote John Bell, "young men should have instilled into their minds that sympathy with the sufferings of their young patients." The hospital was a perfect place to acquire a desire to help those in distress: "To become skillful," asserted Bell, "a man must live among the sick; he must have lively feelings and a sympathizing nature; he must have the inward sympathy with the distresses of his fellow creature."[88]

The general plan of clinical instruction or *Collegium Casuale* first called for the development of examination skills. "Examining the patient," lectured Francis Home, "lays the foundation of all our knowledge."[89] The term applied primarily to what is now considered clinical history taking, not physical examination. A coherent report of the presenting complaints was linked to possible remote and proximate causes, a kind of past and family history elucidated from the patient. Then age, way of life, profession, and especially constitution and temperament (a somewhat vague concept covering hereditary, physical, and psychological variables) were ascertained. The "deserving" poor, of course, were generally believed to have more robust constitutions than the idle rich. The second step of the examination was an inspection of the tongue, throat, and eyes and a quick check of the bodily habit, position, and discharges.[90] The head of the patient was to be kept straight, and to avoid contagion the student was urged to take only a side view of mouth and throat, supplementing this preventive measure with frequent rinsings of his own mouth in a solution of vinegar and water.[91]

After collecting all the particulars volunteered by the patient and further questioning to ascertain "the exact degree in which symptoms occur," students were urged to combine these reports with their findings from the physical inspection. Cullen insisted on "full and proper" observations, telling his pupils that 90% of the recorded clinical histories were incomplete and contained serious errors. In his view many manifestations of sickness passed unnoticed even to the trained professional eye. The patient's own judgment of the presenting problem could be quite misleading, and most symptoms still escaped exact measurement that could establish their degree of importance. "We can measure the frequency of the pulse by a stopwatch," asserted Cullen, "but we have no measure for the hardness and fulness of one pulsation."[92] Most judgments were qualitative, highly speculative, and vague.

After students gathered all this information at the bedside they went on to determine the type of disease affecting each patient and its species and possible class. The contemporary imperfection of classificatory schemes, though freely acknowledged and generously documented by professors like Cullen, was no impediment to attempts to label the patients according to the "true state of physic." Moreover, Cullen's listeners were encouraged to participate in efforts to perfect nosology by making careful observations and writing detailed clinical histories, "collecting the observations of different men, ages, and countries," a program dear to Cullen's vision of the future.[93]

Methods of cure needed to be developed on the basis of more accurate diagnoses and classifications. "Within these fifty years there have been many unusual remedies offered to the public, each of them little short of universal remedies," lectured Cullen, "but however difficult it may be to disprove these in particular, many of them must be fallacious."[94] The problem, as he explained it, was that most clinical phenomena had not been well enough described and differentiated to justify specific therapeutic indications, while useful distinctions between the phenomena of disease and drug effects remained imperfect. "From novelty, omission, mistake, malice, design, our medical histories are necessarily incomplete, erroneous and false, and so not at all sufficient to enable us to distinguish diseases from one another and are unfit for founding a decisive practice."[95]

Such frequent admonitions reflected an attitude and approach that characterized much of the teaching carried out at the infirmary. Indeed, one of the most important goals of clinical instruction was the acquisition of healthy doses of skepticism and caution. "It is of great use in medicine to show that what we trust to does not deserve our confidence," remarked Home.[96] Cullen, in turn, confided, "I still find occasion for more doubts the more I advance in practice and study"; he went on to tell his students that "for the first year of your practice you may have doubts while you are full of your acquired knowledge, but for seven years to come they will be always increasing."[97] Indeed, a perusal of Cullen's candid statements during his frequently informal lectures makes it abundantly clear that he was by far the most outspoken and skeptical teacher visiting the infirmary. Rash conclusions and lack of caution could be hurtful to both the patients' health and the physicians' reputation. "I suppose like most other young doctors that you are very ready and decisive in your judgment," he remarked, but he warned that this false veneer of certainty could be costly at the sickbed.[98]

Cullen indeed insisted that students be fully acquainted with the sources of uncertainty and error in medicine. He repeatedly stressed in his lectures that every pupil should be aware that it was difficult to make complete observations. Lack of attention, bias in favor of certain medical systems, partiality toward specific remedies – all were for Cullen sources of false experience. Above all, Cullen stressed that there was no place for a rigid adherence to the hypotheses and theories of previous medical authorities. In his opinion they merely provided points of departure, temporary platforms from which to view the evidence and gather new facts that could correct or change the old systems.[99] Cullen's antidogmatic attitude was echoed by James Gregory in his own lectures and writings: Theory was merely a connecting medium linking and arranging facts of observation, and no physician was to be "too strongly nor blindly attached to it."[100]

Distrusting the testimony of previous medical authors was as important as guarding against errors in observation. "In the present age where writing is so easy and so much encouraged," asserted Cullen in his concluding clinical lecture of 1773, "there is a great ground for suspecting facts which the vanity of making a book or the interest of vending one give occasion to."[101] For Cullen honesty in acknowledging the limitations of medical art was paramount, and throughout his lectures he repeatedly confessed his own ignorance. "I cannot put you off with a Greek or cramp [difficult to make out] word as I am obliged to do other people," he quipped on one occasion.[102] During reviews of other cases he remarked, "I hope I am very safe in acquainting you with my failures if you are severe critics; I know how to hide them on other occasions,"[103] and "I am not ashamed to say that I do fail in judgment and shall never hide a doubt with regard to a doctrine I advance or a practice I follow; I think candour requires it."[104]

Not as visible in lecture notes from other instructors, such frankness was apparently criticized by Cullen's peers. "Some of my colleagues tell me that I am imprudent in telling you my faults," Cullen acknowledged, arguing, however, that it was better to admit his shortcomings than to have alert students discover the mistakes and be forced to keep silent so as not to embarrass the teacher. This, he insisted, was the only "proper means" of treating the students.[105]

THE DIDACTIC ROLE OF AUTOPSIES

In one of his clinical lectures delivered in 1772 Cullen noted: "It is not improperly said that the earth hides the faults of physicians. If every patient that dies were opened, it would too often discover the frivolity of our conjectures and practice."[106] Cullen's statement reflects the importance he assigned to pathological anatomy and clinicopathological correlations, a topic he occasionally discussed with students. Private practice had hitherto discouraged most attempts to dissect those who died. The statement "my patients being numerous and situated at a great distance from each other, I had no opportunity of obtaining permission to open the body,"[107] was representative of conditions faced by most eighteenth-century British practitioners. Even when the rare occasion of real need arose, it was difficult to secure consent for an autopsy, given the nature of the private patient–physician relationship.

Hospitals, on the other hand, seemed to create favorable conditions for the performance of postmortem dissections. Inpatients belonged to a lower social class than private patients and were indebted for the free medical care received. Many of them were newcomers to the city, living alone without relatives. Under those circumstances, requests for autopsies were frequently unnecessary.

In many European countries, including France and Austria, hospital admissions frequently contained a tacit or formal agreement that a postmortem examination would be performed if the patient died in the institution. The situation was quite different in charitable British establishments like the Edinburgh infirmary. To be sure, managers had authorized dissections since the inception of the hospital, but they followed a series of rules designed to protect the public image of the institution as guardian of the sick poor defending them from coercive demands and abuse by the medical staff. Therefore, according to established infirmary regulations, attending physicians and surgeons interested in autopsies had first to secure permission from relatives or friends of the deceased, "if any such are at hand," to avoid "violation of the feelings of those most nearly concerned." If successful, the practitioners then secured an order signed by at least three current hospital managers before actually scheduling the dissection.[108]

Approval from next of kin was often withheld, "even in cases in which it is most to be wished for the improvement of medicine and the good of mankind," lamented James Gregory.[109] In a fatal case of typhus fever, even Cullen was denied permission: "I was desirous to have a dissection but the interposition of his friends was violent and prevented us."[110] Cultivating a good relationship with relatives of the dying patient could prove beneficial, as in one case during the 1780s. Diagnosed by infirmary surgeons as suffering from an inguinal bubo instead of an incarcerated hernia, the man "eloped" from the hospital and returned to his home a few miles outside Edinburgh, where he died three days later. The "rupturist" faction of surgical consultants, eager to vindicate their diagnostic verdict, traced the patient to his home and persuaded his relatives to bring the body back to the hospital. An autopsy was performed to demonstrate to colleagues and students the true nature of the ailment.[111]

In a reversal of the usual circumstances, relatives during the 1770s actually took the initiative in asking for one dissection. In one of his clinical lectures Cullen related the case of an infant with confluent smallpox, briefly seen at the infirmary in the early stages of the disease but not considered sick enough to warrant hospitalization. "I regret not taking the opportunity the mother offered of examining the child by dissection," he said after the baby died at home some time later. A ten-year-old boy seen by James Gregory in 1785 with a diagnosis of hydrocephalus was discharged without improvement. At the end of his clinical history the student scribbled the following entry: "After continuing sometime at home he died suddenly. Leave was obtained to open the head."[112]

After 1750 the only persons exempted from the requirement of obtaining a dissection warrant from the hospital managers were university professors in charge of the teaching ward.[113] This privilege especially irritated the attending surgeons and became one reason for their criticisms of "the lords of the manor." According to James Gregory, however, autopsy requests were seldom denied by the hospital authorities. In the end, all formalities were designed to signal to the general public that autopsies were not performed merely "for the gratification of idle curiosity, or as making the hospital a school, and the dead patients the subjects of anatomical instruction."[114]

Concern that the public image of the hospital could be tarnished by linkage with a procedure mostly repugnant and incomprehensible to the laity seems to have influenced many official decisions about this matter. In December 1759, for example, one attending surgeon, a Mr. Stratton, conducted a private autopsy in the infirmary's deadroom or morgue without official permission from the managers. As it turned out, the deceased was a soldier who had received a fatal head injury in a fight with a comrade. The surgeon, in the company of two apprentices, not only dissected the head to ascertain the nature of the wound but also amputated the victim's legs, since he was out of practice and scheduled the following day to perform such an operation on a living patient. Sensing that violations of this sort would only provide grist for the rumor mill that the dead were actually dismembered, the authorities dismissed the surgeon from the hospital, indicating that the "welfare of the house is deeply concerned." The managers likewise reaffirmed their policy of being in control of all postmortem authorizations; dissections had to be conducted publicly in the operating theater in "the presence of the licensed students informed of the time by an advertisement put up in the consulting room."[115]

Autopsies were indeed carried out in the third-floor amphitheater before a hastily assembled group of interested students. A set of regulations approved in July 1769 insisted that the actual dissection be done by one of the attending surgeons or a person employed under his direction, usually one of the student assistants. After the examination, the body had to be properly sewed up and dressed before being delivered to relatives for interment. The surgeon or student then wrote a report of his dissection, which was "delivered to the physician's clerk with the injunction to insert it immediately into the ward journal."[116]

Hospital regulations that were approved in 1792 directly assigned the performance of postmortem examinations to the surgical clerk assisted by dressers, thus placing the execution and reporting entirely in the hands of students. The clerk was also enjoined to be "particularly attentive that every thing be conducted decently."[117] However, this stipulation was not always observed. In 1794 a dresser testified that John Bell, one of the attending surgeons, "did in two instances carry off certain parts of the dead bodies of patients on whom he had performed operations."[118] A committee appointed to investigate the charges substantiated them, but Bell, in his defense, insisted that "the preservation of diseased parts might have a real utility in future practice." Although the well-known Edinburgh surgeon apologized for his actions, he was nevertheless dismissed from hospital service. The managers again proclaimed "the utmost delicacy to be necessary in regard to every patient who is received into the house, sensible that if any indecorums of that nature are rumored abroad might be of essential prejudice to the hospital."[119]

Given the low mortality rate of patients admitted to most voluntary British hospitals and especially the Edinburgh infirmary, opportunities for conducting autopsies were rare. Furthermore, since permissions from relatives of the deceased were not always granted, the number of actual dissections was substantially lower. From student casebooks, for example, it appears that during each three-month rotation, only three to five patients hospitalized in the teaching ward died. Barely half of them were subjected to post-

Table 5.4. *Deaths and autopsies at the infirmary, 1770–1800*

Year	Physician	Total no. of deaths	Mortality rate (%)	Autopsies	Autopsy rate (%)
Teaching ward					
1771–1772	John Gregory	4	8.3	2	50
1773–1774	William Cullen	6	7.7	3	50
1779–1780	James Gregory	4	4.7	3	75
1780–1781	Francis Home	5	9.0	3	60
1781–1782	James Gregory	6	5.7	3	50
1785–1786	James Gregory	7	10.5	4	57
1786–1787	Francis Home	3	5.7	0	0
1795	Andrew Duncan, Sr.	4	6.5	4	100
1795–1796	James Gregory	6	9.3	3	50
1796–1797	Thomas C. Hope	5	7.9	2	40
1799	Daniel Rutherford	7	7.4	3	42
		Total: 57		Total: 30	Ave: 52
Non–teaching ward					
1773		3	6.5	1	33.3
1774		1	2.9	0	0
1775		4	8.0	0	0
1776		2	1.7	0	0
1781	John Hope	6	18.1	5	83.3
1784–1785	Henry Cullen	2	4.1	0	0
		Total: 18		Total: 6	Ave: 33.3

Sources: Casebooks and ward ledgers.

mortem examinations. During the late eighteenth century, then, Edinburgh medical students could look forward to witnessing only one or two autopsies during their entire clinical course (see Table 5.4).

However, these dissection rates applied only to medical cases. A perusal of James Russell's 1784–1792 cases and William Brown's 1790–1810 cases gives the impression that surgeons at the Edinburgh infirmary were more successful in obtaining autopsies of their patients, especially those previously subjected to a number of procedures.[120] Attending surgeons were possibly more eager to procure them, since the postmortem findings were of practical importance for their future interventions. In marked contrast with procedure in the medical cases, surgeons went into considerable anatomical detail when writing their reports, describing the local pathological conditions encountered during the dissection. In the case of a man admitted in September 1787 with a shoulder injury and subjected to surgery to repair arterial damage, the surgeons conducted an autopsy to prove the success or failure of their vascular ligatures when the man died five days after his operation. During the final dissection they injected the various arterial trunks in the axilla with liquid wax to determine their patency and the effectiveness of sutures.[121]

In medical cases the postmortem examinations were primarily carried out to ascertain the immediate causes of death. Most of the descriptions contained in student casebooks suggest only partial or restricted examinations. One male patient who had suffered from a diarrhea had only his abdomen inspected; a cancerous growth was found in the stomach.[122] In the case of a servant who succumbed to smallpox, the autopsy simply read, "No praeternatural appearance but lungs in a very inflammed state."[123] The description of a patient who had died of suspected phthisis read, "Thorax, abdomen, and most of the viscera in a very distended state. Many swollen and enlarged glands. Kidneys enlarged and full of tubercules. Pericardium contained an unusual amount of water."[124]

It is of course possible that the surviving casebooks reproduced, in a highly abbreviated form, only the most salient findings of each autopsy, hastily jotted down by students in a great hurry to complete their copying. However, remarks made by Edinburgh professors during their clinical lectures tend to confirm the suspicion that contemporary dissections were fragmentary and superficial. Even Cullen's few clinicopathological correlations were vague and limited.[125] When James Gregory in 1779 reported the autopsy findings of a suspected case of phthisis to his students, he merely pointed out that "the lungs were completely obstructed with tubercles, many of them suppurated." The only other information conveyed was that "much water was found in the pericardium and thorax, 23 ounces by measure," and that this fluid contained "much gluten, so perhaps we should have weighted it."[126]

Duncan, presenting a case of chronic catarrh to his students in 1795, summarized the autopsy findings by simply declaring that "on dissection no particular morbid appearances were found." Moreover, in two cases diagnosed as dropsy, one corpse "was opened up with a view to discover whether any particular organ was diseased," but no abnormalities or excessive bodily fluids were reported. The second dissection focused on the patient's cause of death, with Duncan telling his audience, "It appeared upon dissection that she [the patient] was cut off suddenly by water effused into the thorax and pericardium."[127]

When Edinburgh instructors encountered unexpected postmortem findings, they simply integrated them into their predetermined view of a given disease. Discussing a case with a long history of stomach complaints believed to be gout, Duncan admitted to his students that the surgeon in charge of the dissection had found a contracted stomach with a scirrhous growth suggestive of ulcer or cancer. "How far the scirrhous proceeded from the gout we can by no means satisfactorily say," reasoned Duncan; "we know that the gout will produce tophi, anchyloses, etc." In the end Duncan remained dubious about the results of the autopsy. The possibility that the patient may not have been suffering from gout or may have had two separate diseases was never raised.[128] This approach seems characteristic of all the cases copied into the casebooks or discussed in class and probably reflects the secondary importance ascribed to pathological findings, which were sought merely to illustrate preconceived diagnostic notions rather than to help shape new ones. No serious efforts were made to link the pathology to the patient's clinical manifestations or to use the lesions as criteria for redefining certain diseases.[129]

THE TEACHING OF SURGERY AND MIDWIFERY

All cases admitted to the teaching ward were medical, as were the patients discussed during clinical lectures, which were organized primarily for the benefit of medical students. Yet since its early years the infirmary had also trained a significant number of surgeons under the auspices of the Edinburgh Incorporation of Surgeons. In fact, training simultaneously in both medicine and surgery at the hospital was the goal of a growing number of students who had purchased admission tickets. Such joint education in the same clinical setting was thought to be responsible in good measure for "the very flourishing state of the Edinburgh Medical School for more than half a century past."[130]

At this time, most young men aspiring to become surgeons in the Scottish capital were made provisional members of the incorporation at an early age; a five-year apprenticeship with an established surgeon followed. This arrangement allowed students to accompany their masters to the hospital, where all of them witnessed surgical operations, some qualified as dressers, and a few appointed surgical clerks.[131] Many surgical apprentices also attended regular courses at the university, especially in human anatomy and materia medica.

On completion of their Edinburgh apprenticeship, surgical students generally made extensive trips to England and abroad, especially to France, familiarizing themselves with novel techniques and indications. "For a surgeon, I assure you Edinburgh comes greatly short of either Paris or London," wrote Benjamin Bell to his father in 1771.[132] Bell and James Hamilton, one of the attending physicians, traveled to Paris in 1772 and stayed at the house of Antoine Portal (1742–1832), the famous French surgeon. Others who were less wealthy usually joined the British army or navy for limited tours of duty. Those eventually returning to Edinburgh took three qualifying examinations under the supervision of the Incorporation of Surgeons. Successful candidates became full-fledged members of this organization and were thereby qualified to attend the infirmary as surgical assistants, operators, or consultants.[133]

Stimulated by the success of medical lectures, surgical apprentices repeatedly demanded similar instruction from some of their masters, "but hitherto none of the surgeons have found it proper to spare so much time from their own business as would be necessary for that purpose." In 1769 therefore, the Incorporation of Surgeons requested permission to organize clinical lectures at the Edinburgh infirmary. Reasoning that "it would bring obvious advantages to the Infirmary and the advancement of surgical education in our country," the hospital authorities immediately consented.[134]

The first instructor to give a systematic course of surgical lectures at the infirmary appears to have been James Rae, a prominent Edinburgh surgeon and dentist. Rae was among the sixteen surgeons listed by the incorporation as willing to attend the hospital, and he may have started his teaching as early as 1770. The course carried no official credit at the university, but the instructor followed a format initially developed at Surgeon's Hall, where for several years Rae had given "practical discourses on the cases of importance as they occur in the Royal Infirmary."[135]

"The chirurgical cases of the Royal Infirmary will be discoursed as they occur," an incorporation guidebook explained in November 1772; "the history of each will be given, the treatment as to internal medicines and external applications, the different practice with hospital patients from those who live in a higher sphere." The directory concluded that "practical observations and remarks will be offered on each case. Where operations are determined by the consulting surgeons, the result of their opinions will be mentioned, and the principal reasons on which their final determination was founded."[136]

During the 1770s the Edinburgh Incorporation of Surgeons publicly supported Rae's course of clinical lectures, recommending it "as useful and necessary to the students of physic and surgery" (again a reference to the combined clinical training made possible by the hospital managers). In addition to discussing selected cases admitted to the surgical ward of the infirmary, Rae was to receive from colleagues and present supplementary information concerning interesting and instructive private patients.[137] In the hospital itself, both Rae's lectures and rounds by attending surgeons were designed to foster an interest in pathology. Amputated limbs, for example, were carefullly dissected by the surgical clerk to point out the pertinent lesions, and the most interesting specimens were preserved for future instruction. "Models of some tumors, ulcers, and bad conformation of some parts, are preserved in wax or Paris plaster" and made to appear lifelike through artificial coloring.[138]

According to John Bell, who in 1790 opened his own private school of anatomy and surgery, every young man training for either surgery or medicine needed to be acquainted with the common traumatic ailments: wounds, luxations, and fractures.[139] The Edinburgh infirmary officially sanctioned such requirements and for many years encouraged students to witness the management of incoming surgical emergencies. Because these cases were brought in unexpectedly, no advance announcement could be posted, but the information was quickly communicated to visiting students by word of mouth. A reflection of the importance students ascribed to such instruction is contained in the 1785 controversy between the hospital authorities and the Royal Medical Society. As previously discussed, students vigorously objected to having access to the house curtailed and being "prevented from attending to the accidents that may be brought to the Infirmary."[140]

Finally, discussion of the scope of surgical teaching would be incomplete without a brief mention of the activities of surgical clerks and dressers. In the document in which they protested the curtailment of their access to the hospital, students stressed the usefulness of watching and assisting dressers in their daily chores. "A knowledge of the small operations and of the method of applying electricity is so necessary for every medical gentleman that it would be shameful to be ignorant of them," they wrote, a statement that once more reveals their interest and belief in a broad medicosurgical education.[141]

As a supplement to lectures and practical instruction in the wards, students attending the infirmary were periodically notified about the scheduling of surgical operations and encouraged to be present when they were carried out. "When an operation is performed in the Infirmary, Mr. Russell points out the reasons which render such expedients necessary, and the various proposals which may have been made in the mode of performing it," commented the Edinburgh student guide.[142] Most of the procedures were elective, decided on after extensive consultations, and executed if possible on Sunday afternoons, to accommodate the largest possible number of students, who had presumably fulfilled their religious obligations and enjoyed some free time. Between fifty and one hundred pupils usually attended, all seated in the third-floor amphitheater.[143] The theater also frequently doubled as a lecture hall, autopsy room, and chapel; it had been originally used as an astronomical observatory because of its cupola with ample windows. A visitor touring Britain in 1778 confirmed that "the operating room is excellently well adapted for the purpose of letting a great many persons see the operations there performed. The light is admitted from the top by a large skylight, and ranges of seats are elevated pretty high above each other for the more conveniently seeing the operations."[144]

The impressive surroundings and the large crowd witnessing the procedures were upsetting to both surgeons and patients. James Gregory recalled from his own student days in the early 1770s, "It was not uncommon for the students to bestow very freely their marks of approbation or disapprobation on different operators."[145] When a nervous surgeon with trembling hands attempted a delicate eye operation in 1774, the students' criticism became sufficiently vocal to warrant a severe reprimand from Alexander Wood, one of the attending surgeons. Another incident, also recounted by Gregory, occurred in the late 1780s, when student clapping and hissing during another surgical intervention led to the expulsion from the infirmary of those considered to be the main culprits.[146] In 1758 the managers explicitly banned operations "whereby the privy parts of women are exposed" unless special permission was first granted. Surprisingly for an infirmary manager and university professor who had successfully mediated the conflict between hospital and students, Gregory seemed to disagree with the sanctions imposed on spectators. He apparently believed, with many others, that the students who paid for their privilege of attending the infirmary also had a right to express their opinions, and that violations of hospital rules "never can hinder the students from judging of the real and comparative merits of the different surgeons."[147]

During the 1780s and early 1790s surgical attendance and instruction at the infirmary deteriorated. After 1786 clinical lectures were given by James Russell, a member of the Royal College of Surgeons (the incorporation had received its charter in 1778), but the extracurricular nature of the teaching – the student guide called it an "appendage" to the medical lectures – prevented sufficient academic recognition and provided little professional status to the instructor. The early success of James Rae's lectures had encouraged the incorporation to petition the crown in 1776 for the creation of a chair of clinical surgery at the university. Their candidate for the position was none other than James Russell. The move was designed to provide surgeons with a proper professional position on the medical faculty, since the incorporation viewed neither Alexander Monro secundus nor his teaching (some surgery was included in the regular anatomy course) as adequate. The request was unfortunately denied after a series of political maneuvers. With the support of his medical colleagues, Monro then went on to consolidate his position as a teacher of surgery by persuading the Edinburgh Town Council to authorize him in 1777 "to be professor of medicine and particularly anatomy and surgery."[148]

Little is known about the teaching of midwifery at the infirmary. As early as 1726 the Edinburgh Town Council, following a recommendation from the Incorporation of Surgeons, had created a "city professor of midwifery" with the express purpose of training local midwives. The holder of that position, Joseph Gibson, was a surgeon from the town of Leith, but there is no evidence that he ever lectured to medical students or visited the infirmary. After his death in 1739, Gibson was succeeded by another surgeon, Robert Smith, whose commission read "professor of midwifery at the city's college," an appointment that gave him official faculty status and broader teaching responsibilities, including possibly some lectures to medical students. Smith apparently resigned in 1755 and was replaced by another surgeon, Thomas Young, later deacon of the Incorporation of Surgeons; Young took a medical degree in 1761 and also became a fellow of the Royal College of Physicians.[149]

According to most sources, Young was the first professor of midwifery to organize a systematic course of lectures for medical and surgical students enrolled at the university. Later in the century the course gained in popularity but remained an elective in the official curriculum. To illustrate his instruction Young, who was on the roster of attending surgeons at the infirmary, petitioned the managers in 1755 to create a teaching ward reserved solely for obstetrical cases.[150] At their regular meeting on October 6, 1755, the authorities approved the report of a special committee organized to study the request, "fitting up the ward in the attic story of the east wing of the house." The rooms contained a total of eight beds and were to be kept open six months of the year. Institutional expenses for the first four hospitalized women were to be paid for by the infirmary, but Young was asked to contribute sixpence per day for each subsequent patient. Students enrolled in the midwifery course and interested in attending the new ward were furnished by the treasurer with the proper tickets at the usual price. Since presumably some of the persons observing the deliveries were only sporadic visitors, Young was empowered to make his own selection of participants and to pay the fee of half a guinea to the treasurer for each person without an official ticket.[151]

In 1760 Young sought to shift the expenses of keeping the first six patients lodged in the ward to the hospital authorities, citing the great expenses he was personally incurring. Because of increased revenues from the sale of tickets, the managers, always extremely cautious in financing new ventures, granted the request.[152] Two years later they also extended the occupancy of the lying-in ward to eight months, owing to growing student demand and interest in a summer course while the university was in recess.[153] Then in 1764 the hospital officials rescinded their previous authorization to Young permitting access to individuals without tickets. Believing that the arrangement had an inhibiting effect on attendance and citing the need for more income, the administrators demanded that henceforth all observers purchase admission tickets.[154]

Virtually nothing is known about the pregnant women admitted to Young's ward. They probably did not undergo the usual admission and discharge procedures reserved for patients. However, if complications arose, especially after childbirth, the women could be transferred to the ordinary wards. Cullen, in his 1772 clinical lectures, briefly mentioned palliative measures for one obstetrical patient who suffered from puerperal fever after what was described as a tedious labor.[155]

The 1792 student guide stated that "the practice of midwifery is acquired in the lying-in ward of the Royal Infirmary; but as it is on a very small scale Dr. Hamilton engages to furnish his pupils with *private deliveries* if they are very anxious to see much practice." These students were so-called annual pupils who paid ten guineas and were allowed to accompany the professor in his visits to private patients.[156]

Although the managers seem to have supported the principle of clinical instruction in midwifery at the infirmary, they constantly worried about the irregular hours of student and visitor attendance in that ward. After 1762 no evening visitors, meaning relatives and friends, were allowed. Throughout the 1785 confrontation with members of the Royal Medical Society, however, the authorities maintained that "attendance of students in the ward allotted to the professor of midwifery shall remain the same as formerly."[157] In 1790 a number of new complaints about disruption of hospital routines by the comings and goings of students reached the hospital officials. A committee appointed to study the actual closure of the obstetrical rooms nevertheless reported "that the lying-in ward in the hospital was an expedient establishment which ought not at present to be given up." The favorable report insisted on a strict enforcement of ticket sales to those attending the ward.[158]

Partially as a result of a feud between Daniel Rutherford, a manager and member of the Royal College of Physicians, and Alexander Hamilton, who had replaced Thomas Young as professor of midwifery in 1783, the question of closing the obstetrical ward was back on the managers' agenda the following year. This time the forces hostile to Hamilton and midwifery education prevailed. The modest income derived from the sale of admission tickets was apparently not worth the constant trouble of having students, nurses, and at times the parturient women themselves seeking admission at all hours of the day and night. Furthermore, the care of mothers and delivery of babies were not yet widely perceived as medical problems falling into the purview of charitable organizations devoted to the care of the sick.[159] "Maintaining the lying-in ward is attended with many inconveniences and has long been extremely prejudicial to the good order necessary to be kept in the house"; thus read the official statement issued by the infirmary to justify the closure.[160] Soon thereafter, Hamilton responded by requesting an extension while also presenting to the managers plans for a private lying-in hospital to be erected by private subscriptions in the city of Edinburgh. The ward at the infirmary was actually kept open for another year, until August 1793, when it was converted into a special female fever ward at Hamilton's suggestion.[161]

EDINBURGH AND EUROPE CONTRASTED

The limitations of clinical teaching at Edinburgh

Late eighteenth-century Edinburgh, with its population of about seventy thousand, was incapable of furnishing, in sheer numbers and categories, the panorama of human sickness available in major European centers that were ten times its size, places like London, Paris, or Vienna. Moreover, Edinburgh was not directly affected by the social and economic dislocations of the early Industrial Revolution. Few work-related illnesses and accidents found their way into the infirmary. As noted before, most of the medical admissions represented non–life-threatening diseases housed in the hospital for relatively brief periods of time.

With only about 150–200 beds in use after 1770 and a small teaching ward containing 25–50 patients, there was indeed a shortage of interesting, challenging cases and limited time to observe them. Thus many of the medical students taking courses at the University of Edinburgh supplemented their education by spending several months in London or Paris, "walking the wards" of the teaching hospitals to obtain what they perceived as broader clinical experience. Surgical apprentices, especially, saw the need for study elsewhere, given the paucity of patients requiring such care at the infirmary. Moreover, the hospital's teaching ward was completely shut down during summers until the early 1790s, and no clinical lectures were given then.

Medical education in London hospitals such as Guy's and St. Thomas's was eminently practical at that time and especially designed for surgical apprentices and apothecaries, who came to the wards for periods of six to twelve months and saw patients. Because most institutions lacked their own house staff, students followed only the voluntary attending staff on their rounds scheduled several times a week. "Pupil's business is only to look on and to make such enquiry as he shall choose of the surgeon who is attending," wrote one contemporary making rounds at Guy's Hospital.[162] In spite of this passive role and the difficulties inherent in clinical observations when too many pupils crowded around the sickbeds, students seem to have benefited from these experiences in London hospitals and kept recommending them to younger classmates.

The same lack of bedside responsibility hampered medical education at the Edinburgh infirmary. As in other British voluntary hospitals, professional interests remained subservient to the benevolent image and economic conditions influencing such charitable institutions. Hence student access to patients remained restricted, enforced by a set of regulations seeking to protect patient privacy and institutional routines. Indeed, students had barely one hour per day to visit and inspect patients on their own. For the rest of the time they just followed in the footsteps of professors, ordinary physicians, and student dressers making their daily rounds. In addition they climbed the amphitheater seats to witness operations and autopsies or listened to the biweekly clinical lectures.

When the Austrian physician Joseph Frank – son of the famous medical reformer Johann P. Frank – briefly visited Edinburgh in the summer of 1803, he commented on the fact that medical students at the infirmary were merely spectators at the sickbed.[163] Except for those few seniors hired as hospital clerks and the volunteer dressers, no Edinburgh student made decisions about the management of hospitalized patients. Even the clerks had primarily accounting duties and were quite busy taking dictation from the physicians, keeping ward journals and registers, or collecting money from paying patients. Surgical dressers and clerks were, of course, the exception. They could assist in the treatment of wounds, perform bleedings and cuppings, administer electricity, help out during operations, and carry out postmortem examinations.

The passive role dictated by the constraints of most charitable British organizations involved in hospital care was perhaps the most serious flaw of clinical instruction at the Edinburgh infirmary. Additionally, the paucity of autopsies hampered the development of pathological anatomy as a discipline that could furnish important criteria for the description and classification of diseases. As previously noted, low institutional mortality rates and frequent refusal by relatives of the dead to grant permission for dissections combined to provide students and professors with only rare opportunities to establish clinicopathological correlations. Because the actual dissection was a distasteful manual task unworthy of British gentlemen-physicians and a potential source of contagion, it was always delegated to relatively inexperienced surgical apprentices unfamiliar with the previous clinical evolution of the individual being examined. Thus professional barriers certainly compounded the problem originally created by the scarcity of corpses for dissection, preventing Edinburgh physicians and their students from assimilating lessons that could have been obtained from the deceased hospital patients.

On the other hand, Frank praised Edinburgh's educational system for having designed a comprehensive course of clinical lectures and having forced students attending the sessions to copy complete case histories of the patients to be discussed by the professor.[164] Compelling students to keep a diary of bedside events or to reproduce entire histories that were later reviewed in greater detail by those in charge of patient management was the next best thing if most pupils were barred from employing a direct, hands-on approach in their education. Clinical lectures and case copying were indeed compromises that reduced instruction at the bedside, often quite uncomfortable and frightening to the patients if many students attended. These evening discussions, in turn, allowed those who had failed to position themselves close to the professor or patient during rounds to listen and take comprehensive notes from a discussion of all therapeutic indications.

Other European models of clinical instruction

Frank's critique of clinical teaching at the Edinburgh infirmary was to a great extent based on his belief that senior students and recent medical graduates should be given direct responsibilities for patient care under the supervision of a professor. In expressing this aim Frank closely followed the opinions of his father and their shared educational experiences at the Universities of Pavia and Vienna. Selected students assigned to teaching wards of university-affiliated hospitals in both these cities did indeed assume duties for patient care.[165] There students' clinical histories were not merely copies from physician-dictated ward journals, as they were at Edinburgh, but individually composed narratives based on their own observations, judgments, and therapeutic decisions.

To understand this development it is necessary to examine briefly a series of proposals made by Johann P. Frank and his predecessor at the University of Pavia, the Swiss physician Samuel A. Tissot. In 1781 Tissot accepted an offer from the Austrian emperor Joseph II to become professor of clinical medicine at Pavia. His educational plans, first outlined on November 26, 1781, during the inaugural lecture, were at least partially implemented by the Archduke Ferdinand during Tissot's two-year tenure and were finally published in 1785.[166] His proposals took as their point of reference the activities of the "clinical hospital of Edinburgh," in Tissot's words "one of the best practical schools in existence in Europe."[167] To begin with, the new professor sought to reorganize the university-linked Ospedale di San Mateo in Pavia according to the Edinburgh infirmary model. The teaching-ward was to contain a total of twenty-four beds, equally divided between men and women. However, Tissot was quick to recommend that the functions of hospital director and chief of the teaching unit be combined, thereby ensuring that medical and pedagogical interests would receive the highest priority, rather than remain subservient to administrative and economic factors, as at Edinburgh.[168]

Tissot saw his teaching functions in the specially reserved "clinical" ward as mainly supervisory. He wanted to admit only acute cases to the hospital because he thought that they alone possessed enough educational value. Patients with chronic problems were simply not to be accepted. Tissot wanted each new arrival assigned directly after admission to two medical students, a senior acting as *chef* in charge of the case and a junior functioning as his assistant. The students had not only to conduct the initial interview and physical inspection but to compose their own clinical histories. After a diagnosis was established, the students prescribed the necessary therapeutic measures and followed the case until discharge, all under the immediate supervision of the clinical professor.[169]

In Tissot's opinion, such individualized assignments of incoming cases would not only protect the patients from large troops of students descending on their beds but give both the student *chef* and his assistant invaluable firsthand experience in patient management. Finally, those taking care of patients who died in the hospital were encouraged to perform their own dissections, the postmortem to be preceded by a brief review of the entire clinical history. To what degree Tissot's recommendations became reality still remains unclear. From remarks by his successor, Johann P. Frank, it appears that by 1783, the year of Tissot's departure, only twenty-four medical students were training at Pavia, although there were at least as many graduates from other universities attending the clinical rounds to acquire further experience.[170]

Frank, on his accession to the directorship at Pavia, brought ideas regarding clinical instruction quite similar to Tissot's. In addition to performing multiple administrative duties for the Austrian government in Lombardy, Frank became a very successful clinical teacher at Pavia. In his ten years there, student enrollment seems to have expanded, and he was able to implement most of Tissot's recommendations as well as some of his own. Like Tissot, Frank was impressed by the Edinburgh teaching program, and soon after his arrival he sought to establish a comprehensive patient registration system in the teaching ward, including some bedside charts with information usually reserved in Edinburgh for ward journals.[171]

Although Frank was also interested in the infirmary's biweekly clinical lectures – they gave professors enough time to prepare reasonably polished and learned presentations – he preferred that students acquire most of their experience directly at the bedside. Frank strongly believed that the more spontaneous discussions during ward rounds, all conducted in Latin in deference to the patients and foreign visitors, generated greater interest among the attending medical students. For Frank it was very important that students should observe the unrehearsed reactions of their professor, faced with changing conditions in his patients, trying to justify the use or cutoff of drugs.[172]

Like Tissot before him, Frank sought to restrict clinical instruction to students who had completed their theoretical medical courses, and he shared the conviction that selected seniors should gain firsthand knowledge concerning history taking, inspection of the patient, diagnosis, and treatment. Students were to respect the confidentiality of the hospitalized patients, conduct all bedside discussions in Latin, and ensure the modesty of the women housed in the teaching ward. Together with their professor, they assumed responsibilities for patient management.

Such a program of instruction, headed by Frank in his dual role of hospital director and clinical professor, was transferred in 1795 to the Allgemeines Krankenhaus in Vienna, the teaching hospital of the Vienna Medical School. Here Frank also managed to extend the total number of years spent on medical studies to five, the last one completely devoted to clinical training in the hospital. Between 1796 and his departure in 1804, Frank taught about three hundred medical students per year, allowing seniors to carry out diagnostic and therapeutic activities, the latter only with his prior approval. Although postmortem dissections were fairly common, Frank supplemented his pathological lectures through demonstrations[173] with a large number of preserved specimens depicting prominent lesions.

Finally, in contrast with Britain, surgery in prerevolutionary France flourished under royal patronage during the eighteenth century. In Paris surgeons made up almost all the medical staffs of the numerous city hospitals, and clinical instruction carried out in these institutions became quite traditional.[174] At the Hôtel-Dieu, for example, about a hundred positions for apprenticed surgeons were available after the 1720s. Similar organizational schemes existed at La Charité. The entire surgical house staff kept careful records and composed clinical histories. Working under the supervision of senior surgeons, the students examined, diagnosed, and treated the patients. Moreover, the students not only had direct patient responsibilities but also attended regular courses in anatomy and carried out postmortem examinations of those inmates who died.[175] Valuable clinicopathological correlations could be established and an awareness of local organic lesions fostered.[176] In contrast, medical students before the Revolution visited the wards sporadically, since such clinical training was not formally required by the university. If they came to the hospitals, however, they remained mere spectators watching their surgical colleagues carry out the clinical chores.

Given the high professional and social stature of French surgery before 1789, postrevolutionary reformers were quick to suggest a merger between medicine and surgery. Indeed, the new Paris School of Health, established in 1794, adopted and expanded the surgical organization and training program already functioning in hospitals. Philippe Pinel, one of the early figures of the new school, was very emphatic in proposing that third-year medical students be directly entrusted with the care of individual patients. Writing in his 1793 essay on medical instruction, Pinel sought to move students beyond their previous passive role, recommending that they begin to undertake the bedside activities that surgical apprentices had been in the habit of performing for decades. Like Johann P. Frank in Vienna, Pinel recommended that henceforth in Paris the periodic rounds by attending professors be simply occasions during which students presented their own reports. Standing at the bedside and in front of the entire group, the pupils should engage in informal discussions and receive comprehensive critiques of their performance from the professor before their therapeutic recommendations were implemented.[177]

CONCLUSION

In spite of the described shortcomings, clinical instruction at the Royal Infirmary of Edinburgh during the last decades of the eighteenth century was perceived to be among the best in all of Europe. What had begun as a modest, somewhat disorganized effort, because of the small number of hospital beds, gradually evolved into quite an important component of the educational opportunities available at the Edinburgh Medical School. The combination of daily bedside instruction during rounds and biweekly evening lectures linked the spontaneous responses in the ward with more polished review sessions filling in details and providing needed overviews. Although barred from managing patient care on their own because of the nature of British voluntary hospitals, students kept meticulous clinical notes and copied entire cases from ward journals. Such activities undoubtedly instilled in them a keen sense for bedside observation and fostered the idea that the events they observed ought to be organized and preserved in casebooks.

How important were such clinical experiences for the future careers of medical students enrolled at the Edinburgh Medical School? In addition to gaining opportunities for a direct observation of the most common diseases afflicting the population, students learned the basics of history taking, diagnosis, and therapeutic intervention. They also studied side by side with surgical apprentices in an atmosphere of relative tolerance and collegiality that certainly helped break down the age-old professional and social barriers separating them in Britain.

More important, students – most of them for the first time – were confronted with the plight of lower-class patients as they interrogated and examined them. The migrant farmer suffering periodic paroxysms of ague after weeks of traveling in a wagon from England, the feverish servant girl, exhausted from "watching" and surviving on meager fish scraps, the phthisic carter wasting away in a small tenement with a large, dependent family – all these cases unfolded before the eyes of the students. They indeed raised serious questions about the relationship between environment and disease and motivated many future physicians to play active roles in social reform movements.[178]

Above all, however, students attending the Edinburgh infirmary were exposed to the skepticism of William Cullen and James Gregory. Cullen's position was based in part on Hume's philosophical tenets; as noted, Cullen questioned every observation, judgment, and conclusion made at the bed-side.[179] When it came to patient care, he adopted an almost empirical attitude and remained his own harshest critic, freely acknowledging errors and omissions in lectures. Yet medical theory, he insisted, was a necessary organizing instrument employed to link and arrange facts.

While stressing the primacy of clinical experience, both Cullen and Gregory went to great lengths trying to explain it with the help of a neuropathological framework. Thus students listening to Cullen's lectures came away with the impression that such theories and disease classifications were hypothetical and heuristic devices employed to rationalize clinical events and make sense of the rapidly changing events at the sickbed. What ultimately mattered was the direct clinical experience as the *only* guide to diagnostic judgments and therapeutic indications. Medical theory and nosology, for their part, offered convenient explanations and categories for organizing and expressing information, not guidelines for bedside action.

Despite repeated complaints by students and professors that the Edinburgh infirmary failed to admit adequate numbers of instructive patients, student attendance during rounds and enrollment in the clinical lecture course rose steadily in the 1770s and 1780s. The primary reason, of course, was that a greater number of medical students made their way to Edinburgh to take courses from famous teachers such as Monro, Cullen, and Gregory. In addition, after midcentury, future physicians considered it increasingly important to receive exposure to clinical matters and acquire practical therapeutic skills, following the earlier example of their surgical brethren. In Edinburgh the only opportunities for education of this sort remained the infirmary and the public dispensary, the latter seeing only ambulatory outpatients.

As the university authorities officially recognized the importance of clinical experience and after 1783 included it in the curriculum as a requirement for graduation, enrollment in clinical lectures at the infirmary continued to climb. Eventually, to avoid the exodus of students to London hospitals during summers, the managers authorized a third course of lectures to be given between May and July.

In sum, there is no question that during the last decades of the century clinical teaching at the Edinburgh infirmary significantly contributed to the success and reputation of the local medical school. Foreign visitors and local professors, students guides and scholarly writings, all extolled the virtues of an instructional system that effectively integrated clinical matters into the rest of the curriculum. More important, the Edinburgh Medical School allowed its most prominent faculty members to teach at the bedside, surgical amphitheater, and clinical lecture room, thereby conferring on these activities the importance and prestige that ultimately ensured their success.

Epilogue

GENERAL CONSIDERATIONS

The eighteenth-century establishment of hospitals in the modern sense of the word – meaning institutions exclusively devoted to the care of sick people – constituted one of the most critical developments in the history of medicine. As noted in the preceding chapters, hospital practice gradually but decisively changed the character, content, and direction of medicine.[1] Although developments at Edinburgh were perhaps unique, all similar British institutions played significant roles in the transformation of medical care and education.

Enlightenment ideals and policies allowed the medical profession throughout Europe to reach sectors of the population hitherto more dependent on domestic healing measures. Operating under the banner of "medical police," the new mission to restore and preserve the health of lower-class people became a political and economic goal. For the benefit of the entire nation, the poor were to be placed back on their feet and made once more productive members of society. One prominent tool used to implement such policies was the hospital, a place that could hasten the recovery of those affected with curable diseases.

In Britain eighteenth-century hospital foundations became a tangible expression of private philanthropy and civic-mindedness, a visible product of compassion and voluntarism. Thus British medical professionals, physicians and surgeons alike, saw hospital work as a personal commitment to charity, an honorable task widely appreciated by like-minded humanitarians that quickly became a status symbol for furthering a lucrative private career.[2] This certainly was the situation in Edinburgh before the 1740s, when members of the local College of Physicians and Incorporation of Surgeons pledged their free services to the fledgling infirmary.

As the Edinburgh hospital expanded its scope and established more formal ties with the local university faculty in the late 1740s, medical professionals quickly realized the social and intellectual advantages inherent in a continuing association. Recurrent conflicts between the physician-dominated hospital administration and the Incorporation of Surgeons seeking an expanded role for its members were part of an obvious power struggle for greater professional and social recognition through association with the infirmary's staff. Several hospital physicians, in fact, became employees of the institution, thereby giving up some of the authority and freedom of private, entrepreneurial activities.

So great, apparently, was the prestige conferred on the "ordinary" physicians of the Edinburgh infirmary that prominent graduates from the local university applied for these positions, usually with the support of powerful relatives who could apply useful pressure on the board of managers making the appointments. One example was the selection in 1776 of Henry Cullen, a son of the famous William Cullen, as physician-in-ordinary. His replacement in 1791 was Daniel Rutherford, son of John Rutherford, the first clinical professor. Daniel actually exchanged his status of clinical professor for that of attending physician. All were fellows of the local College of Physicians.

After nomination each of these men took an oath of allegiance to the hospital and promised to follow its statutes and regulations strictly. Like the house surgeons, attending physicians made almost no budgetary or policy decisions. They were forced to prescribe specific institutional diets and in-house remedies listed in the infirmary's pharmacopoeia. Most important, the salaried physicians were barred from hiring or dismissing ancillary personnel, especially nurses, a prerogative jealously guarded by the matron.

In exchange, infirmary practitioners acquired a fair amount of authority and control in medical matters over hospitalized patients – a significant shift of power from the patient-controlled relationship operating in private practice. Such domination allowed professionals to follow up individual cases closely by making rounds through the wards at least once or twice a day, more often if circumstances warranted. These advantages were rarely available in private practice, since physicians depended on calls from their patrons for return visits.

The issue of continuity in bedside observation and therapy needs special emphasis. Extending the practitioner's opportunities to visit with the sick eventually revolutionized clinical medicine. On one level it played a decisive role in the development of examination skills and in learning to recognize clinical signs. In spite of language barriers, physicians sharpened their interviewing skills, getting away from the practice of suggesting answers while probing for discrepancies between the history and the physical findings. Bodily inspection and examination gradually expanded, especially decades later, as new pathological knowledge spurred physicians into correlating the observed lesions with clinical manifestations.

Another important consequence of serial hospital observations was a revision of the criteria used in the definition and description of particular diseases, especially their institutional evolution. Although eighteenth-century practitioners were apprehensive that the hospital environment would distort the "normal" development of a given disease, some set out to record meticulously every change in symptomatology and physical appearance, correlating each one to environmental conditions in the hospital and the use of specific remedies. With new insights about the role of ventilation and hygiene in the progress of fevers, for example, physicians modified their notions about "typhus" fever and its prognosis and treatment.[3] The only trouble, also frequent in private practice, was the loss of diagnostic clues present from the onset of illness until the patient sought medical help. Treatment in the hospital setting robbed the physician of critical opportunities to observe the early "unfolding" of a disease. Treatments prior to admission could further complicate the clinical picture by obliterating the pathognomonic "markers" needed for diagnosis.

Basing their judgments entirely on clinical manifestations in the form of specified symptom complexes, Edinburgh hospital physicians sought to diagnose each disease encountered in the wards. The diagnostic process then in vogue prescribed, through interrogation and inspection, the collection from the sick of symptoms and signs that matched those included in the "natural history" of a particular disease. The specific label assigned to the sickness in question was based on a contemporary nosology or disease classification. In Edinburgh William Cullen's *Synopsis Nosologiae* dominated medical practice after its publication in 1769. His categories, based on hypothetical notions of neuropathology and personal clinical knowledge, helped shape medical experiences at the infirmary.

Notably absent from Cullen's nosology were diagnostic criteria based on pathological anatomy, soon to become in France the deciding yardsticks employed to characterize individual diseases. Their absence did not mean that Edinburgh physicians, including Cullen, ignored the value of autopsies and the possibilities of establishing clinicopathological correlations, as exemplified by the work of the Italian author Giovanni B. Morgagni, published in 1761. The truth was that hospital practitioners in Edinburgh had few opportunities to witness dissections because of the low institutional mortality rate and the frequent withholding of autopsy permissions by relatives and friends of the deceased. Moreover, the actual postmortem examination was judged an unpleasant manual task and therefore delegated to relatively inexperienced surgical apprentices, who were necessarily unfamiliar with the patient's clinical evolution.

These professional barriers certainly prevented Edinburgh physicians from assimilating the lessons that surgeons routinely obtained from the dead. At the infirmary surgeons were eager to ascertain the effects of their work, checking the accuracy of their diagnoses and the extent of postoperative complications. Consequently, autopsies were of great practical importance, and permissions to carry them out were aggressively pursued. The protocols were generally explicit and even detailed about the findings.

The paucity of postmortem observations in Edinburgh was responsible for the physicians' impression that such local changes were of secondary importance. In their view these abnormalities were simply additional effects of a particular disease already sufficiently characterized through clinical signs. Since the lesions usually remained hidden and were possibly late in developing, physicians who had pressing diagnostic, prognostic, and therapeutic matters to decide continued to look for more accessible criteria available while the patient was still alive. As expected, they settled on phenomena readily discernible at the bedside instead of waiting for unexpected postmortem revelations.

The availability of numerous diagnostic categories or "species" and their placement in complex taxonomies allowed hospital physicians in Edinburgh to provide patients with labels that carried significant prognostic implications. Such information was in itself quite therapeutic, decreasing the patient's fears if the illness was benign, as was mostly the case with infirmary admissions. As expected, nature almost invariably took its course regardless of medical intervention. In fact, given the growing skepticism about the value of their medical treatments, practitioners spent increasingly more time honing their observational skills and improving their diagnostic acumen.

Thus, regardless of the effects of medical treatment, hospital patients at the Edinburgh infirmary received a great deal of psychological reassurance from their doctors, who were recognized as competent leaders of their craft. "We are firmly persuaded that next to professional skill the manner of prescribing remedies and of addressing and conversing with the patient is one of the best sedators of pain and one of the most potent cathartics of the mind," observed one author writing in 1801 for *Scots Magazine*.[4] Daily medical rounds and the attention bestowed on patients by students and teachers became welcome healing rituals. Such symbolic actions provided a great deal of confidence to persons who for the most part had reluctantly resorted to hospital treatment. To receive personal attention from the most famous physicians and surgeons of the city – some of them, like Cullen and the Gregories, with international reputation – was probably for many an uplifting experience.

Much has been written about the depersonalizing effects of hospital admission on patients, and the inhumanity pervading the institutions. Eighteenth-century infirmaries were bureaucratically run with the help of detailed regulations and precise accounting practices. The goal was to bring order and achieve a measure of control over the ravages of disease threatening large sectors of the population. But here again, present conditions and values have somewhat distorted the interpretation of past events. To be sure, those who gained entrance into the Edinburgh infirmary lost their original support network of relatives and friends. Anxious and frightened, they were exposed to the noises and smells of disease as well as the occasional brutality of nurses. Zealous administrators and cold-hearted practitioners who saw illness as an opportunity for moral reform could also make things unpleasant for hospital inmates.

Under the circumstances, however, most patients seem to have fared quite well. Many cultivated new friendships within the institution. Doing a number of cleaning chores, watching and feeding one another, talking about their problems and fears, hospitalized people forged strong bonds of solidarity and fellowship, as evidenced by the contemporary experiences of Joseph Wilde.[5] Moreover, in eighteenth-century Edinburgh, ambulatory patients could temporarily leave the infirmary and return home; the bedridden were allowed to receive daily visitors, many of them bearing presents of food.

From the evidence it appears that the managers earnestly tried to keep the patients' interests ahead of other considerations in spite of the powerless state of the "deserving" poor. Repeated admonitions to members of the house and attending staff demanding that they respect the feelings of the patients and treat them with "delicacy and kindness" may suggest occasional abuses, but they also reveal a genuine concern. John Gregory's recommendations for the establishment of a bond of "sympathy" between patient and practitioner were part of a protective and paternalistic attitude that transcended self-serving efforts toward improved relations with the public. As for the presumed moralizing, the evidence is lacking. Physicians in their writings and lectures tried to focus on the purely physical problems of their patients. James Gregory, for example, declared in one case of induced abortion, "I did not inquire into her situation with respect to matrimony because our views are purely physical; it would in this case be [un]necessary and improper to give any offense."[6]

MEDICAL THERAPEUTICS

The observational continuity that helped practitioners understand the progress of particular diseases also had a profound effect on medical therapeutics. Rather than the touted "blind empiricism," denoting an arbitrary and confused approach toward treatment, Edinburgh hospital practitioners developed a series of specific clinical guidelines for the use of drugs and physical methods. These measures were not direct applications of new medical theories but procedures traditionally employed to help patients "go through their diseases" by assisting the body's natural healing tendencies. The primary goal of therapy at Edinburgh was to help "carry off" the patient's disease without causing additional harm.

In this context it needs to be emphasized once more that Edinburgh physicians such as Cullen, Gregory, and Home were empiricists at the bedside, establishing their criteria for therapeutic intervention on purely observational grounds. Among such guidelines were the Hippocratic doctrine of "critical days" and an improved science of semiotics or knowledge of clinical signs. These practitioners accepted the gulf between contemporary medical theory and practice, realizing that clinical medicine was definitely not an applied science but a series of inductions derived from bedside events.

The trouble, of course, was that several theories of human health and disease, carefully systematized by famous eighteenth-century physicians including Boerhaave, Hoffmann, Stahl, and Cullen, became successively obsolete as new developments in biology and chemistry were reported.[7] Because of their inherent instability and speculative nature, these frameworks failed to provide useful guidelines for diagnosis and treatment. As James Gregory admitted, "Much more than ninety-nine parts in the hundred of all that has been written on the theory and practice of physic for more than 2000 years is absolutely useless."[8]

Although medical theories proved incapable of determining clinical decisions, they nevertheless were extremely useful in ordering and explaining *post hoc* some of the complex events occurring at the bedside. Cullen himself, for example, after 1770 vigorously promoted his own neuropathology, eventually publishing his ideas in the *Institutions of Medicine* (1777) and *First Lines of the Practice of Physic* (1778–1779). The new physiological and pathological views pointed to the brain and nervous system as centers of organic control and dysfunction,[9] whereas Boerhaave, in contrast, had located mechanical disorders in bodily fibers and blood vessels.

Cullen's theories, even though they were speculative and lacked clinical value, offered a coherent set of explanations without placing bedside developments in a conceptual strait jacket. When Cullen's disciple John Brown attempted in the early 1780s to create a closer link between these somewhat simplified theoretical views and medical practice, he was strongly attacked for ignoring or seriously distorting clinical phenomena.[10] The consensus among the leading medical men of Edinburgh was that clinical activities remained an art to be learned and executed at the bedside using the time-honored observations and descriptions of individual cases as foundations. Theory definitely did not dictate practice; it merely explained and justified it after the fact.

While the casebooks reveal among the various Edinburgh professors great similarities in therapeutic approach, treatment of individual patients remained distinct. Not knowing their charges beforehand, physicians began by prescribing standardized recipes taken mostly from the in-house drug formulary. However, as hospitalization proceeded, the practitioners specifically adjusted both remedies and dosages in response to the patients' peculiarities and reactions. Thus one cannot speak of an emergence of stereotyped healing formulas within the context of institutional care.

Moreover, the infirmary data clearly suggest that most medical treatments, with the possible exception of mercurial use in venereal ailments, were not overly aggressive. Indeed, for many infirmary patients, healing took place almost exclusively because of bed rest, a cleaner environment, and regular meals. Drugs and physical therapies merely provided symptomatic relief under the watchful eye of hospital practitioners. The longer physicians observed the effects of various drugs, the more skeptical they became regarding their usefulness. Whether the late eighteenth-century reduction in pharmaceutical expenses at the Edinburgh infirmary reflects a decline in drug use remains to be explored. There is no question, however, that practitioners during the 1770s and 1780s eliminated a series of ineffectual compounds from the official pharmacopoeias.[11]

It has been alleged that patients at this time were being subjected to "the most frivolous and irresponsible kind of human experimentation."[12] To be sure, medical practitioners at Edinburgh and elsewhere began very tentatively to test certain drugs in hospital wards, army barracks, and naval vessels. Some of the medicines were new, others well known but compounded in new ways or administered in novel dosages. James Gregory's remark about physicians "playing with the human hide" reflects his bewilderment, shared by others, about a new medical activity replacing traditional autoexperimentation. Moreover, the comment reveals that at least some contemporary practitioners were fearful of violating the Hippocratic principle of avoiding harm. Given the tenor of his concerns, Gregory's misgivings were probably justified, but a study of Francis Home's clinical investigations discloses little that was truly "experimental" in his labors. In addition, all treatments were carefully monitored by lay managers, professors, apothecaries, and house officers who would not tolerate any interference with the hospital's benevolent designs.

However, not all medical treatments prescribed at the Edinburgh infirmary were harmless. The widespread use of mercurial preparations frequently caused obvious symptoms of mercurial poisoning, especially when employed for extended periods in the treatment of venereal disease. During the eighteenth century Edinburgh physicians certainly recognized the relationship between the ingestion of mercury and the appearance of sores in the mouth, salivation, and loose teeth, and some practitioners tried hard to space their doses and keep the complication rate low. In this attempt, unfortunately, they were only partially successful. Forced to choose between curing what appeared to be a dreadful disease with the only therapy considered effective and using substitutes unable to stop the ravages of syphilis, and thereby further compromising individual and public health, practitioners opted for mercury.

Bloodletting, although already extensively discussed, deserves a parting comment since it always figures prominently in the litany of harmful medical treatments of yesteryear. Also a traditional measure originally employed in both folk and professional cures, the withdrawal of blood had over the centuries become one of the most common and dramatic procedures in the treatment of febrile illnesses. In the form of venesection, it temporarily lowered the body temperature, decreased other inflammatory symptoms, and induced faintness, relaxation, or sleep. Piercing veins required a degree of technical proficiency eagerly supplied by surgeons and their apprentices. It could produce a number of complications ranging from infection at the extraction site to general debility from excessive blood loss.

However, under the skeptical eyes of their peers, Edinburgh infirmary physicians substantially refined their indications for the extraction of blood and became much more selective about the people subjected to it. Patients with typhus fever were completely excluded, and those suffering from other types of fever were bled sparingly. During the three decades of this study, only one in five patients admitted to the teaching ward endured a venesection; the average amount of blood ordered withdrawn was not greater than one quart. In a significant number of instances, only about half of the prescribed quantity was actually taken. Case records suggest that bloodletting at the infirmary did not prolong hospitalization or precipitate the death of a single person admitted to the teaching ward.

If sustained, the use of emetics and cathartics may have retarded recovery by weakening the patients though these measures were seldom fatal. Such usage was extensive in both domestic healing and medical circles because of the popular notion that food and stool remaining in the gastrointestinal tract created a natural obstacle to the restoration of health. For millennia, the traditional imperative to cleanse the "prima via" survived in European folklore, justified and legitimized by medical theories such as humoralism and, in the late eighteenth century, Cullen's neurophysiology. The practice was ultimately derived from the observation of natural phenomena occurring in fevers. Nausea, vomiting, and diarrhea spontaneously accompanied a great number of febrile illnesses. Nature, it seemed, pointed the way, and healers were only too eager to imitate or supplement what they believed were necessary steps toward recovery. They ascribed most drug effects and patient weakness to the actions of the disease rather than their treatments, an assumption not exclusive with eighteenth-century practitioners.

Certain treatments, especially if they were frequently instituted, undoubtedly caused harmful side effects. Like their modern counterparts, eighteenth-century physicians remained ignorant of the dangers posed by many measures or, if dimly aware, could not or would not change their prescriptions. As today, practitioners went ahead, convinced that the benefits to be derived from the use of these therapies outweighed possible complications. Then as now, such judgments were based on the contemporary state of the medical art and were offered as more helpful than not.

In view of the subsequent therapeutic activism known as "heroic medicine," which led, especially in the United States, to an almost indiscriminate use of bloodletting and purging with mercurials,[13] the moderation shown by eighteenth-century physicians at the Edinburgh infirmary needs to be particularly stressed. Perhaps public image and lay administrative supervision, peer control, and educational objectives all combined to exert considerable restraint. Experienced clinicians such as Cullen, the Gregories, Duncan, and to a lesser extent Francis Home and Daniel Rutherford were able to make sober analyses of the options then available in the treatment of diseases. Most of the prescriptions written by these attending physicians contained only single drugs, not the usual ineffective mixtures. Instead of having to act precipitously because of strong patient pressure, hospital physicians could afford to temporize and be cautious. There was time for official and informal consultations to discuss problems and correct errors. In what other setting could a physician of Cullen's stature publicly admit, "I think I was wrong in the case of this poor man, but the aftergame [new plan of treatment] allows me and other people to correct me"?[14] It seems that scientific curiosity and professional honesty could flourish in such an institutional setting, shielded from the pressures of private practice.

EIGHTEENTH–CENTURY HOSPITALS: FOR BETTER OR WORSE?

For all these reasons, even when measured against modern standards, the balance sheet of eighteenth-century hospital care ceases to be "so unrelievedly deplorable a story."[15] Patients unable to be properly cared for at home could be removed from crowded, filthy quarters into ventilated wards where they usually got clean sheets and clothes. Instead of being forced by masters to continue performing assigned tasks, hospitalized workers were exempted from their usual obligations and allowed to rest. Though the prescribed diets – especially in fevers – were rather meager, still patients were fed regularly. Often they received wine and meat during extended periods of convalescence.

The observation that eighteenth-century hospitals were incapable of reducing mortality rates in the immediate population they served is probably correct but hardly a meaningful issue. Decisions about cases considered proper for hospital treatment relied on contemporary clinical experience and judgments of medical effectiveness. Criteria for admittance tended to favor young and productive members of the labor force, affected by usually acute but brief and self-limited illnesses from which rapid recovery was expected. These criteria did not coincide with the major causes of death in cities sur-

rounding the voluntary hospital, particularly since half of the mortality occurred in infants and small children barred from admission, except into special hospitals. The best that can be said for voluntary hospitals on this score
is that they made indirect contributions to the welfare of families whose
breadwinners fell ill and were nursed back to health in infirmaries.[16] Likewise, removing a significant number of sick servants from upper-class
households decreased the threat of contagious diseases for that level of society.

Compared to similar establishments in the British provinces, the Edinburgh infirmary obviously possessed in the late eighteenth century a more
liberal admissions policy. As noted, it allowed the entrance of people bearing a number of contagious diseases, including smallpox, consumption, and
venereal disorders. Occasionally parents were permitted to bring their sick
children into the institution. Such tolerance was due partly to fiscal considerations, since it was a factor in negotiating contracts for the admission of
soldiers, seamen, and servants. On the other hand, given the needs of an
expanding teaching ward, the boundaries of what were proper cases for
admission necessarily remained flexible in order to give students opportunities for observing patients with unusual problems. Always struggling to
maintain financial solvency, the Edinburgh infirmary was forced to display
at all times its public image of benevolence. This posture led to its embel-
lishment of discharge categories and its restrictions on student access.

Like similar institutions throughout Britain, the Edinburgh infirmary was
not very responsive to the medical needs of the immediate community.
Yearly admissions in the 1780s constituted about 3% of the total Edinburgh
population, a figure that dropped to about 2% a decade later. The statutes
stressed the admission of "diseased people of all countries or nations," although most patients came from Scotland. Moreover, the infirmary never
followed the example of Manchester in setting up a dispensary, a home
visiting program, or a health board. In the late eighteenth century, of course,
Edinburgh remained a medium-sized provincial city outflanked by the Industrial Revolution and thus seemingly without pressing needs for a comprehensive welfare program.

The infirmary did, however, show considerable sensitivity toward the
educational needs of medical students matriculated at the university. Their
training was stressed in spite of clear signals that patient care was the institution's top priority. Although managers repeatedly assured the public that
the charitable goals commanded their highest attention, scientific and pedagogical objectives were far from ignored, particularly since the sale of
admission tickets to students in the 1790s generated about a fifth of the
hospital's income. As described, university professors in charge of the teaching
ward were given considerable discretion in their admissions, internal transfers, and delayed discharges, even though such actions could adversely af-

fect the infirmary's statistics. From time to time the hospital's apothecary even furnished for therapeutic experiments exotic products obtained from the physic garden, which were especially favored by Andrew Duncan, Sr.

Another notion needing further explanation is the charge that eighteenth-century hospitals were "death traps" or "gateways to death." The dangers of hospital-acquired disease were unquestionably real: They were frequently discussed by contemporary medical authors. Hospital-based epidemics of "fever" – mostly of the "typhus" variety – certainly occurred in Edinburgh and elsewhere, although there is no direct evidence in the student notebooks that any of those affected contracted the disease while in the hospital. By repeatedly stressing institutional pathology, authors like Michel Foucault and Thomas McKeown have unnecessarily exaggerated and distorted this problem, perhaps because they have paid inordinate attention to the writings of one French surgeon, Jacques R. Tenon.

In a 1788 report about hospital conditions in France, Tenon dramatically exposed the insalubrious conditions then prevailing in certain Parisian hospitals; the 25% mortality rate of the infamous Hôtel-Dieu was considered at the time the highest in all of Europe.[17] Tenon's document was written for the Parisian Academy of Sciences as a great debate raged throughout France regarding the desirability of maintaining such large hospitals. His account prominently featured the Hôtel-Dieu, because it was the target of contemporary criticisms and many members of the academy were seeking to replace it with four smaller institutions, to be located in the outskirts of the city.[18] Tenon's depressing observations should not be considered typical for all eighteenth-century European hospitals. In fact, all his suggested improvements were based on conditions observed in English hospitals that he visited in 1787.[19]

Many of the insights obtained from military experiences, especially the importance of ventilation, influenced British hospital construction and remodeling in the period under study. Walls were whitewashed periodically, and attention to cleanliness included floors, beds, and other articles of furniture. New guidelines for institutional isolation led to revised admission criteria, restricting entrance to those capable of speedy relief before any "hospital distemper would creep in."[20] Other people were shifted to outpatient facilities or dispensaries or simply visited in their own homes. Like fields, certain wards remained fallow for weeks, subjected to ventilation and cleansing measures to root out contagion. Wards exclusively devoted to the admission and isolation of patients affected with fevers sprang up in numerous voluntary hospitals, a development followed by the rise of actual "fever hospitals" after 1800.[21]

Although there were no official reports, eighteenth-century infirmary physicians in Edinburgh certainly remained alert to the danger of hospital-based infections and blamed such outbreaks for a small number of deaths, including those of a few medical students. In general, however, the problem was minor during the period under study because the hospital authorities avoided overcrowding and had the financial resources to ensure an acceptable level of institutional hygiene.

On the other hand, the risk of contracting hospital diseases did increase in London and other provincial centers toward the end of the century and in the early 1800s as voluntary institutions became excessively crowded, their resources inadequate to cope with greater demands for care from swelling urban centers affected by the Industrial Revolution. At that point some hospitals sustained in-house epidemics and mortality rates more typical of nineteenth-century London.

We cannot simply assume that hospital conditions must have been worse in earlier times. Before 1800, overcrowding and breakdowns of hygienic conditions were infrequent in British voluntary hospitals, particularly in provincial infirmaries. One could successfully argue that the low, 4%–5% mortality figures listed by these institutions in their annual reports were products of very selective admissions systems as well as early discharge practices for those about to die. Yet the Edinburgh teaching ward, which housed more acute and serious cases, never exceeded a death rate of 8% between 1770 and 1800, a figure that hardly supports a view of the infirmary as a "death trap."

A brief comment about discharge statistics: During the second half of the eighteenth century these figures acquired great importance as true indexes of hospital performance, especially for British voluntary hospitals vying for subscribers. Mortality rates for French hospitals – in particular, the Hôtel-Dieu of Paris – were repeatedly quoted to stress the superiority of care provided across the Channel. By 1775 the Hôtel-Dieu and St. Louis Hospital in Paris reportedly had death rates of about 13%, these figures worsened to 15%–20% just before the French Revolution. Amsterdam Hospital reported that 12% of its patients hospitalized in 1774 had died. In London inpatient mortality at St. Bartholomew's and St. Thomas's was estimated at around 7.6%; the 1751–1754 figures for Manchester and Newcastle were 2.8% and 6.5%, respectively.[22]

The closest comparison can be made by analyzing the statistics of the Aberdeen Infirmary for the period 1770–1786, also published in *Scots Magazine*. In general, the figures are quite similar to those reported for Edinburgh. Aberdeen's "perfectly cured" rate was 68%; a "recovered" category corresponding to Edinburgh's "relieved" was 12.5%. Significantly lower were Aberdeen's discharges labeled "by desire," "improper," and "deserted," lumped together and constituting only 7% of the total. The higher Edinburgh figures, especially the "irregular" and "by desire" dismissals, probably reflect the presence of unruly soldiers and seamen.[23]

In contrast to Edinburgh, the Aberdeen Infirmary retained a category listed as "incurable after a long trial," but only 1.3% of the patients were placed under this heading. Finally, Aberdeen's mortality rates also were somewhat lower: an average of 3.5% for the entire period, only 3% for the 1780s. Given the usual inaccuracies and distortions in hospital reporting, the 1% difference is probably not significant, but it might well reflect the higher death rates experienced in Edinburgh's teaching ward. In any event, mortality at the Edinburgh infirmary was probably average for contemporary British provincial hospitals but significantly lower than for similar institutions with educational responsibilities in London and Paris.

THE "BIRTH" OF THE CLINIC

In his three brief references to the Edinburgh Medical School, Michel Foucault indicated that he viewed its program of instruction as a typical example of the "protoclinic" reaching back to Herman Boerhaave's teaching at Leyden earlier in the century. In Foucault's definition, protoclinics were institutions teaching their students a more or less static body of knowledge – a "medicine of morbid species" – based on speculative views of bodily function that also found expression in rigid disease classifications resembling botanical taxonomies. At the bedside these educational efforts were used merely to illustrate contemporary medical learning rather than to stimulate a search for new knowledge. In sharp contrast, Foucault portrayed postrevolutionary clinical education in France as a radically new and dynamic research program transcending the medicine of species. Differences between Edinburgh, for example, and France were said to be so great as to constitute an "essential mutation in medical knowledge" – indeed, an "epistemological break" leading to what Foucault called the "birth" of the modern clinic.[24]

A review of his other works makes it clear that Foucault was primarily interested in broad, unconscious changes affecting the perception and organization of knowledge in Western societies. However, his outline of sharp conceptual and methodological discontinuities between the "old" clinics in Leyden, Edinburgh, and Vienna and the "new" ones in Paris after the Revolution poses for medical historians a number of challenges as well as problems. Among the difficulties is, of course, Foucault's lack of proper historical documentation to substantiate the postulated break and the employment of a vague, idiosyncratic terminology in describing it. One recent historian has taken up the challenge, describing at least for France a lengthy "gestation period" preceding the so-called birth and presenting surgical training in hospitals of the ancien régime as a worthy antecedent of later developments.[25] Other writers, while accepting the importance of early nineteenth-century medicine in France, have concentrated more on the historical continuities and intellectual ancestors that may have facilitated this birth.

The foregoing analysis of medical activities at the Edinburgh infirmary cannot completely ignore Foucault's notion of a *coupure épistémologique* between late eighteenth-century European medicine and the new French clinic developed after 1794. In fact, the evidence uncovered in student casebooks and lecture notes helps us understand the sudden and profound change in medical thought. As outlined before, Edinburgh medicine remained in many ways a protoclinic in Foucault's sense, while at the same time displaying characteristics that would place it within the gestational period that has been posited for France. Like most of its counterparts in other European medical centers, Edinburgh offered a picture of medicine in transition, at the threshold of a new era while still doggedly clinging to traditional concepts and methods.

Among the major characteristics of Foucault's protoclinic were its efforts merely to confirm and illustrate existing knowledge. This description does to some extent apply to Edinburgh, where Cullen's medicine of species, based on rigid disease classification and speculative pathology, was certainly the rule. However, prominent teachers such as Cullen himself and James Gregory insisted that these frameworks were temporary, to be challenged and corrected if new bedside experiences warranted. In fact, Cullen freely admitted the deficiencies of his nosology, encouraging students to observe patients directly and keep detailed records about their findings that eventually could improve the prevailing nosological categories. This was certainly more than illustration; Edinburgh medicine seems to have actively promoted the search for new knowledge at the bedside. One of Cullen's students, Thomas Fowler, collected about five thousand complete cases in his ten years at the Stafford Infirmary.[26] Many of these data found their way into contemporary medical journals and books in the form of tables, reports, and disease descriptions.

The major conceptual hurdle to further developments that would ultimately establish the new modern clinic was a somewhat vague but wholistic view of disease as a concrete reality to be described and classified as any other natural object would be. Its contours were defined exclusively by clinical criteria in the form of a symptom sequence that provided a distinctive "natural history." As the disease clashed with the individual patient, a battle ensured within the body, pitting the forces of the invading sickness against the natural healing powers brought into action by the patient's constitution. Physicians called to witness this struggle carefully set out to collect symptoms and signs that could possibly reveal the nature of the intruder. In doing so, practitioners paid great attention to the total impact of particular diseases on the functional state of the sick person, rather than focusing on local disturbances or possible anatomical lesions.

But here again, changes were in the offing, as confirmed by Cullen's discussions of clinicopathological correlations. Indeed, certain diseases became increasingly linked to specific organic lesions discovered during postmortem examinations.[27] A beginning seems to have been made with the frequent discovery of tubercles in the lungs of patients labeled as suffering from phthisis. If no purulent expectoration suggesting the presence of such tubercles could be elicited, phthisis in Edinburgh was labeled "incipient" and therefore proper for hospital care. However, if the sign occurred, it was a phthisis "confirmata," deemed incurable.

For all its fame, however, hospital medicine in late eighteenth-century Edinburgh remained in transition. Evidently the key for transcending the basic tenets of the medicine of species was pathological anatomy. As France reorganized its medical education after 1794, reformers adopted the surgical model, with its hospital-based instructional program. Students henceforth were to spend substantial portions of their medical studies in hospital settings observing patients and dissecting those who died there.[28]

Such a comprehensive instructional program was possible in Paris because of the abundance of hospitalized patients. Since medieval times a large number of "hospitals" or charitable institutions had dotted France, in the country and in the capital city, which possessed forty-eight by the late 1700s, most of them housing a fair number of people who could be characterized as sick.[29] On the eve of the Revolution Paris, with its population of nearly 700,000, harbored over 20,000 hospital inmates – the infirm, old, indigent, orphans, and so on – about half of them sick.[30] In comparison, late eighteenth-century London, with a population of nearly 720,000, had only 1,500 sick patients housed in infirmaries; and Edinburgh, with 75,000 people, allowed only 150–200 patients into its hospital.

Whereas the British establishments were governed by private boards trying to impress private subscribers, French hospitals after 1794 operated under the auspices of the central government, which financed their upkeep. In Britain permission for autopsies was always necessary; in France postmortem examinations were at times mandatory for all patients dying while hospitalized. Strict control of admissions kept mortality rates low in British institutions – around 4% – whereas French hospitals, especially the notorious Hôtel-Dieu, practiced open admissions policies. As previously noted, because of the ensuing overcrowding, institutional infection, and prolonged hospitalization, mortality rates climbed to 15%–25%.[31]

Aided by such social, professional, and institutional factors, the newly founded Paris Medical School quickly departed from the epistemological foundations of the previous medicine of species. Gradual inclusion of pathological findings as criteria for the diagnosis and classification of disease caused a complete revolution in the way sickness was perceived by physicians. A whole new set of diagnostic signs made their appearance as the richness of organ pathology unfolded before the dissecting knife: the hard edge of a cirrhotic liver, the dullness of a pneumonic lung, the peculiar sounds made by a calcified valve. As French hospital physicians systematically began dissecting all institutional casualties, virtually every patient revealed tangible evidences of the struggle with disease. The bedside and autopsy room became sites for the performance of clinical research rather than for simple demonstration. As Laennec proudly announced a decade later, pathological anatomy had quickly become the new basis for nosology and the true guide to medical diagnosis. Henceforth diseases were to be characterized only by the specific lesions they produced and the functional abnormalities stemming from their presence.[32]

As Ludwig Fleck has proposed, particular styles of thought emerge from specific cultural contexts that define and allow only a certain range of observations.[33] Such a model certainly seems to explain better than Foucault's philosophical prose the profound differences between medicine in Edinburgh and Paris, the so-called epistemological break or further pathological reductionism. As the preceding analysis makes clear, Edinburgh was just a provincial British city with a secure and prosperous medical profession adhering to the ideals of the traditional gentleman-physician. Surgeons remained in an inferior social and professional position, charged with the manual and untidy aspects of healing and dissection. Although hospital practice, particularly after 1760, gradually forced a number of significant conceptual and social readjustments of the original patient-dominated model of private practice, these changes failed to produce a major reorientation of medicine in Scotland. In Edinburgh, at least, practitioners advocated increasing skepticism toward medical systems, strict attention to bedside phenomena, and growing therapeutic restraint. Caution, however, should be exercised in applying these findings to other voluntary institutions or to British medicine in general.

Paris, on the other hand, was a large metropolis, the capital of a nation in revolutionary turmoil. After a temporary abolition of the legal and educational foundations of a discredited medical profession in the early 1790s, surgeons and physicians united and together adopted a program of professional and social rehabilitation.[34] Its blueprints called for a comprehensive plan of care and instruction that would take advantage of the extended system of French public assistance, including numerous hospitals. Unfettered by professional and institutional barriers, practitioners went to observe the large urban hospital population, which offered a rich panorama of human sickness. Expanding previous routine autopsy practices established on a smaller scale by prerevolutionary surgeons, Parisian physicians set up a research program of systematic clinicopathological correlations. The result was a complete reorientation of medical thought and action around anatomical pathology.

THE FINAL BLESSING

On Friday, February 1, 1780, twenty-four days after entering the infirmary in a delirium, Margaret ("Peggy") Carmichael finally went home "cured."

James Gregory's clinical rotation had ended the day before, and the teaching ward needed to be emptied of patients to give Francis Home, his successor, a chance to select his own cases. Peggy's father, Andrew, and her sister, Mary, had left about a week earlier, similarly "cured" of their encounters with typhus fever. Little is known of three-year-old brother Pat, who was not officially entered in the General Register but apparently was dismissed from the teaching ward on January 17. He also recovered and was perhaps placed in the custody of a neighbor or friend of the family. Peggy's grandmother, Margaret Clunie, left January 31, "relieved" according to the notebooks, "cured" in the register. For the Carmichaels, hospitalization was over. They all had survived the typhus and probably returned to their home in Grass Market, ready to resume their places in society.[35]

Whether the family kept in touch with their physicians remained unrecorded, but the practice was not infrequent. In spite of its steady growth, the old town of Edinburgh remained a close-knit community, and Cullen and Duncan, at least, kept tabs on their ex-patients' progress.[36] Duncan, who for almost two generations was a popular figure in the clubs and alleys of Edinburgh, met many of them in his daily walks. In the early 1800s he recalled, "I have a hundred times in the street got the blessing of patients for the care they had met with in the Infirmary."[37] On being discharged from the hospital, one such grateful patient wrote to his physician:

> Wherever I languish, or whatever my fate,
> This still shall be my prayer: long may you live
> To serve at once your country and your God,
> And when late time shall call you to your rest,
> May bliss eternal be your great reward.[38]

APPENDIX A

Sources

Student casebooks, 1771–1799

With the appointment of a "clerk of the house" according to the 1743 statutes, the hospital acquired a permanent house officer whose duties included dictating clinical case histories to students attending the infirmary. The practice was originally reserved for Saturday afternoons, when

> the whole of the practice in the house is read leisurely by him from the ledger to the whole of the students in the operating room, to give them an opportunity of taking notes of every cure they think worthwhile; yea he has orders to give them full copies of every cure they call for upon their paying a trifle for writing it out for them.[1]

Why would students want to copy hospital cases? The question seems relevant because most contemporary practitioners were indifferent about recording the clinical fortunes of their private patients unless an individual case proved to be particularly puzzling or unusual. Ledgers were generally kept for accounting purposes. The previously decried lack of continuity in observing the evolution of private patients was the rule rather than the exception, and it frustrated most efforts at documentation.

Yet repeated admonitions by eighteenth-century medical authors to abandon armchair speculations and actually observe the sick began having effects. "If a set of physicians of sufficient abilities would undertake it heartily and confine themselves to *observations* in the plainest and simplest manner," wrote Francis Clifton, "they would be able in a few years to write as well upon the diseases of England as ever Hippocrates did upon those of Greece."[2] The gradual emergence of medical journals devoted to the presentation of single or a limited series of clinical cases demonstrated the value of a closer look at the evolution of disease. What better place to study such developments than in a hospital filled with submissive patients who could be daily interrogated and observed?

When John Rutherford (1695–1779), professor of the practice of medicine at the University of Edinburgh, applied in 1748 to the managers of the infirmary, offering to give a formal course of clinical lectures, he was explicit about the content of his conferences: the presenting symptoms, management, and progress of selected hospital patients.[3] Thus students attending these lectures flocked to copy the details of cases discussed in class for immediate and later references. In fact, Rutherford's son Daniel, a chemistry professor but also physician-in-ordinary at the infirmary, lectured on the importance of collecting case histories, encouraging students to "read over this case" once again after the patient had been presented in class.[4]

In 1783 the University of Edinburgh published its new statutes spelling out requirements for the M.D. degree. Among them was an examination in which "the cases of two patients with questions relative to them are given to the candidate which he is required to illustrate in writing with proper solutions of the questions." The document also made the clinical lectures a compulsory course and indicated to the students that they could inspect and make "extracts" from the hospital chronicles to learn "the progress of the disease" and "the effect of the medicines."[5]

When hospital officials decided in 1750 to establish a special teaching ward to house only patients chosen by the visiting university professor, interest in acquiring a complete record of their management increased. By 1755 this practice had become popular enough to motivate administrators to expand the copying hours. Newly appointed medical students who replaced the clerk of the house were to continue the dictation, Wednesdays from 5:00 p.m. to 8:00 p.m. and Saturday afternoons.[6]

From the 1780s onward, students were allowed to copy from the hospital's journals on a daily basis, from 11:00 a.m. to 12:00 noon and from 6:00 p.m. to 7:00 p.m. Because the clerks were overwhelmed with duties, dictation was suspended and the original documents had to be individually checked out. New regulations enacted in 1792 stipulated that students borrowing ward journals and ledgers "shall be considered answerable for them till they are restored, and the books shall not on any account or pretext whatever be carried out of the hospital, or be scrawled upon or otherwise defaced."[7]

Despite restrictions, a majority of students took advantage of the copying opportunities. Having invested considerable time and money in attending the infirmary, they reproduced complete cases, reports, and prescriptions and even took notes of the clinical lectures in shorthand. At the end of their rotations, many of them possessed "complete and regular journals of every prescription and symptom from the hour that the patient entered the ward till he was dismissed."[8]

Fourteen student casebooks form the core of the present study.[9] Most of the authors remain anonymous, most likely busy students attending the infirmary and taking the course of clinical lectures. The casebooks cover chronologically almost three decades of hospital practice in Edinburgh; all but two follow the progress of so-called clinical patients who were housed in the teaching ward of the infirmary. Because this ward was under the management of a university professor, most patients listed in the notes were seen between November and the January of the following year, a three-month period that corresponded to the winter semester at the university. Other cases belonged to the spring semester, February to April.

In the absence of surving hospital ward ledgers, student casebooks are the key documents for reconstruction of hospital practice at the Royal Infirmary of Edinburgh. Each case copied from the ledgers began with a brief history mentioning circumstances that surrounded the onset of illness, followed by a description of the most prominent symptoms and a note indicating whether the patient had any treatment prior to admission. Next came the actual daily management of the patient, with a list of dietary recommendations, drug prescriptions, and orders for the application of physical methods. By closely following the everyday progress of each patient, the reader of these chronicles can understand the entire clinical evolution, as well as the adjustments to the therapeutic regimen made by the medical staff in response to bedside events.

The first casebook contains details about the hospitalization of 50 patients, 30 men and 20 women, who were under the care of John Gregory (1724–1773), professor of the theory of medicine, from Nov. 18, 1771, to Jan. 31, 1772.[10] The second one lists 52 patients, all women, treated by William Cullen (1710–1790), professor of the practice of medicine, between Nov. 1, 1772, and Apr. 8, 1773.[11] Cullen was also in charge of another group of 79 patients, 44 men and 35 women, seen from Nov. 1, 1773, to Apr. 8, 1774, whose records were collected in a third notebook.[12] As mentioned, Gregory and Cullen shared the clinical teaching at the infirmary after the death of Robert Whytt in 1766, and each of them lectured for three months. Gregory was forced to retire because of illness in Feb. 1772, leaving Cullen as the sole instructor until Gregory's son James (1753–1821) assumed teaching duties in 1776. The fourth manuscript lists the cases of 85 patients, 38 men and 47 women, who were treated in the clinical ward from Nov. 8, 1779, to Jan. 31, 1780, by James Gregory.[13]

The next volume has 55 case histories depicting the hospitalization of 25 men and 30 women from Nov. 1, 1780, until Jan. 31, 1781, under the care of Francis Home (1719–1813), since 1768 the first professor of materia medica at the university.[14] The sixth volume collects records of 33 patients, 25 men and 8 women, whose progress in the hospital was extracted from a book kept by John Hope (1725–1786), one of the physicians-in-ordinary. In contrast with the preceding documents, Hope's journal contained cases admitted to the ordinary medical ward from Aug. to Oct. 1781.[15] In 1768 Hope had replaced David Clerk, one of the original attending physicians, and he concurrently held the professorship of botany at the university.

Hope's ordinary cases are followed by a document divided into two separate volumes. Together they list 104 patients, 58 men and 46 women, seen by James Gregory in the teaching ward between Nov. 9, 1781, and Feb. 8, 1782.[16] Another group of 57 patients also under the care of James Gregory, makes up the ninth sample. The owner of the casebook, Nathan Thomas, selected only female patients who were hospitalized from Nov. 17, 1785, to Jan. 31, 1786.[17]

The next casebook, composed by Robert Dunlop, covers 52 patients, 24 men and 28 women, also under the supervision of Francis Home, from Nov. 10, 1786, until Jan. 31,1787.[18] Next comes a student record listing 65 patients, 30 men and 35 women, whose daily care was entrusted between Feb. 1 and Apr. 25, 1795, to Andrew Duncan, Sr. (1744–1828). In 1790 Duncan had been appointed professor of the theory of medicine at the university, succeeding James Gregory, who transferred to the chair of practical medicine previously held by William Cullen. The anonymous student who copied these cases arranged them according to William Cullen's disease classification and inserted notes from Duncan's clinical lectures specifically referring to the management of the patients.[19]

The next two manuscripts contain cases from the teaching ward under the control of James Gregory and Thomas C. Hope (1766–1844). Gregory's 64 patients, 32 men and an equal number of women, were admitted from Nov. 1, 1795, to Jan. 31, 1796.[20] A year later Hope treated 63 patients, 32 men and 31 women.[21] He was at the time teaching chemistry for Joseph Black at the university while sharing the clinical lectureship at the infirmary with James Gregory. Finally, another student assembled data on Daniel Rutherford's 94 patients, 54 men and 40 women, who were admitted during the summer session, May 7 to July 31, 1799.[22] In 1791 Rutherford had become one of the ordinary physicians of the hospital, although he also occupied the chair in botany left vacant by John Hope's death in 1786. Like his predecessor in the infirmary, Henry Cullen, Rutherford was authorized by the managers to conduct courses of clinical lectures based on patients in his own care while the teaching ward remained closed for the summer. Together the fourteen casebooks furnish a total of 853 individual clinical histories with a wealth of detail unparalleled in other medical publications of the period.

To be sure, these student notes were somewhat selective in the cases they contained. The first choice was made by the attending physicians in the admissions room, who screened the applicants and allowed entrance only to those who had diseases "proper" for hospital care and who produced letters from infirmary subscribers. The next selection occurred when the university professor in charge of the teaching ward descended to the admissions room and chose those patients who in his judgment would make "good teaching" cases because of either the nature or the circumstances of their ailments. A third determination was made by the medical students enrolled in the course of clinical lectures and attending the infirmary. Students most likely copied those cases that were slated for discussion during a forthcoming lecture or simply wrote down as many as their limited time would allow them to transcribe. Richard W. Hall, who copied the 1772–1773 Cullen cases, reproduced only the records of women suffering from fever and rheumatism. Judging from the sloppy handwriting and frequent abbreviations used in some notebooks, time constraints must have been frequent. Copying hours were limited, and who would want to spend his Saturday afternoon transcribing hospital cases instead of taking a welcome break from studies in an Edinburgh pub?

Errors and omissions, however, were rather uncommon. In some books the occasional entry of a prescription or progress report is followed by the statement "the above report ought not to have been written as it belongs to another case." In the casebook containing James Gregory's patients for 1779 –1780, certain clinical histories were completely omitted toward the end and only lists of drugs copied. With Francis Home's clinical charges, the student-author began his notes by transcribing four 1783 histories but then stopped for unknown reasons and resumed his copying of patient records only during the 1786–1787 winter session.

Discrepancies in the spelling of Scottish surnames reflected a contemporary lack of consistency common in other documents, including the General Register of Patients. Minor differences between admission dates in casebooks and in the register can be explained by the practice of transferring certain patients from other parts of the hospital into the teaching ward, at the request of either the ordinary physicians or the university professor in charge of the clinical ward. In most cases those patients remaining at the end of the professor's three-month rotation in the teaching ward were "remitted to the ordinary physicians" to give the clinical successor freedom in selecting his own patients.

What the casebooks also disclose are several serious deficiencies in the General Register. On the average, about 10% of all the patients described in the student documents do not appear at all in the register. The records for others show significant discrepancies, especially in diagnosis and discharge status. A case in point is Alexander Lawson, a patient who was under the care of John Gregory in 1771 with a severe case of jaundice. Because the therapeutic measures did not seem helpful enough to Mr. Lawson, he simply ran away on Dec. 15, but the General Register listed him as suffering from "hypochondriasis" and on that date indicated his discharge status as "relieved."

If medical practice at the Royal Infirmary can indeed be closely followed through the study of cases from the teaching ward, surgery is much more difficult to reconstruct. Surgical lectures delivered at the hospital lacked official status, and there was no special teaching ward to house patients afflicted with problems requiring care from surgeons. Surgical casebooks were kept by several of the practitioners who rotated through the infirmary as voluntary surgeons. Although less systematic and detailed than those of their medical counterparts, these journals – especially the ones made by William Brown (1757–1818) and James Russell (1754–1836) – contain a select number of cases seen in the daily surgical practice of the hospital.[23]

Ward ledgers, 1773–1776

The only surviving example of an infirmary ward ledger contains hospitalization details for 245 men, almost half of them soldiers, for the years 1773 –1776.[24] The first volume covers 46 patients admitted between Sept. and Dec. 1773; the second lists 34 patients hospitalized from Jan. to June 1774; the third gives information for 50 patients treated between Jan. and Dec. 1775; and the final volume enumerates 115 men admitted from Jan. to Aug 1776. Each entry is relatively brief, beginning with name and age of the patient, date of admission, a very brief history, and initial prescriptions. The notations restrict themselves to a sentence or two listing new medications. The last entry generally announces the patient's dismissal, and discharge status.

Entries in the ledgers, unlike those in student casebooks, were arranged in strict chronological order of admission. Their brevity and the occasional stylish handwriting clearly suggest that these documents contain data carefully abstracted from a much more comprehensive source, presumably the ward journal, of which unfortunately no samples survive. Again, as with student casebooks, 10%–15% of the patients listed in this ledger cannot be found in the General Register of Patients. Occupation is usually given only for those patients who were soldiers.

Clinical lectures, 1771–1799

Several students also took extensive notes from the lectures delivered by Edinburgh professors as part of their teaching obligation during rotations at the Royal Infirmary. The lectures were reproduced in greater or lesser detail, with the comments and judgments the teachers made while reviewing the evolution of patients admitted to the clinical ward. Fast-writing students took down numerous professorial assertions almost verbatim, a procedure which suggests that perhaps many lectures were first written down in shorthand (a few have survived in this form) and then later recopied in full from the abbreviated original notes.[25] Like the casebooks, these carefully bound lecture notes were considered very valuable clinical guides and became sought-after items that occupied a special place in a physician's professional library.

The most detailed notes used in the present study were taken from the lectures delivered by William Cullen between Nov. 18, 1772, and Apr. 23, 1773.[26] After an introductory lecture, Cullen discussed before the Christmas recess a great variety of diseases, especially several cases of catarrh. Most of January was devoted to a study of fevers – their types and different approaches to treatment. In March Cullen discussed acute and chronic rheumatism. His dedication, sagacity, and candid statements reveal a superb teacher and role model for medical students, one who contributed decisively to the prominence of medical education in contemporary Scotland.

Another set of clinical lectures employed in this study was delivered by John Gregory from Nov. 28, 1771, to Feb. 19, 1772,[27] when he resigned because of ill health and was replaced by William Cullen, who continued the lectures until the end of April of that same year.[28] Lectures given by Francis Home during the summer of 1769 were also examined, particularly the preliminary address of May 15, 1769, which laid down for the students the fundamentals of the Edinburgh *Collegium Casuale,* a methodology for history taking and physical examination formulated by the medical faculty.[29]

Also available were notes taken during James Gregory's regular rotation at the infirmary between Nov. 16, 1779, and Jan. 28, 1780.[30] Like Cullen, Gregory began by discussing a variety of diseases but settled down to talk about fevers for nearly three weeks after Christmas. Andrew Duncan's "clinical reports," on the other hand, were not complete lectures but valuable commentaries about the management of specific patients, arranged by the note-taking student according to Cullen's nosology and inserted before each clinical case.[31]

Hastily jotted-down information from James Gregory's 1796 lectures was found difficult to decipher but yielded some insights into the condition of patients hospitalized under his care between Nov. 1796 and Jan. 1797.[32] More useful were notes taken from Daniel Rutherford's clinical lectures delivered between May 7 and July 24, 1799, during a special summer series jointly organized by the infirmary and the University of Edinburgh.[33]

In general, the clinical lectures failed to offer startling new opinions not already expressed by the various lecturers in printed sources. However, the less formal discussions provided additional details about diagnoses and therapeutic rationales; and they also contained a number of admonitions and behavioral recommendations that allow a better understanding of the pedagogical objectives pursued by the Edinburgh Medical School.[34]

Selected clinical cases

The following cases, which are representative of the most common diseases seen at the infirmary, were copied in their entirety from the various student casebooks. Here they are preceded by a brief commentary concerning the evolution of the case, the rationale for treatment, and the choice of dismissal category. Slight editorial changes have been found necessary to help the reader along, such as writing out the numerous abbreviations and translating into English all therapeutic indications originally written in Latin. Fortunately, most of the drugs employed are recognizable; their amounts are included if the student who copied the records gave the information.

Case 1

Patient:	J.M.
Notebook:	Andrew Duncan, Sr., Clinical reports and commentaries, Feb.–Apr. 1795, presented by Alexander Blackhall Morison, Edinburgh, 1795
Location:	MSS Collection, Royal College of Physicians, Edinburgh
Age:	32
Sex and status:	Male, a wright
Admitted:	Feb. 13, 1795, during Duncan's clinical rotation from Feb. 1 to Apr. 25, 1795.
Diagnosis:	Syphilis

Although patients suffering from venereal diseases were frequently hospitalized in the ordinary medical ward and the unit reserved for soldiers, only a handful were allowed into the teaching ward for demonstration purposes. In this instance the daily accounts of the patient's progress copied by the student are followed by a commentary probably delivered by the attending professor, Andrew Duncan, during his clinical lectures.

Duncan's remarks allow us to follow his reasoning leading up to a diagnosis of syphilis. He assumed that all ulcerations occurring around the genitals, even those already healed, signaled the presence of a systemic disease in need of extensive treatment to accomplish a definitive cure. Like other practitioners, Duncan was suspicious of throat ulcerations as being venereal, and his ultimate test concerning the venereal character of a lesion consisted in observing it "yield" to treatment with mercury, an assumption that must have increased the use of the drug and probably led physicians astray on several occasions.

In the case of this tradesman, the history of a genital chancre and presence of ulcerations (which could have been produced by the caustic ointment previously employed) determined the diagnosis. The patient was then immediately subjected to an additional eight-week course of mercury, using a topical preparation for the genital ulcers and pills for systemic action. Duncan kept the man's constitution generously "charged" with mercury throughout his lengthy stay,[1] to the extent that a number of typical side effects appeared on Mar. 2, about two weeks after the therapy had been instituted. Soreness of the gums and salivation, both signs of mercurial poisoning, gradually increased for the next ten days and then slowly abated after Duncan halted the daily use of the ointment, while insisting on the administration of the mercurial pills. A month later, toward the end of the patient's stay, the mercury produced an ulcer inside his cheek that was quickly treated with a liniment.

In all, the treatment outlined in the notebook was straightforward and standard for its day. Gargles were given for the throat and gum complaints, and purgatives administered as the mercury did no longer "run off by stool." According to Duncan, salivation had to be kept at a minimum.[2] A milk diet supplemented by meat and the use in the later stages of a tonic, the Peruvian bark, were designed to increase the patient's strength.

Feb. 13, 1795   About six months ago got a small chancre on the prepuce which soon disappeared by use of a caustic lotion and mercurial pills which produced a soreness of mouth and spitting for two months when he desisted from their use. Has on the scrotum and perineum extensive excoriations, not hard or elevated at the edges covered with a whitish crust and discharging a considerable quantity of white, thick matter.

These lesions began three months ago with itching, followed by very slight excoriation which gradually acquired the present extent. Has also considerable swelling and some redness of the tonsils with very slight ulcerations and some pain on swallowing.

Pulse and other functions natural. Has for six months taken two mercurial pills every night which produced no sensible effect.

14   Mercurial ointment to be applied to scrotal lesions

15	Excoriated parts of scrotum easier from application of ointment – otherwise easier
16	Excoriated parts of scrotum easier. Milk diet and bit of meat daily
18	Excoriation almost healed – gums not affected – no copper taste in his mouth
20	Ulcerations at the scrotum now healed. No obvious affection of gums no any copper taste in his mouth.
23	Continues free from ulcerations of scrotum. Throat nearly as before. Gums not affected nor does he complain of copper taste in his mouth. Continue ointment and give mercury pills 2 gr
24	Two stools since he took the pills – as yesterday
25	No more looseness – still griped – gums not affected – nor has he copper taste in mouth.
26	Throat nearly as at admission – continue medications. Gargles with Peruvian bark and rose water infusions
27	Slight pain in his throat from use of gargle. In other respects as yesterday.
Mar. 1	Some sickness from pills last night but without vomiting. In other respects as before.
2	Some soreness of his gums and copper taste in the mouth.
3	Soreness of gums rather augmented and complains today of gripes but without looseness.
4	Mouth nearly as before – free from gripes today – pulse 85 – bowels regular
5	Soreness of the gums increased and he spits a little. Pulse 100 – bowels regular.
6	Sweated profusely in the night. Gums and spitting as before. Pulse 84 – bowels rather bound – Continue medications – give aloetic pills 10 gr at bedtime
9	Spits a little – bowels regular; continue gargles – use aloetic pills intermittently
10	Still spits a little – pulse 96 – bowels regular
11	Continues to spit a little and complains today of more soreness in his gums. Pulse 92 – bowels regular – continue gargles – use mercurial ointment intermittently
12	Gums rather easier – spitting diminished – continue gargles and repeat ointment
13	Mouth easier, spitting diminished. Pulse and bowels natural
17	No spitting – has still soreness of gums
21	Soreness of gums and sweated a good deal during the night. Pulse 82 – bowels regular – continue gargles – use ointment intermittently
25	Still some soreness of gums but no spitting. Pulse 90 – bowels regular
29	Still some soreness of gums but no spitting. Pulse 94

Apr.	2	Mouth as before – continue gargles but omit ointment
	3	Mouth nearly as before – pulse 90 – bowels regular. Take salts of phosphor
	5	Salts have not operated – Still some uneasiness of jaws; pulse 78; inject in evening a domestic enema. Give jalap powder
	6	Had but one stool from powders yesterday but had several loose stools this morning. Pulse 82 – repeat jalap powders
	7	Has had frequent stools from purgation. Give Peruvian bark powders
	8	Gums still sore – bowels regular – no spitting – Pulse 82 – continue Peruvian bark
	9	Very little affection of gums
	15	No spitting – but has much pain from a small ulcer on the inside of right cheek near the last of the molars; continue Peruvian bark and apply liniment containing diluted sulphuric acid
	16	Slight pain from application of liniment
	17	Ulcer in cheek almost healed. Pulse 84 – bowels regular
	20	The ulceration of the cheek is now healed and there has been no affection of throat or scrotum some time past. Let him be dismissed *cured*

Dr. Duncan's comments

In the case of this patient, the symptoms are neither numerous or distressing, and are such as to leave us little room to doubt of its being a venereal affection. The symptoms when he came into the house might have arisen from different causes but the local affection which had taken place in the genitals and throat had as much the appearance of syphilis as of any other disease.

When we add that he was under the influence of contagion some time ago, there is no reason to doubt of venereal virus. He had, sometime ago, a chancre and though this was cured by proper means, we may yet suppose that the malady was not eradicated from the constitution. The healing of topical ulcers has often produced ulcers in different parts of the body. For my own part, I am not acquainted with any test which proves that the contagion is eradicated when it has been once received.

It is not difficult, we imagine, to cure this disease when it makes its appearance in the form of ulcers in the throat. This may be done in some instances in a short time, in others there is nothing more improper than to consider as laboring under a latent pox every person who has once had it, or again, to neglect such symptoms when they appear in a person who has been exposed to the affection.

In the present case though, the symptoms did not clearly mark the disease, yet we certainly had presumption for supposing it to be venereal. As the syphilitic appearances were not transitory, I think it is highly probably that during the time they would have been more violent if the disease had not been kept down by mercury.

As to the prognosis, I think the termination will be favorable. It would appear from what we have seen, from the quantity of mercury thrown in that he is of a constitution on which mercury will not act with ease. Hence, it will be more difficult to effect a cure. No considerable local affections have taken place, and as far as we can judge, the disease has only attacked the softer solids; there is no reason to believe that the bones are affected.

There is no disease with which syphilis may be so often confounded as scrofula, but when it is doubtful which disease it may be, the yielding of a syphilitic complaint to mercury will characterize them. For there are few diseases the cure of which can be so well depended upon as syphilis, so that there is little reason to doubt of our being able to eradicate this disease. The eradication, however, must depend on proper observance of the remedies for some time.

As to the cause of syphilis, there are some particulars on which all practitioners are agreed, as that it is produced by a specific contagion, although they may differ in their opinion whether this is the same disease that produces gonorrhea. It certainly is propagated in the same way.

There are three modes in which mercury may be said to act on the system and cure the disease. 1) by preventing the virus from acting, 2) by expelling it from the system, and 3) by allaying its acrimony. On these three suppositions it may be overcome and on all recourse is had to mercury. The two last opinions are supported by many very ingenious authors as Cullen and Hunter, but that which is the oldest and has, I think, the greatest probability, is the first.

We may suppose mercury to act as sulphur does on mercury or acids on alkalines. It would be foreign to my purpose to enter into a longer discussion of this subject, but I may refer you, for my opinion, to the observations I have published. There is no doubt but that mercury is an effectual mode of cure, and of all the modes adopted in this country it answers best. I have no experience about what has been said of opium and other remedies, but mercury is certainly the most powerful. It very rarely fails, therefore, except in very particular cases it is employed.

To a mercurial drug, therefore, I had recourse, but there is no urgent symptom which requires that it should be precipitated, and indeed it is more on its slow progress that we can depend on it eradicating a syphilitic taint. There can be no doubt but when mercury produces a looseness that its action is retarded. I am inclined to hold the same opinion with respect to the use of salivation. This is indeed a proof that the mercury has entered the system and it is a means of restraining patients from irregularities which might be improper. Therefore, it should be proper to induce a state of salivation, yet I by no means think that it is necessary to the cure. It also prevents us from the use of mercury for some patients, yet on the continuance of which the cure sometimes depends.

The most effectual way is to keep the constitution charged for some time which is not to be judged of by the length of time but by the peculiar marks of fetid breath, sore gums, and copper taste in the mouth. It will be proper to keep them thus charged and on the verge of salivation for some time. This is difficult to be done on account of its affecting the mouth. It is on this plan I have proceeded with the present patient and as it seemed to have a tendency to have run off by the bowels, I have not pushed it. I shall defer any remarks on the mercurial used or its mode of operation.

I formerly stated my sentiments at considerable length on this patient and mentioned those circumstances which pointed out a venereal taint. I therefore subjected him to a mercurial course for nearly the space of two months. Under this regimen, the patient was kept constantly charged with mercury and on the verge of salivation, and all the symptoms disappeared. There was afterwards an affection of the gums, an ulcer, but the latter was not syphilitic – rather what may be called a mercurial ulcer. It was soon cured by the application of honey and vitriolic acid. After the cure of this, he left us free from an affection either of throat or scrotum, and I think what was before his admission a venereal disease, is now radically cured.

Case 2

Patient:	M.R.
Notebook:	Francis Home, Clinical cases from the Royal Infirmary and reports with notes as delivered by Francis Home, by Robert Dunlop, Edinburgh, 1783 and 1786–1787
Location:	MSS Collection, Edinburgh Room, Edinburgh City Library
Age:	26
Sex and status:	Female, a widow
Admitted:	Jan. 11, 1787, during Home's clinical rotation from Nov. 1, 1786, to Jan. 31, 1787
Diagnosis:	Lues Venerea

Female patients suffering from venereal diseases usually were "locked up" in the infirmary's "high" or "salivation" ward or if it was filled, admitted to the medical ordinary wing. This woman, however, was sent to the teaching ward, presumably for instructing the students in the use of mercury and because her pains in the bones were suggestive of a later clinical stage of syphilis. The diagnosis was apparently made on the basis of genital ulcers and warts, followed by a skin rash that was interpreted as reflecting systemic disease.

In contrast to other histories, most progress notes on this case were brief, concentrating especially on the effects of treatment. Like Duncan's patient, the woman received the standard mercurial treatment consisting of an ointment and a bolus or large pill, the latter made with corrosive mercurial sublimate and mucilage, a popular combination also known as Plenck's solution if both items were mixed with a syrup.[3] The addition of mucilagenous substances was thought to prevent excessive diarrhea and salivation, although the latter occurred to a considerable degree in this case. The ointment contained a powder made from the leaf of savin, an evergreen, used extensively in the eighteenth century to "consume" the venereal warts.[4]

The treatment ordered for this patient was based on the well-known actions of two drugs, one of them used externally on the lesions, the other given by mouth to act systemically. The amount of salivation was closely monitored to avoid excessive inflammation of the gums followed by the loss of teeth. Throughout the hospitalization the patient was kept on a milk diet supposed to moderate the mercurialism. Modest improvement was noted in a relatively short time, and the patient was discharged "cured" – clearly an exaggeration – at the end of Home's clinical rotation to make room for new arrivals selected by his colleague, James Gregory.

Although not recorded, it is likely that the woman received on discharge sufficient mercurial pills to complete her treatment at home, since most courses of therapy with this drug lasted about six to eight weeks. By discharging the patient prematurely for bureaucratic reasons, the attending professor clearly risked the likelihood that she would promptly discontinue taking her medicine because of the considerable discomfort in her mouth. Stopping the mercury too soon would probably result in only the temporary arrest of the disease, with the patient gradually progressing to a more severe stage and perhaps still capable of infecting her subsequent sexual partners.

Jan. 11, 1787   Complains of severe pains in the middle of the bones of all her extremities especially in those of the lower extremity and says these are always most severe when warm in bed. No eminences can be felt on either. Says that about 12 months ago when giving suck to a child her breasts became affected with foul ulcers which continued to discharge for about a month and were succeeded by blotches all over her body about the size of half a crown. All of which disappeared again in two months except one which still remains on the outside of her right thigh. Soon after drying up of the blotches a number of warty excrescences appeared about the anus and perineum. These have become now ulcerated and discharge a quantity of acrid fetid substance. About six months ago two large livid blotches appeared on the naturalia and now the whole labia externally are affected with a continued ulceration. Since then at different times several other ulcerations have appeared about the top of the thigh which appear much inflamed and discharge sanies.

The whole of her body at present is affected with small florid blotches of three weeks' standing but which have disappeared twice before on using Glauber's salts. Her throat at present is not affected but she says it was sore about five months ago.

Pulse natural – bowels bound – menses have appeared but only these past four months – last one occurred four weeks ago

Give bolus composed of gum arabic and mercury precipitate – bathe lesions in tepid water – apply powder of savin to the warts.

12   Nausea after the bolus; had the bath this morning. Repeat bath & bolus – milk diet.

13   No sensible effect from the bolus – repeat

14   Brassy taste in her mouth which waters a little. Continue bolus – stop bath

15   No effect except nausea – continue medication

16   No sensible effect from medicine

17   Began to spit yesterday afternoon and has spit 2 boxfuls – Omit bolus

18   Has spit 2 boxfuls – All symptoms much abated – continue medication

19   Mouth sore – has spit one boxful

21   Nocturnal pains – ulcerations and the excrescences on the anus better – mouth sore – repeat bolus

23   Has spit a boxful and half; omit bolus

24   2½ boxfuls – symptoms are all better

25   1½ boxfuls

26   All the venereal symptoms are gone except the warty excrescences on the anus. Spit 2 boxfuls last night but has no spitting today – Repeat bolus.

27   Has spit ½ boxful – repeat bolus

28   No spitting – repeat bolus

30   Warty excrescences look better since the application of the savin powder – Spits none – repeat bolus

Feb. 1   Spits a little – repeat bolus

2   Purged twice; warty excrescence much diminished. Dismissed *cured*

Case 3

Patient:	J.W.
Notebook:	William Cullen, Clinical cases and reports taken at the Royal Infirmary of Edinburgh from Dr. Cullen, taken by Richard W. Hall, Edinburgh, 1772–1773
Location:	MSS Collection, National Library of Medicine, Bethesda, MD
Age:	17
Sex:	Female
Admitted:	Dec. 13, 1772, during Cullen's rotation from Nov. 1, 1772, to Jan. 31, 1773
Diagnosis:	Fever

This patient is a good example of the inflammatory fever cases handled at the infirmary. Young and female, with acute symptoms for barely one week prior to admission and a record of previous treatment, the typical fever patient was immediately placed on an "antiphlogistic" regimen that included a low diet, emetics and purgatives, and bloodletting. Cullen preferred the use of ipecac powder for swift emesis and then continued with antimony preparations, especially the tartar emetic or potassium tartrate, which acted as both an emetic and a purgative.[5] His bloodletting orders came during the early stages of this patient's inflammatory condition and amounted to a total of sixteen ounces, although less was probably extracted because of technical problems. Secondary infection ensued around the incision about two weeks after the phlebotomy, prompting a surgical consultation and local treatment with a poultice.

For the first ten days the patient's temperature fluctuated greatly, and she was frequently delirious at night in spite of the hourly fomentations of her feet and legs. Temporary deafness, a persistent cough, and chest pain suggested a respiratory infection, inducing the administration of expectorants and diaphoretics, such as the mucilagenous and saline mixtures, and the production of a blister on her back. The golden root or virga aurea *(Jacobea palustris)* was employed as an astringent and bitter medicine designed to counteract the systemic debility produced by the fever after all overt inflammatory symptoms abated on Dec. 19, signaling recovery.[6] The last ten days of hospitalization – almost a third of her total stay – were devoted to total recovery and were entered into the ward ledger as a convalescent period. This protracted convalescence was not uncommon if the patients came into the teaching ward during the winter months in the middle of a professor's clinical rotation or around the holidays when there were fewer demands for beds.

Dec. 13, 1772	Complains of pains in her head and in general over her body with great debility, sensation of heat, restlessness and oppression about the precordia, thirst, bad taste in her mouth – anorexia; Skin hot, pulse 120, complaints of 8 days standing and were preceded by a sensation of excessive cold and great debility. She was bled 3 days ago and after it served with a vomit and purging which continued all that night, but she has had not stool since. Inject a saline enema and give ipecac powder 1½ gr
15	Pulse 126 and pretty full – skin not very warm but she is thirsty and still complaining of pain all over her body; gets little sleep and was delirious in the night; has still a frequent cough; powders made her vomit a little and she has had several stools since. Remove 8 oz of blood – repeat Ipecac powders. Before and after the powders use mucilagenous mixture every two hours
16	Pulse 128, it was difficult to find a vein in any part of her arm or hand, and therefore the blood was drawn from her foot, from which she felt some relief, but still complains a

great deal of her head; has had one stool since last night, has slept little, been delirious and takes very little food. Withdraw another 8 oz blood from arm at 7 pm. Give solution of tartar emetic – alternate every 2 hours with mucilagenous mixture and nitrous mixture

17   Pulse 120. Was bled at the arm yesterday but seemed little relieved by it – as it did not flow freely, it is not sizy – solution did not make her vomit but has purged her twice – continues very delirious – has slept very little but has taken some food; thirst still great; pulse though frequent is without any perceptible quickness, soft and regular. Cough less frequent. Repeat solution of tartar emetic – continue mixtures; fomentations of feet and legs hourly. Apply blister to interscapular area of back

18   Pulse 120 but still soft and regular. Was very delirious in the night and is deaf today – thirst continues but tongue quite moist. Four doses of the solution last night did not make her vomit but have purged her several times – has no appetite; cough less frequent. Repeat solution of tartar emetic 1 ounce per dose – Continue mixture. 3 doses at 10 pm

19   Pulse 120, slept all yesterday afternoon and evening but awakened between 9 and 10 o'clock as delirious as before, and she continued very delirious during the whole night – got some sleep again this morning and afternoon, but now the delirium appears to be very abated – three doses of the solution as ordered last night did not make her vomit but have purged her four or five times. She has taken some food this morning. Her feet and legs were fomented during the night but with no effect in quieting her delirium; there is now some moisture on her skin; her deafness is much as before. In afternoon give golden root powder gr X and continue mixture

20   Pulse 110. Powder last night did not make her vomit or even seem to make her sick; has had some stools since, but how many is not known as she gives no notice of them to the nurse, but they do not appear to have been very many; she has slept considerably at different times but, in the intervals, she is as delirious as before; thirst continues but tongue moist and soft; has very little appetite; the blister applied on the 17th did not appear risen till this morning when it has discharged pretty well. Continue mixture.

21   Pulse 106 – slept much, but in the intervals is as delirious as before; has taken some food; still drinks a good deal; has had no stool since yesterday afternoon. Repeat golden root powder

22   Pulse 110 – Powder last night occasioned some wretching

but she did not vomit, has purged since as the nurse thinks, three times but the patient gives no notice of it and the nurse cannot be exact; slept none in the night but has slept this morning; delirium continues but it is of a less restless and more cheerful kind; has still no appetite. Omit powders – continue mixture

23   Pulse 108, slept a good deal in the night, delirium abated; has had one stool and has taken some food this morning. Continue mixture – Let her have a sweet orange to take a little of now and then as she desires it.

24   Pulse 98, slept little in the night but much this morning; delirium abated and takes food; belly regular. Continue mixture

25   Pulse 104, rested well a great part of the night but was restless this morning, though she was very little delirious; she takes a little food; has had no stool; cough rather more frequent.
      1) Inject saline enema using 2 oz salt at 7 pm
      2) Omit mixture of nitre salts
      3) Use mucilagenous mixture
      4) Fomentation to feet and legs every hour

26   Had a stool by the glyster last night, was put to sleep by the fomentation and slept a good deal after it and would have slept more had it not been for the frequency of her cough. Delirium almost gone; takes food. Repeat fomentations in the evening and continue mucilagenous mixture as desired.

27   All her symptoms easier – continue

28   Pulse 80. Has a swelling and suppuration on the part of her arm where last bled. Otherwise continues to recover. Continue medications.

29   Sleeps and takes food pretty well. Complains of pain in her arm. The surgeon has ordered a poultice of bread and milk to be applied to it. Continue medications.

30, 31–Jan. 1–5 Convalescent
Jan. 6–8 Convalescent
9   Dismissed *cured*

Case 4

Patient:	P.M.
Notebook:	Daniel Rutherford, Clinical cases, Edinburgh, 1799
Location:	MSS Collection, Royal College of Physicians, Edinburgh
Age:	17
Sex:	Female

Admitted: June 28, 1799, during Rutherford's special summer lectures, from May 7 to July 26, 1799
Diagnosis: Typhus fever

In contrast to inflammatory fevers, so-called nervous fevers also known as typhus began insidiously and lingered on, getting progressively worse with bouts of fever, tremors, and delirium recurring during the second and third weeks of the disease. Physicians at the time recognized that this type of fever could not be effectively treated with conventional antiphlogistic measures, and therefore they instituted from the onset a stimulating regimen designed to strengthen the patient's constitution.

The young woman under Rutherford's care was managed in a typical way. She was treated with painkillers, notably a draft containing laudanum, and she received a number of tonic drugs, including a camphorated solution and wine mixed with diluted sulfuric acid. Frequent fomentations were ordered to counteract her delirium, and a blister was applied to the neck because of severe headaches. An initial diarrhea was stopped by the use of a chalk potion,[7] but the bowels were "kept open" with the help of rhubarb powder and occasional enemas. Generous doses of fluids were given in the face of a continuous fever that parched her lips and mouth.

The patient had quite a stormy and lengthy hospitalization, frequently delirious and restless during nights, unruly enough to require restraints, including a waistcoat. When she was awake, her mental state was periodically checked by nurses and physicians. As Rutherford commented, "delirium is always attended with great inconvenience; the worst circumstance is when one cannot get direct answers from the patient which prevents us from judging so accurately of the patient's situation."[8]

In time, from the rubbing of bedclothes or simply the pressure on her skin, the woman developed an extensive bedsore on her back that called for the application of poultices. She remained in the teaching unit for a month and was remitted to the ordinary medical ward at the end of Rutherford's summer session. Omissions in the General Register of Patients do not allow us to ascertain her final disposition, although it is quite probable that she remained in the hospital for only a few days convalescing before being dismissed. Indeed, Rutherford commented that her symptoms were "augmented by her great desire to go home to her friends."[9]

June 28, 1799   Complains of general sense of soreness through the body with frequent nausea and at times severe headaches. She is also much affected with diarrhea – appetite very bad – much thirst – tongue furred but moist – pulse quick and weak – Menses did not appear at the last period – A fortnight ago she was seized with shivering, headache and sickness attended with a considerable degree of soreness of the throat, but she is now quite recovered from the latter. Knows no cause for these complaints except exposure to cold – has used no medications

29 Has passed a very restless night. The diarrhea continues to be severe – pulse quick and small – skin hot and dry – tongue extremely furred – headache constant and severe – Give rhubarb powder [as purgative]. Mucilage gum arabic. For diarrhea chalk potion

30 She has been extremely restless and delirious throughout the night – at present she is distinct and the heat of the body is not considerable. The pulse is however very quick and rather small and feeble – headache severe and the purging continues. Apply blister to the nape of the neck. Continue chalk potion. Anodyne draft for evening administration

July 1 Was extremely restless and delirious throughout the night, in so much that she could hardly be confined to bed and caused great disturbance by her constant screams. Today the pulse is not remarkably quick nor strong. Skin is hot and dry – she does not seem to feel much uneasiness – the bowels are rather loose. Rhubarb powder – continued. Anodyne draft with 40 drops laudanum at bedtime

2 She continued very restless and unruly all evening but she became calmer presently after she was fomented. Passed a quiet night and slept much though at times she moaned considerably. At present she is rather languid. Skin cool – pulse moderate in velocity and quite soft – tongue rather foul but moist. Evening enema. Continue fomentations. Anodyne draft with 30 drops of laudanum

3 Was again restless last night and at times very delirious and unruly. At present she is quite distinct but seems much distressed with general uneasiness yet specifies no particular complaint except that of headache. Eyes are very heavy – but she does not seem very languid – Pulse quick and rather small but is regular – Skin rather hotter than natural – tongue considerably furred – thirst urgent. Repeat enema & fomentations. Saline mixture. Draft with 40 drops of laudanum at bedtime

4 She was again restless last night though not so considerably as the night before. Today the febrile symptoms are by no means great. She is perfectly distinct – roused by questions proposed to her; at other times she seems incoherent. She has neither headache nor pain in any part of the body. Pulse moderate – tongue and skin continue parched – the belly is very loose – Omit saline mixture and anodyne draft

5 Was just as delirious last night as she has been in the two preceding ones, yet at present she answers questions quite distinctly. The general febrile symptoms are not increased,

only the tongue is extremely dry – she occasionally takes a little food and drinks plentifully – the bowels are loose – Administer a camphor solution

6   She was not just so restless last night and this morning seems considerably better. The skin is pretty cool – pulse is more natural – tongue moist except for a small streak through the middle – bowels pretty regular

7   In the course of the night she was distressed and is represented to have passed some blood by stool. At present, she is very drowsy, yet answers apparently to the questions that are proposed to her. The pulse is very little quicker than natural – Skin rather dry but of natural warmth. Evening enema with linseed infusion. Repeat camphorated draft and fomentations

8   Has passed a quiet night though at present in a profound sleep. The skin is moderately cool and the pulse reduced in frequency. She takes very little food but drinks plentifully. Omit camphorated draft. Give 4 oz of wine daily

9   Has had a quiet night. At present the pulse of nearly natural velocity, though rather feeble. Skin is cool but the tongue is still loaded and the appetite very bad. Continue wine

10   She has continued extremely drowsy yet when aroused, she seems quite distinct and says she is quite free from pain or uneasiness in the head. The pulse is feeble but is reduced to natural frequency. The skin is quite cool. In many places the scarfskin seems to separate. Tongue is dry – the countenance is not expressive of particular languor nor is it remarkably pale. She is still reluctant at taking food though has had two loose stools this morning. Continue wine

11   All the febrile symptoms are very much abated, but the tongue is still slightly furred in the middle, it is however moist and clean at the edges, and she has little thirst. Continue wine

12   Skin and pulse are quite natural, but the tongue is still foul, and at times she is very incoherent. Vitriolated elixir 20 drops in infusion of chamomile

13   Has been at times extremely restless and at times unruly and incoherent, but skin and belly are pretty regular. Tincture of opium 25 drops

14   Has slept calmly the whole night and is at present asleep. There is a pretty considerable gangrenous spot on the back. She does not complain of pain, however. The pulse is of natural velocity but rather feeble. The skin is rough from the separation of the cuticle but of natural warmth. Yesterday and today she has been very averse to taking food. Double the wine dosage

15   Was so extremely unruly through the night that to prevent her from exasperating the sore on the back, it was necessary to restrain her by means of a strait waist coat. She is now quite quiet. The draft was accidently omitted. Takes food with less reluctance than formerly. Continue medications

16   She was very restless during the greater part of the night. Since morning she has been quiet. This morning she took some food with appetite. Her skin is quite cool and general febrile symptoms are altogether gone. Continue all medications

17   She was uncommonly restless and unruly last night and continued so in the morning in so much that she could hardly be kept in bed. At present she is quiet. The pulse and skin are quite natural and the tongue is clean. Her appetite seems to return. She occasionally calls for food and takes what is brought her seemingly with relish. The bowels are regular. Tincture of opium 40 drops – continue fomentations – camphorated draft

18   She was out of bed for about half an hour in the evening and apparently without much uneasiness. Yet she was very restless again in the night but now she is quite calm and disposed to sleep. There is no appearance of a return of febrile symptoms and she does not show reluctance at her food. Continue medications

19   Had a very good night and seems in all respects greatly recruited. Complains of pains in the hollows of her side and the gangrenous spot on the back seems to penetrate deeper than it did, but it is not extended in breadth. Continue medications

20   Continues to recover but the sore on the back is represented to be rather extended. Continue medications

21   Seems very weak and the mind is much enfeebled, but in general she is very quiet. The sore on the back is enlarged and a very thick slough begins to separate from it. Continue all prescriptions

22   No bad symptoms appear though she is at times restless and even delirious. Continue

23   She seems to recover but the sore does not heal – continue medications

24   She continues to recover

25   She continues to recover but the sore of the back gives her very great uneasiness – it is very deep and though a thick slough has been separated, the ulcer looks very foul. Apply poultice to ulcer

26   It was impossible to procure carrots proper for the poul-

tice. Turnips were substituted for them. She still complains
of pain but the appearance of the ulcer is rather improved.
Continue poultice and remit to ordinary physicians

Case 5

Patient:	K.K.
Notebook:	Thomas C. Hope, Clinical casebook, Edinburgh, 1796–1797
Location:	MSS Collection, Royal College of Physicians, Edinburgh
Age:	15
Sex:	Female
Admitted:	Dec. 15, 1796, during Hope's clinical rotation from Nov. 1, 1796, to Jan. 31, 1796
Diagnosis:	Phthisis

Phthisis or tuberculosis, as it was later called, was a frequent ailment in eighteenth-century Edinburgh according to the city's mortality figures. Only cases considered incipient and therefore potentially curable were viewed as proper for hospital treatment. This young woman gave a history of respiratory and digestive symptoms that had bothered her for about eight months, with hemoptysis, cough, weight loss, and progressive debility suggesting a serious if not fatal disease. Some of her symptoms, such as the cough, dyspnea, and chest pain, were promptly treated with expectorants, vapor inhalations, blisters, and even leeches to remove local congestion.

Pills containing aloes were given as mild laxatives to keep the bowels open; the ferrous sulfate, half baths, and electricity were designed to stimulate the bodily system, confer strength, and thus, it was hoped, help her overcome the disease. The deleterious effects of submitting patients daily to electrical sparks were noted; but all these measures were thought to act as emmenagogues to restore the patient's menstrual flow, always considered a sensitive indicator of impaired health. Also used for this purpose was asafetida, a gum resin from a Persian plant then being cultivated in the hothouses of Edinburgh's botanical gardens, thanks to the efforts of Thomas C. Hope's father, former professor of botany John Hope.[10] Cullen and others employed it as an antispasmodic drug in suspected cases of hysteria.[11] In this instance it was administered to the patient on Jan. 9, 1797, after she complained of an oppression in her throat that prevented swallowing food.

In the eyes of the attending professor, the protracted medical treatment was at least partially successful in helping the sick adolescent regain a measure of strength while simultaneously ameliorating some of the respiratory symptoms. At the end of Hope's rotation the patient was sent to the ordinary medical ward; the General Register of Patients listed her as dismissed "relieved" on Feb. 14, 1797, two months after her admittance to the teaching ward. The case points out the limited role of medicine in the management of pulmonary tuberculosis and the dangers of confining such patients in hospitals lacking "fresh country air."

Dec. 15, 1796	Is affected with a violent cough attended with scanty and difficult expectoration; much dyspnea, considerable pain in both sides, and under the unciform cartilage, increased by cough and somewhat by a full inspiration. She has also much vertigo, particularly on going from the recumbent posture on sitting to an erect posture. Pain in the right side, constant headache, pain of the back and only pain in the loins and lower part of the abdomen, stretching down the thighs. Nausea and vomiting, frequently induced by the cough, which is most severe at night. Says she often coughs up a small quantity of blood which she describes as black and not frothy. Has occasionally epistaxis; her feet and legs swell towards the night and she is very much debilitated and depressed.
	Pulse 104 – tongue clean – appetite bad – very costive – sleeps ill from violent cough. Menstrual periods appeared for the first time about 8 months ago and returned at regular intervals but [were] stopped by exposure to cold and moisture, to which she also attributes her other complaints which have since been on the increase. Says she was very much affected but less so some time past with a vomit of blood which though black and grumous, she never observed mixed with her food. Has ineffectually taken various remedies.
16	Apply blister to sternum. Aloetic pills – 8 gr
17	Blister rose well, cough with expectoration as usual – vomited her supper last night – pain in breast and other parts of the body abated. Semicupium bath – frictions of abdomen and back. Expectorant bolus. Ferrous sulfate 4 gr
18	Cough much relieved – vomited her breakfast this morning – no change of her symptoms. Repeat partial bath and medications
19	Headache gone – no vomiting since yesterday – other symptoms as formerly – thinks herself rather weaker – omit partial bath, – instead full cold bath. Continue expectorant bolus
20	No report
21	Vomited her supper and breakfast. Continue medications and cold bath
22	Vomited her supper – pain of breast – little change – other pains easier

23	No vomiting – pains continue. Electrical machine – sparks over lumbar and abdominal regions
25	Cough and pain as formerly – was not electrified till this morning and for 2 hours. Has not used the cold bath. Electrical machine treatments twice a day. Repeat cold bath
26	Did not get the bath – still pain of head and breast
27	No vomiting – breast, head and stomach somewhat more uneasy in the afternoon
28	Cough unchanged. Troches with glycerin and opium
29	Complains of more pain about the back and loins, and even the stomach. Vomited her dinner and supper immediately after taking them. Her cough has been troublesome. Has not been electrified above once a day. To exercise with the chamber-horse – continue electrification twice a day – To have steak for dinner
31	The electrifying produced so much uneasiness as to cause her to faint. Since then the pains of her back and abdomen have been severe. Has taken but little food but no vomiting. Pulse 108 – fuller and stronger than usual. Omit electricity – Half bath in evening – continue expectorant bolus
Jan. 1, 1797	In the afternoon all her pains became much easier and they continue so. Vomited her breakfast – pulse 110, not so full or strong as yesterday. Repeat half bath in evening
2	No vomiting – continues free from pain
3	Says she is a great deal better – also stronger
4	Vomited during the night – all her pains have quitted her except that of the stomach
5	No report
6	No vomiting – coughed a good deal during the night – her strength improves daily – her ankles now swell at night
8	No vomiting – cough continues to diminish – cramp in her stomach still continues – pulse 102
9	The uneasiness about the stomach was not abated – pain between middle of sternum and unciform cartilage – it was much increased by placement of a blister – no vomiting – less cough – the uneasiness she now feels she compares to that of a swelling under the sternum which prevents her from taking food or drink. Asafetida 12 gr
10	After second dose of asafetida, pain and uneasiness under the sternum was relieved – cough more urgent and the former pain returned to her back – pulse 112
13	Sickness continues – pain in back and limbs – fomentations – evening half-bath
17	Pains abated – cough still urgent – some dyspnea. Vapor inhalations at bedtime
22	Cough still troublesome. Apply 8 leeches to painful area of chest
23	Seven leeches fixed – Previous blister has not yet risen –

says her cough has been as troublesome as formerly

26   Cough continues to abate – uneasiness of the stomach has plagued her repeatedly though she had considerable temporary relief from taking the solution of asafetida

30   Complains of headaches – uneasiness of stomach and back troublesome during the night – strength considerably improved – remit to the ordinary physicians

Case 6

Patient:	K.S.
Notebook:	John Hope, Cases of patients in the Royal Infirmary under the care of John Hope, M.D., Edinburgh, 1781
Location:	MSS Collection, University of Edinburgh
Age:	28
Sex and status:	Male, a laborer
Admitted:	Sept. 10, 1781, to the ordinary medical ward under the care of both attending physicians
Diagnosis:	Ague or intermittent fever

This seasonal farm worker was hospitalized twice in the fall of 1781 for a disease he apparently acquired six weeks earlier during the late summer harvest in one of the fen counties of southeastern England. His febrile paroxysms at the outset occurred every third day but had become daily before the initial admission, which lasted three weeks. In addition to traditional antiphlogistic measures, such as emetics (ipecac powder), purgatives (rhubarb powder), and fomentations, the patient received antimony drafts to stimulate diaphoresis and an expectorant, julep of squill.

After the disappearance of fever fits ten days later, the physicians abandoned their sedative regimen and began a stimulating course of treatment that included Peruvian bark extract, the specific tonic widely employed in intermittent fevers. Before the man was discharged, he also received a full diet containing meat.

The second admission occurred six days later, when the patient returned to the hospital with a number of symptoms suggestive of an acute respiratory ailment. Again, he was initially given emetics and purgatives, his chest was cupped and blistered, and he also received bedtime sedation in the form of a drink containing laudanum. Both antimony solutions and a saline mixture were used to promote further sweating. As the patient gradually became more debilitated and emaciated, he received a more stimulating regimen that included a cordial julep (*Julapium cardiacum*) with saffron and aromatic spirits,[12] wine, Peruvian bark, and a meat diet. Unfortunately, he died a month after readmission in spite of all efforts made to save him. Presumably his debilitated body, which already had endured severe febrile fits in England and an exhausting trip back home in a wagon, could not resist the additional burdens of a respiratory disease.

A dissection of the body was authorized. Among the findings described by the physicians were signs of cerebral and pulmonary congestion, extreme emaciation, and bowel changes that could well have occurred after death. No comments about the size and condition of the spleen were recorded.

Sept. 10, 1781	Complains of constant headache, sickness and at times cough with viscid expectoration. When he attempts to cough he feels his breast uneasy and sore. He sweats copiously every morning with apparent relief of headache and sickness but always finds himself considerably weakened by it. About six weeks ago while at harvest work in England after being very warm and perspiring very freely, he was seized with coldness to which the headache, cough and pain of breast succeeded without heat but in a day or two the morning sweat supervened. These complaints have continued nearly the same ever since. Pulse about 100 – bowels regular – appetite at times tolerably good. Ipecac powder. Anodyne draft with antimony at bedtime
11	Vomit operated well – a good night – sweated much. Cupping of both temples – Repeat anodyne draft
12	Headache and all his other complaints gone
13	Pretty frequent cough. Infusion of linseed – Julep of squill
14	Yesterday after the visit was seized with chilliness and shivering succeeded by heat – at present easy
15	About seven in the morning seemed confused and indistinct towards forenoon. He became quite stupid and even insane and at intervals slept a little from 3 to 4 p.m. He was very unmanageable afterward, fell asleep and did not fully awake till this evening when he became totally distinct. He then took a draft of small beer, and slept very well through the night
16	Today there is no marker of insanity and he appears as distinct as when he came into the house. Complains still of headache – pulse 100 – no fit since the 14th
17	No sleep during the night – sometime ago seems to have been affected with a feverish paroxysm – pulse 100. At 2 p.m. became exceedingly sick and threw up a good deal of yellow, bitter stuff and complained of general uneasiness and soreness over his whole body. Pulse 136 – skin hot. At 4 p.m., skin hot – pulse 160 and full – no appetite – no return of vomiting – still sickly – complains of general soreness. At 6 p.m., has slept upwards of an hour and says he is

somewhat easier – pulse 136 – tongue dry – thirsty and
still sick.

At 8 p.m., pulse 116 – has slept almost since 6 o'clock –
still complains of general soreness and thirst – tongue
moister – skin very hot – has eaten little or nothing today.
Inject saline enema. Fomentation of legs. Antimony solution at bedtime

18   8 a.m. – slept well during the night and sweated a good
deal – says he is pretty easy – pulse 100 and soft – tongue
rather dry – still thirsty and has a desire for a small beer –
had a natural stool from the injection

19   a.m., pulse 96 – skin of natural heat – continues easy – is
thirsty but has no appetite at visit, skin pretty cool, pulse
about 92 – feels himself easy. Give Peruvian cortex powder and rhubarb powder

In the afternoon and evening, pulse from 100 to 112 – skin
of natural heat – has no hectic complaint

20   Had a antimonial anodyne last night – slept tolerably well
and sweated some in the night. Pulse 116 and pretty full –
skin hot – tongue dry – complains much of thirst – is
desirous to have small beer – no appetite – says he has not
eaten anything last 5 days – during the forenoon he felt
very weak and complained of general uneasiness and sickness – great thirst – pulse 100 – had a plentiful loose stool
last night – At the visit, pulse 96 – skin hot – tongue
moist – to have one bottle of small beer daily. Repeat antimonial anodyne

In the afternoon and evening very distressed – had several
loose stools – seems somewhat delirious – pulse 120 –
skin hot – thirsty

21   Got the antimonial anodyne last night – slept a little but
was watchful great part of the night – had a loose stool
this morning – complains much of weakness – tongue dry
and somewhat blackish – great thirst – pulse about 84 –
today as distinct as usual – At visit, pulse about 104 –
continue Peruvian cortex

22   Skin cool, pulse 96 – tongue moist – to have milk morning and evening. Peruvian cortex powder continued – no
rhubarb

23   Finds himself considerably easier – pulse 96 – continue
medication

24   Countenance more natural – is considerably relieved – no
fit

25   Continues better – is sensible in every respect – pulse 84
– continue Peruvian cortex

26   Recovering his looks – no fits

29   A bit of meat daily

Oct. 1	Dismissed *cured*
Readmission Oct. 6, 1781	Complains of headache and sickness, short tickling cough and difficulty of breathing. About 6 weeks ago when at harvest in a fen county in England, was seized with headaches, sickness, and general pains. He says he never but once had a chilly fit but has frequent hot fits succeeded by sweating, especially in the night. At times his distress seems to assume somewhat of the tertian type, at others that of the quotidian.
	Pulse upwards of 100. Skin cool. Tongue whitish. Little appetite – bowels at present pretty regular though costive for some time past – complains of pain in his left side which he attributes to riding from England in a wagon. Had a brother who died of an intermittent fever on his way from England. Ipecac powder, 1 scruple
7	Pulse 76 – on pressure feels pain in the region of the spleen. Saline julep. Cupping over painful side
8	Pulse 96 – pain of the side relieved. Is very weak and complains much of want of sleep. Repeat saline julep. Anodyne draft with 20 drops of laudanum at bedtime.
9	A better night – no pain in his left side. Repeat anodyne draft
10	Yesterday afternoon a chilly fit succeeded by sweating
11	Omit saline julep. Instead give solution of antimony 3 oz three times
12	Yesterday had a regular paroxysm consisting of cold, hot, and sweating stages
14	For 3 days after admission had no fit – Regular paroxysm at the visit – skin cool now, pulse 72. Peruvian cortex powder
16	Yesterday had neither cold, hot, nor sweating fit – bowels open and frequent – troublesome dry cough. Anodyne draft with 20 drops laudanum at bedtime and in the morning
17	Pulse varies, about 100. Tongue dry and crusted – was slightly delirious in the night. Complains of general weakness and uneasiness. Has not taken the bark since last night. Region of the stomach tense. Inject saline enema and give acidulated drinks. Saline infusion. Continue Peruvian cortex intermittently
18	Pulse as yesterday. Feels easier, skin softer. Tongue moist – still delirious in the night. Is remarkably deaf – in the night passed insensibly 2 or 3 copious, thin stools. Rhubarb powder 15 gr. Saline julep
19	Pulse feeble, from 112 to 120 – 3 stools – urine with a color – no delirium. Cordial julep 6 oz with 9 oz of water

20	4 stools – a good deal of delirium – tongue soft and moist – great feebleness and torpor. Cordial julep 12 oz with 18 oz of water. To have daily 4 oz of sago with a little wine
21	Pulse 100 – tongue still crusted – was highly delirious in the night – 3 stools. Fomentations of head with tepid vinegar
22	Was highly delirious in the night – one stool – refuses food and medicines. 1 pound of beer – 4 oz of white wine. To have a shirt from the house – pulse about 100
23	Pulse rather undistinct – seems under 100. Has taken his drink and medicine – is much more sensible. Continue wine and beer
24	Pulse 100 – Tongue moist and cleaner. Rhubarb powder 12 gr – Ipecac powder 1 gr with water
25	No delirium – many small stools. Skin pretty cool – pulse 84 – respiration natural. Continue medications
26	Pulse about 90 – slept tolerably – tongue moist and much clearer than formerly – complains of soreness of his eyes which seem to be impatient of light. Repeat medications – is desirous to have a little bit of beef – to have sowens as he has repeatedly asked for them
27	Slept tolerably in the night – complaining of pain in his left knee – Pulse 84 – tongue pretty clean – no delirium – skin rather hot – about six stools since last visit
28	Pulse about 90 – tongue cleaner but somehow dry – two stools – continue medications
29	Pulse about 96 – complains of general soreness – tongue dry – one stool. To have sowens 3 times a day. A clean shirt from the house
30	Countenance more natural – has not raved – tongue softer – skin pretty cool – respiration natural – pulse feeble, under 100 – continue medications
31	A good night – no delirium – takes a little food – tongue moist on the edges – pulse feeble, rather indistinct
Nov. 1	Last night for an hour and a half, copious sweat over his head and breast – rested well, takes a little food – skin pretty cool – pulse still feeble, under 90 – tongue on the edges moist
2	Tongue moist and pretty clean – no delirium – urine deposits a sediment – pulse still feeble, indistinct – slight sphacelations on his sides and back. Peruvian cortex 2 scruples. Inject saline enema
3	Has not been so easy since last visit – at times delirium with heat – thirst and dyspnea – pulse feeble and indistinct – has taken only two doses of the bark. Apply blister to sternum

4   Since last visit symptoms increased, particularly dyspnea
         and debility
5   *Died* yesterday evening

Appearances on dissection

On opening the head a large quantity of a serous fluid was found at the base of the brain, and in the sheath of the spinal marrow. The ventricles were likewise fuller than usual and both contained a small quantity of a white mucus resembling the albumin of very fresh eggs when coagulated. The arterial ramifications upon the surface of the brain were more distinct than common and there were some small partial adhesions of the dura mater. There was also upon its surface between the several convolutions a quantity of very limpid, colorless fluid. The lungs appeared to be natural but their follicles contained an unusual amount of mucus. Upon inspecting the abdomen, there were several sphacelated spots upon the ilium and the whole of the mesenteric glands were swelled and indurated. The other abdominal viscera were sound – not the smallest vestige of fat could be seen upon any of them.

Case 7

Patient: D.R.
Notebook: John Gregory, Clinical cases of the Royal Infirmary of
                  Edinburgh, Edinburgh, 1771–1772
Location: MSS Collection, Medical Archives, University of Edin-
                  burgh
Age: 48
Sex and status: Male, a "niger"
Admitted: Nov. 29, 1771, during Gregory's clinical rotation from
                  Nov. 1, 1771, to Jan. 31, 1772.
Diagnosis: Smallpox

Because of the dangers of institutional contagion, patients suffering from smallpox were usually not admitted to general hospitals. Presumably this man was accepted into the teaching ward because he could be properly isolated, with his bed placed next to the door or fireplace to prevent the bodily exhalations from reaching other patients. From all indications the patient was an older black servant, but the source of his infection was not revealed.

From the outset, Gregory tried to "conduct him through the disease" as well as possible with a supportive regimen featuring generous administrations of fluids, sedatives such as opium in the form of liquid laudanum, and enemas to cleanse the bowels. A poultice was applied to his throat, expectoration facilitated by a mucilagenous mixture, and a blister applied to the foot in the belief that it would help the indispensable discharge of purulent matter from the body contained in most of the pustules. In the later stages of hospitalization, the patient had his skin lesions anointed with oil, and additional poultices and ointments were repeatedly applied to the smallpox pustules covering the extremities in the hope that they would drain the pus.

In spite of further supportive measures such as the administration of a tonic, the Peruvian bark, and a diet containing beef tea and port wine, the man's condition gradually deteriorated and he died almost three weeks after admission. The extremely terse autopsy report revealed only the presence of pneumonia, a common complication of smallpox.

Nov. 29, 1771	Was taken ill last Monday with several symptoms such as headache, shivering, pain in the small of his back, great nausea, thirst, belly natural though rather costive; the eruption appeared yesterday, has also a slight cough with expectoration.
	Got a vomit on Tuesday, drank something warm at bedtime which for two nights produced sweat, has used no other remedy.
	Pulse 100 – pustules pretty distinct on his face, complains chiefly of weakness in his limbs. Let him have some beer from time to time with a toast in it, but let barley water be his chief drink. Saline julep 1½ oz, at 4 and 9 p.m.
30	Pulse 90 – belly bound, slept ill – urine deposits no sediment
	1) Inject common enema & give liquid laudanum 25 drops at bedtime
	2) Continue saline julep
	3) Let him have barley and currants, or rice and milk for dinner
Dec. 1	Pulse 76 – enema operated well – no particular complaints today, only complaining of sore throat and difficulty swallowing; is not sensible of his face being swelled – did not sleep well with the anodyne but slept in the morning – little swelling of face. Let him have apples roasted or boiled – repeat at bedtime and inject another common enema
2	Pulse 66 – face beginning to swell – was a little delirious in the night – complains of sore throat today. Give common gargle – omit saline julep and give mucilagenous mixture every 2nd hr. Let a cataplasma of bread and milk be applied to his throat
3	Poultice was not applied to his throat, as the gargles relieved him – slept well – face continues to swell – had a loose stool last night – continue medicaments
4	Slept well, no particular complaint – swelling of his face keeps up. Inject common enema
5	Pustules on his face begin to harden – slept well last night

– had an easy stool with the enema – no perceptible swelling of his hands, spits freely – repeat enema

6   Pulse 92 – enema griped him a good deal and produced 3 stools – had a restless night – hands begin to swell – Liquid laudanum 25 drops at bedtime, when faintish let him have a little wine and water – let him also have rice and currants with a little warm wine in it and also apples.

7   Pulse 104 – slept well – had no stool yesterday
1) Inject common enema at 7 P.M. – had only one stool from the enema
2) Inject another enema – liquid laudanum, 25 drops at bedtime – has a blister on his foot – let it be opened and dressed with basil and a poultice of chamomile flowers in milk

8   Pulse 130, considerable difficulty in breathing, does not expectorate freely – very little swelling in his hands and pustules of his hands don't seem filled with matter. Let cataplasma of bread and milk with a little of bruised mustard seed be applied to his feet immediately; apply blister to neck and head. Solution of tartar emetic – and repeat at 5 p.m. – let him have a little wine and water and use the gargle frequently

9   Pulse 108 – solution did not vomit him but produced some loose stools – was ordered last night to breathe over the steam of warm water with a pint of vinegar
Let plasters be applied to his legs, thighs, and arms, spread a little ointment with ⅛ pound of yellow wax – At 7 o'clock, pulse 124 – let his nose be rubbed with fresh butter. The blister produced some degree of strangury which still continues.
Inject another enema with an infusion of linseed, and again liquid laudanum 40 drops.

10   Pulse 120 – passed a restless night – was a little delirious – has no particular complaint – had a loose stool last night and more since. Inject common enema with 40 drops of liquid laudanum

11   Injection not operating last night – got another with one ounce of Glauber salts in it – passed the injection without any stool. Senna leaf 1 oz – Glauber salts – cream of tartar 1½ oz. Let his face be anointed with oil of almonds

12   Pulse 114 – took only ⅓ of his physic – had but one loose stool and another last night. Let him have a little wine, boiled barley and rice as he pleases.

13   Pulse 120 – very feeble, was ordered port wine last night and beef tea – to take 4 oz of a very strong decoction of bark every 3 hrs. Had 3 loose stools in the night, let him have an anodyne with the port wine, also calf-foot jelly.

14	At 6 p.m. last night pulse 104 and much easier, just now 112, very feeble – had no stool since yesterday morning. Let him have some wine and water and inject domestic enema – immediately
15	Pulse 115, very feeble and irregular, had a very loose stool with the enema last night, extremely fetid. Skin very dry – let his mouth be well washed with honey and water; may take currant jelly
16	An injection was ordered last night but the patient refused to take it. Was given another enema this morning without any effect. Pulse 140, extremely feeble – to have wine from time to time. Feet very cold, let them be fomented in warm water
17	*Died* at 3 p.m. On dissection no praeternatural appearance, but the lungs in a very inflamed state

Case 8

Patient:	J.B.
Notebook:	James Gregory, Cases of patients under the care of James Gregory, M.D., Edinburgh, 1781–1782
Location:	MSS Collection, Royal College of Physicians, Edinburgh
Age:	30
Sex and status:	Male, a painter
Admitted:	Nov. 21, 1781, during Gregory's clinical rotation from Nov. 1, 1781, to Jan. 31, 1782
Diagnosis:	Chronic rheumatism

Attending physicians and professors called into the admissions room were hesitant to accept protracted cases into the house, largely because they had little to offer such patients by way of medicines. They recognized that their limited efforts had a better chance to succeed in acute, usually self-limited conditions, and they knew that lengthy stays in the wards were hazardous because of the chances of contracting contagious diseases there.

This particular patient was probably admitted to acquaint medical students with a disease then very common in Scotland, whose long-term management everybody had to learn in spite of Cullen's pessimistic pronouncements regarding a cure. Another possible reason for agreeing to take the patient was the availability of an electrical machine in the infirmary: At this time physicians were still quite optimistic about the usefulness of electrical sparks in the treatment of stiff joints and paralytic limbs, and there are indications that even private patients were occasionally directed to the hospital for such treatments.

Although the man claimed to be a painter at the time of admission, his history disclosed that he had been a migrant laborer who had worked in the malaria-infested fields of Lincolnshire and contracted the ague there. From the start, James Gregory based his entire treatment of the patient on a stimulating regimen that included daily electrical sparks, a full diet containing meat, and a number of tonic drugs such as camphor and copper sulfate. Several narcotics, including hemlock powder and laudanum drafts, were given periodically to ameliorate the rheumatic pains. Later the patient also received agents to promote sweat, such as antimonial wine and a diaphoretic julep listed in the hospital's dispensatory.[13] Localized topical treatments were not neglected. Leeches were employed to diminish local discomfort, and a sweat box was applied to one of the legs. In the end, after five weeks of hospitalization, the patient acknowledged some improvement and was promptly dismissed as "relieved."

Nov. 21, 1781   Complains of an almost constant pain in the large joints, especially in the knees and ankles with some degree of swelling and inability of motion. The small joints of his right hand, especially the thumb, are swollen and very uneasy. During the first part of the night is never able to obtain any sleep on account of the increased pain. He observes that a partial sweat always breaks out, the large joints remaining below their natural heat and quite dry. Warmth of friction afford him considerable relief. The muscles of the legs and arms are much wasted, though the pain stretching down from them is but trivial.

While in Lincolnshire about a year and a half ago, was seized with an intermittent fever which lasted ten months. Scarcely had he got rid of this ailment in consequence of exposure to diet, he was attacked with the acute rheumatism in a violent degree for which he was only bled and repeatedly purged till he found himself very weak. After the inflammatory symptoms disappeared, the present complaints continued and of late have become much aggravated. Has been electrified and made use of a great variety of spirits and oils with little benefit. Has also taken guaiacum with little effect. Does not know that any of his family were ever affected with the gout, nor has he from the first had any complaints in his stomach.

Has been much used to paint in oil colors but never perceived any ill effects from them. Pulse 96 – weak – belly regular – appetite natural

Hemlock powder 10 gr. Place on electrical machine daily and direct sparks to the affected parts

24   Motion of the limbs much freer and easier after being electrified, but they soon grow stiff again. Repeat hemlock extract. To have a bit of meat for dinner

25	No change of symptoms. Omit hemlock – Give camphor and rectified spirits of wine in a bolus in the evening. Continue electricity
26	Felt a kind of heat pervading his body followed by a copious sweat all night. Pains easier today. Repeat bolus of camphor
27	Sweated again all night from his bolus. Double dose of camphor bolus
28	Sweated much – pains easier and he moves better. Continue medications
29	By mistake did not get his medicine last night and is worse today. Administer evening bolus as prescribed
30	Took his bolus – much better – did not sweat. Repeat bolus of camphor
Dec. 2	Finds himself better in the morning but his pains return at night. He complains of weakness and wasting. Repeat bolus
3	Little change of symptoms. Anodyne draft with 25 drops of laudanum and antimonial wine 40 drops at bedtime
4	Slept well and sweated much – pain relieved. Repeat bolus of camphor and evening draft with 40 drops of laudanum and 1 oz of antimonial wine
5	Sweated pretty well and slept after his draft till disturbed by *Richard Aldridge* [another patient hospitalized with epileptic fits]. Pains relieved and motion freer. Repeat bolus and evening draft
7	Take diaphoretic julep
9	Complains still of great weakness, flying pains and sweating. Pains almost gone from his knee where they were formerly worst. Take a copper sulfate mixture
11	A great deal better – let him have a dumbbell to exercise his hands. Continue mixture
14	Complains of severe pain, especially in the left knee which is a good deal swelled. Apply 6 leeches to the affected knee
15	Pain but not swelling removed from his knee since the leeches were applied. Let his right leg be put in the box and sweated.
16	Right ankle freed from pain. Pain still severe in the left. Let the left leg be sweated in the box for two complete hours.
17	Pain almost gone from his feet – relieved everywhere else – continue medications
19	Convalescent
20	To have a bottle of porter daily
26	Dismissed *relieved*

Case 9

Patient:	M.B.
Notebook:	Andrew Duncan, Sr., Clinical reports and commentaries, Feb.–Apr. 1795, presented by Alexander Blackhall Morison, Edinburgh, 1795
Location:	MSS Collection, Royal College of Physicians, Edinburgh
Age:	20
Sex and status:	Female, a servant
Admitted:	Jan. 29, 1795, just before Duncan's clinical rotation from Feb. 1 to Apr. 25, 1795
Diagnosis:	Dyspepsia

This case is representative of "dyspepsia," then a frequently employed diagnostic label for a number of digestive complaints, including anorexia, nausea and vomiting, and burning sensations or pain in the stomach before or after meals. Most patients were young women, and if the symptoms included any oppression of the chest or throat, hysteria was seriously suspected.

Dyspepsia was seen as essentially a disease of systemic debility requiring a stimulating treatment, an approach confirmed by Duncan's remarks concerning this case. At the same time, however, the professor took pains to prevent constipation, viewed as an obstacle to recovery and a source of further digestive troubles. Because she was menstruating, the young woman received only a mild laxative, the electuary of senna, eventually changed to the more aggressive rhubarb powder after the menses had stopped.

The tonic drugs employed almost throughout her hospitalization were powders obtained from the Angostura bark and the Colomba root, two items of frequent use at that time. The former, introduced in England during 1788, was promoted as a stimulant of the digestive organs with powers considered superior to those of the popular Peruvian bark.[14] The Colomba root, another aromatic bitter, popularized by Thomas Percival of Manchester, was thought to possess antiseptic qualities effectual in preventing vomiting and settling the stomach.[15]

Although the initial history disclosed an episode of vomiting blood, the patient suffered no recurrence of this symptom during her three-week stay in the teaching ward. She seems to have had a mild fever suggestive of an incipient tuberculosis but apparently recovered quickly from it and had an uneventful convalescence.

Jan. 29, 1795   Five days since after symptoms of pyrexia and headache she was seized with pain in her right side to which immediately succeeded severe vomiting and the contents of her stomach were mixed with blood of a dark color. The vomiting is easily excited on taking food. Is affected also with dyspnea which with the other symptoms is aggravated towards evening. Takes little food by reason of her inclination to vomit. Has likewise pain in the abdomen which is sore to the touch and some pain in passing her urine.

Pulse 90 – skin and tongue dry – thirst – has taken some medicines which purged her. Ascribed her complaints to cold; experienced two similar attacks before, one six months, the other 3 weeks ago – Menstruating

30   Had not been vomiting since admission but has slept little and taken no food. Still complains of sickness at stomach. Pulse 96 – heat moderate – tongue moist – bowels bound – Give immediately electuary of senna

31   Had two stools from the electuary and no return of the vomit. Still complains of nausea, particularly in an erect posture. Appetite remains bad. Pulse and skin natural. Continue electuary intermittently. Give three times daily powder of Angostura bark

Feb. 1   Powder sits easy on her stomach and she has had no return of vomiting. Appetite somewhat mended and in other respects easier. Has had no stool since she took the electuary. Pulse 96 – heat natural. Continue Angostura bark. Pills with rhubarb 10 gr at bedtime

2   Had stool from pills and continues in every respect easier. Pulse 96 at the fire. Heat natural. Continue Angostura bark. Rhubarb pills as needed

3   Had uneasiness at stomach after dinner yesterday and vomited her powder in the evening, but it sat easy this morning. Is in other respects relieved. Pulse 90 – heat natural

4   Had pain in abdomen during the night with vomiting and continues upon the whole easier. Pulse 96 – heat natural – no stool since taking the pill. Continue Angostura bark & rhubarb pills

5   Had a stool from the pills and is easier. Continue

6   Was much affected yesterday afternoon with pain and swelling in the region of the stomach, but without vomiting; is at present easier – pulse 80. Continue Angostura & repeat rhubarb pills. Let her have meat daily

7   Pills have operated once and she has had some return of uneasiness at the stomach – Vomiting since breakfast. Pulse 82 – heat natural

8   Free from nausea and vomiting. Pulse 82 – heat natural. Continue medications intermittently

9   Two stools from pills and continues free from pain in stomach. Continue

10   Pills have not operated and much affected in night with headache and pain of stomach but no vomiting. Pulse 82 – heat natural. Continue

11 Free from headache and vomiting. Pulse 90 – bowels regular – menses flow done. Continue

12 Attacked last night after going to bed with shivering fit followed by augmented heat and sweating, which continued till this morning. Is freer at present from febrile anxiety

13 Had some return of coldness yesterday followed by heat and sweat. Pulse 115 – skin moist – tongue clean – bowels regular. Saline julep every third hour

14 No return of febrile paradox last night but complains more today of uneasiness at stomach but without vomiting. Pulse 96 – bowels natural. Saline julep – give also powder of Colomba root

15 Powders agree – no febrile symptoms nor affection of the stomach. Pulse 92 – heat and bowels natural. Continue powders

16 Pulse 83 – bowels natural – Continues easier

17 Continues easier

18 Continues free from any return of complaints. Let her be dismissed – *cured*

Dr. Duncan's comments

If we may credit the account this patient gave, her complaints appeared about 5 days before she came in. Symptoms of pyrexia followed by vomiting of a black colored matter. She told us also that this was not her first attack. If this is true, it would constitute a particular disease, but it is difficult to give her disease a name because the hematemesis may be symptomatic of fever or, vice versa, perhaps there is still greater reason to doubt the existence of the hematemesis. For, both the patient and attendants are apt to be mistaken with regard to the vomiting of blood.

Here, however, we must not consider what happened prior to her coming into the hospital but what we have observed since, which have been symptoms of dyspepsia. She was also subjected when she came, to febrile anxiety – some degree of thirst and want of appetite for solid food. These symptoms no longer remain but all her complaints are dyspeptic as flatulence and vomiting. There is no particular appearance in the vomited matter so that her complaints are of short duration and in slight degree unless we consider them as the sequel of a more formidable disease.

There has been some irregularity in her menstrual discharge, it having returned in ten days but this was merely accidental. I have not observed it to take place in similar cases. At present she has no alarming symptoms and the principal complaint is considerably diminished, particularly a return of appetite. Within these two days past she has had some febrile symptoms. If this should continue to diminish with the other symptoms, we may hope that she will soon be able to leave the hospital.

The great object with us has been to restore the tone and vigor of the stomach and to give a due action to the intestines. For the first, we gave the Angostura, and for the second the stomachic powder. I hope these will be sufficient. If they should not, we may refer to others of a similar nature which will often succeed though a more powerful one has failed. For Angostura I may substitute Colomba – for the rhubarb, aloes. If more violent symptoms occur, our remedies must be adapted to the circumstances.

When I formerly spoke of this patient, I expressed some doubt about the origin of her complaint, particularly of the dyspeptic appearance which it had put on. It was with me a matter of doubt whether the fever was symptomatic of her hematemesis or the hematemesis of the fever. It was no less a matter of doubt whether the hematemesis had ever existed. I rather considered it as a case of dyspepsia attended with some febrile symptoms. Therefore, I expected a favorable termination and she was indeed soon discharged. It may, however, return on any irregularity or improper exposure but I think for the present it has been removed by the medicines.

At her admission she had a recurrence of the menstrual flux which was certainly an objection to violent medicines but did not prevent us from using gentle laxatives. I attributed much of her complaints to costiveness and therefore ordered the electuary sennae to be taken every two hours when the catamenia disappeared. I judged it necessary to restore vigor to her stomach and for this purpose had recourse to the Angostura bark which I think I have used with great advantage. The tree which yields it is unknown but it has its name from its place of growth. Angostura is in South America. It is useful in some conditions of fever. The cinchona is recommended in other diseases where tonics are of use. I have, I think, seen it of service as in dyspepsia where Colomba has disagreed. It was here used with benefit and it immediately acted on the patient without producing any uneasiness – she had a better appetite. This was not of long continuance nor was there a regular discharge of feces. I ordered her the rhubarb powder – she remained from the 1st to the 7th with some mitigation of her vomiting, but a circumstance rather particular now occurred, namely a return of the menstrual discharge. To what cause this is to be attributed is difficult to conjecture. It was not attended with any alarming appearance and was much less so than might be expected.

During their continuance, she continued the use of the rhubarb and she afterwards resumed the bark, but on the 18th she had a pretty severe return of the febrile symptoms. A sweat was now on the skin which I thought should be encouraged. I therefore ordered the saline julep which is fixed vegetable alkali neutralized with lemon juice. By this the moisture was supported for a certain time and on the next report she was free from febrile symptoms.

I now preferred giving the Colomba as a tonic. This is obtained from the island of Ceylon in the East Indies, but of this vegetable as well as the tree of Angostura we are ignorant. We have no proper botanical description. The root is a very useful stomachic. We had recourse to it and during its use her body was not bound. Under this treatment she was soon free from all complaints. We have no certain evidence of the benefit from these medicines; yet I think the *Angostura* and *Colomba* were of some service.

Case 10

Patient:	R.M.
Notebook:	James Gregory, Cases of patients under the care of James Gregory, M.D., Edinburgh, 1781–1782
Location:	MSS Collection, Royal College of Physicians, Edinburgh
Age:	19
Sex:	Female
Admitted:	Nov. 14, 1781, during Gregory's clinical rotation from Nov. 1, 1781, to Jan. 31, 1782
Diagnosis:	Hysteria

According to the notebook, the patient gave a typical history of dyspeptic symptoms coupled with a sensation of "heavy balls ascending from the pit of the stomach," which characterized most episodes diagnosed as hysteric fits. Each episode of "swooning" or unconsciousness lasted between twenty and sixty minutes and was preceded or followed by convulsive muscular movements.

Because physicians believed that hysteria was a manifestation of excessive nervous irritability occurring in feeble women of "delicate habit," the goal of therapy was to strengthen the bodily constitution and thus ameliorate the muscular, digestive, and cardiovascular weakness. Authors such as William Cullen and James Gregory also linked hysteria to an irritability of the sexual organs and paid much attention to concurrent menstrual irregularities that could be playing major roles in the genesis of the disease.

In this particular case, Gregory began his stimulating regimen with the administration of vitriolated ether, a powerful antispasmodic drug,[16] and a strengthening electuary of the Peruvian bark, the *elect. Peruvianum roborans* listed in the hospital's dispensatory.[17] The young woman was placed on a full diet containing meat and eggs, which she tolerated poorly, and was ordered to exercise daily on a special bench. To keep the bowels open and settle her stomach, a laxative bolus containing white magnesia and rhubarb powder was also prescribed. A few days later she received aloetic pills and wine as laxatives and a bedtime narcotic draft containing laudanum.

Since the patient claimed to have missed her last two menstrual periods, Gregory sought vigorously to promote their return, in the belief that the interruption was directly linked to the hysteric fits. Thus the lower abdomen was exposed to daily electrical sparks, and she received a number of warm evening footbaths designed to shift the circulation to the lower part of the body. Among the emmenagogues prescribed by the professor were gum pills composed of asafetida and galbanum[18] and powder of madder root or *rubia tinctorum*.[19]

However, two weeks after her admission, the woman suddenly developed a respiratory infection with fever, chest pain, cough, and apparently some sputum tinged with blood. Gregory immediately ordered a purga-tive–emetic combination containing antimony and Glauber's salts, an expec-torant, and a blister to be placed on the painful area of the chest. As her fever increased, she quickly became restless and delirious and received sed-atives as well as hourly fomentations. The hair on her head was cut off and blisters applied to both temples, measures employed in cases of intense headaches, stupor, or delirium. A number of stimulating measures includ-ing red wine were also prescribed.

Fortunately, the patient responded quickly, and her fever went away. At this point she also started her menstrual period and was believed to be re-covering. Therefore she received more wine and again a full diet. That no further hysterical fits were reported probably confirmed Gregory's impres-sion that these episodes were directly related to her previous menstrual suppression.

Nov. 14, 1781	Has for a long time at intervals complained of pain and swelling in the epigastric region, especially after taking food. Nausea, cardialgia, and pyrosis. A small quantity of food after she has swallowed it often returns suddenly into her mouth, bringing with it a sour and disagreeable taste. These complaints have much increased of late. She says also that she is affected several times with a sense of sick-ness, heaviness and slight trembling, at which time a sense of weight as if from a heavy ball seems to ascend from the pit of the stomach and she faints away. The pulsation of the arteries still continue although sometimes faintly in-termitting. Her respiration little impaired. She is quite in-sensible while in the fit. After remaining in this state about twenty minutes, her extremities begin to twitch and she gradually recovers. There are often at this period consid-erable discharges of wind from the stomach which she thinks afford her some relief. Belly and menses regular – appearance good – has taken a variety of medicines with-out any permanent relief. For hysterical paroxysm vitriolated ether 2 oz in 4 oz of water – Electuary of the Peruvian bark. A bit of meat for dinner and an egg for supper. Exercise every day on the bank
16	Headache and sickness easier since she took the ether but had three fits yesterday afternoon and two today. Con-tinue medications
17	Only one fit since yesterday of about an hour duration. Acid vomiting always after taking food. Omit electuary. Give bolus with white magnesia and rhubarb powder. Re-peat ether instantly if paroxysm occurs.
18	Has had a great many fits since yesterday generally pre-

ceded by hiccups. No return of pyrosis since she took her first bolus – belly natural – Omit ether and bolus. Give anodyne draft with 25 drops of laudanum at bedtime and also gum pills

19   One fit yesterday afternoon – slept hardly any these three nights. Complains much of sickness and headache today. No appetite. Pulse 100 – tongue and skin natural – Menses suppressed for the last two periods. Ipecac powder as emetic. Combine with infusion of chamomile. Repeat gum pills and evening anodyne draft

20   Pulse natural – vomit operated well – nausea and headache gone – slept well – two slight fits since last report. Place on electrical machine daily. Evening footbath

21   No fit – complains of nausea – slept well – no menstrual discharge. Repeat medications and electuary

22   One fit last night of half an hour, beginning with syncope and ending with convulsions of the extremities. Complains much of nausea and weakness. No menses. Omit gum pills – Give the root of madder. Continue this medication

23   No fits – no complaints but headaches

24   No change of symptoms. Continue medications

25   No fit – headache gone – no menses. Repeat foot bath for 1 hour in evening. Aloetic pills at bedtime

26   No fits and no complaint but some little pain and swelling about her stomach – no effect from the pills – no menses.

27   No fits but some coldness, sickness and headache about her. Physic operated well – Repeat powder of madder root and electricity

28   Vomited pretty freely last night with infusion of chamomile – slept very ill – has sweated much but is not relieved by it. Pulse 114, of moderate strength. Complains of pain in her breast increased on coughing – Coughed up some blood this morning. Glauber salts and crystals of tartar dissolved in water. Apply blister on painful area of chest this evening. Mucilagenous julep with spirit of vitriol

29   Was attacked yesterday afternoon with gripes and tenesmus, and discharged at repeated efforts some blood and slime after which she got one dose of the solution. Had an anodyne at 5 P.M. and another near midnight and was fomented with immediate relief to the pain in her bowels – great stupor and delirium – constant moaning – pulse 130 – tongue natural – little cough – no more hemoptysis. Cut hair on her head – apply blister to the temples. Red wine in water 8 oz – Fomentations hourly

30   Pulse natural – tongue clean and moist. She slept well –

appetite still bad. Release of vaginal discharge – catamenia present. Repeat wine

Dec. 1 Febrile symptoms gone – slept well last night. Two hysteric fits last night – appetite returns. Let her have a bit of steak for dinner today. Continue wine

2 Convalescent – repeat electuary of the Peruvian bark. Continue wine and diet as before

3 Convalescent

4 Free of complaints – dismissed *cured*

APPENDIX C

Clinical teaching

Statutes for the regulation of the M.D. degree established by the Senatus Academicus of the University of Edinburgh, December 8, 1783

I. No person shall be received as a candidate for a degree in medicine unless he has applied during three complete years, to the study of medicine in this or some other University. It is expected of candidates to attend the University of Edinburgh at least one of these years, that the professors may be acquainted with their character, conduct and diligence in prosecuting their studies.

II. Every candidate for a degree in medicine must signify his intention to the Dean of the faculty of medicine at least 3 months before one of the two stated days of public graduation each year, and shall then undergo, in the house of one of the professors, the first and most private examination in all the branches of medicine, viz. anatomy and surgery, chemistry, botany, and materia medica and pharmacy, theory of medicine and practice of medicine, each of the professors proposing questions to him in order.

As the professors consider themselves bound in honor not to divulge the unfavorable result of an examination, a candidate may be remitted to his studies, in this stage of his trials without injury to his reputation or interest.

III. Each candidate six weeks before one of the stated days of public graduation shall deliver to one of the professors a dissertation on a subject in medicine that it may be revised by the professor and then subjected to the consideration of the faculty of medicine.

IV. The candidate shall then take a second examination upon all the branches of medicine in the library of the University particularly with respect to points not touched in his former examination.

V. An aphorism of Hippocrates is selected of which the candidate is to deliver explanation and illustration in writing. At the same time a question in medicine is proposed to him, to which he shall return an answer in writing, illustrated with a commentary and with respect to both these, he is examined *in the library by the professors*.

Edinburgh College Minutes, 1773–1790, pp. 321–324, MSS Collection, University of Edinburgh

VI. The cases of two patients with questions relative to them are given to the candidate which he is required to illustrate in writing with proper solutions of the questions.

VII. Upon a report from the medical faculty of all these proceedings with the approbation of the candidate, his dissertation is published by authority of the Senatus Academicus; he is required to defend it in the common hall of the University against the professors appointed to impugn it, and then by act of the Senatus Academicus, he is promoted to the highest academical honors with the usual solemnities.

VIII. All these different exercises are performed and each part of the trials carried out in the Latin tongue.

The public will judge with respect to the degree of accuracy and strictness in conducting these various parts of trial from being informed that there is seldom any year in which more than one candidate is not remitted to his studies. At the same time the professors mention with much satisfaction that it is not uncommon for candidates who have been found unqualified to apply afterwards to their studies with such diligence and success that they have acquitted themselves with great applause in a subsequent examination, to which they cannot be admitted till a year elapse from the time of their former trial.

Though a person may offer himself as a candidate for a degree in medicine after applying to the study of that science during three years in this or in some other university, it is to be observed that a considerable proportion of the graduates in the University of Edinburgh attend the college of Medicine several years behind that period.

Besides the lectures on the various branches of medicine in the University, clinical lectures are delivered each year by two of the professors of medicine on the cases of certain select patients in the Royal Infirmary entrusted to their care by the governors of the hospital, whom the professors visit and for whom they prescribe in the presence of the students. No person is admitted as a candidate for a degree in medicine unless he has attended these clinical lectures.

Students have likewise an opportunity of attending the ordinary physicians of the Royal Infirmary, who visit the patients every day, examine their cases and prescribe in presence of the students, keeping regular journals of the progress of the disease, of the various prescriptions, of the effect of the medicines, and of the final issue of the case, all which are open to the inspection of the students, and from which they may make extracts.

The medium number of students of medicine in the University of Edinburgh for the seven last years has been annually four hundred. This year their number exceeds five hundred. About twenty-two are promoted annually to the degree of doctor of medicine.

Lecture on how to take a clinical history, by William Cullen

In taking cases the following particulars are to be marked:

1. The person's *NAME:* note the proper spelling of the surname to be studied.
2. *AGE.* Young women give their age as less than it really is and among the vulgar of this country women above forty appear older than they really are. The vulgar of both sexes often don't know their age exactly, but a tolerable chronologist will find it out, by examining their memory of public transactions or the steps in the progress of the person's own life.
3. *TEMPERAMENT,* whenever distinctly marked as sanguine or melancholic, or by complexion, eyes, hair or habits of body. This is not necessary to the physician but useful to the student.
4. *PROFESSION,* or other circumstances in the manner of life which may have modified their constitution, as habitation, labour, diet, sobriety or intemperance.

   In married women, the number of their children, the circumstances of their deliveries, their nursing, their present state with regard to pregnancy or otherwise.

   Of all persons their parentage, their hereditary dispositions and former diseases.
5. *REMOTE CAUSE.* Of this patients are generally bad judges and are ready to mention the universal circumstances which last occurred to them; their account, however, must be taken but it requires knowledge to judge of this and to expiscate the true cause.
6. *BEGINNING OF THE DISEASE,* often carefully marked by patients and often forgotten, commonly better marked by their friends.

   Inequality of spirits and strength not commonly observed by labouring people.

   Some defect in the exercise of the functions not observed till some more considerable uneasiness or pain arises and these arising make smaller previous ailments to be forgotten. Falling off of appetite the most frequent beginning of chronic diseases.

   In febrile diseases the horror which determines their beginning is often inconsiderable and forgotten but to be expiscated. The taking to lying in bed does not determine the beginning of fevers.
7. *SYMPTOMS.* The symptoms are of two kinds: those which consist in the feelings of the patients themselves and those which consist in circumstances that may be observed by the physician. In the reports of the first there is much fallacy both from the difference of sensibility in different persons and from this that every person is disposed to aggravate their uneasy feelings, and hospital patients in particular to secure their reception and engage attention.

Fragment from the Cullen papers, MSS Collection, University of Glasgow

At first examination the patient's own account is to be taken and that upon the most general question, for particular questions are ready to be echoed back and every symptom reported that is inquired after.

Particular questions therefore to be put only after some interval. Inconsistencies or what may seem to be such not to be readily admitted but there are exceptions to this.

The exact state to be learned only by cross questions and these with observation only after some days.

The symptoms falling under the physician's observation are to be fully and accurately marked, but a young man must be cautious in marking the degrees of symptoms, the distinction of which is not to be acquired but by much experience.

In collecting the symptoms of any case a commonplace of the several heads to which symptoms may be referred is useful, as otherwise by young persons many questions may be omitted. But this does not lead to make long cases. The positive symptoms indeed are always to be marked, but if we can suppose the proper inquiries to have been made, all negatives may be omitted except in cases where positive symptoms were to be expected. For a commonplace you may take the following: SYMPTOMS are referred to the three heads of functions, excretions and qualities. The functions are

vital in pulse and respiration

natural in appetite and digestion

animal in external and internal senses, and in voluntary motions

The excretions are those of stool, urine, sweat, saliva, mucus expectoration, halitus, air and in women milk and menses. The qualities to be observed are those of colour, odour, bulk, heat and cold, changes in the skin.

It would be very troublesome to question every patient by this commonplace and a physician of any experience generally takes hold of some leading symptom or symptoms of disease by which he may either confirm or reject his supposition. This must proceed upon a knowledge of nosology and of the history of diseases. In imitating this, a young practitioner should have the nosology by heart and be acquainted with the history of diseases as fully as he can and for that purpose consult the writers referred to in the nosology. But still aware of the defects and ambiguities of both nosology and history he will often employ his commonplace, make his cases full and leave it to the physician to lop off the superfluities.

8. PERIOD of the diseases when it is of any standing. The series of symptoms and remedies which have been employed.

Clinico-pathological correlations, by William Cullen:
Observations about the autopsy of J.C., a case of pulmonary
tuberculosis, made on March 2, 1773

Formerly I spoke of this case and considered it in general, but I can now
resume consideration with regard to it because we can speak of it with more
certainty and clearness. I gave you my opinion that the case was to be considered as desperate; however the appellation of the term might be disputed.
I say it was a *phthisis confirmata* which very seldom admits of remedies, and
if it does admit of any, they are such as we cannot employ in this house.
Here, we could do nothing but palliate matters, and in all such cases among
poor persons our chief means of palliating their ailments is to keep them
under the shelter of this house. Therefore, I allowed him to remain in the
hospital since we were not pressed at the time for room, and also because I
thought that you might wish to have the opportunity of observing the
progress of such a disease, and especially the after course of it.

With regard to what we might have observed when the patient was alive,
we have since had an opportunity of dissection, and I have a few remarks
to make upon that. What occurred at first view was a considerable difference in the size of the two sides of the thorax. This must have been a matter
of original configuration. We need not inquire into what might give occasion to this; we only observe that it was probably the defect that disposed
this man to have his lungs more readily liable to the disease he laboured
under. We have other instances of a faulty proportion of the thorax as the
effect of rickets, predisposing persons to various afflictions of the lungs and
particularly phthisis. In this man it certainly disposed the left side which
was the smallest, to be affected to a more considerable degree than the right,
as we have found to be the case.

There was also a general adhesion of the surface of the lungs to the costal
pleura, and this occurring in a young man, does presume some inflammatory state. It is, at least, the most frequent occasion of such an adhesion.
Indeed, it may be questioned whether the adhesion was not owing to the
small size of that left cavity. Both the blood and air continued to be impelled
into that lobe [of the lung] and in consequence of that its surface applied to
the costal pleura. Yet I imagine that this supposition is not well founded
because we were saying not long ago that both the air and blood can be
entirely prevented from entering a lobe. Therefore, I suppose that the lobes
of the lungs will only have the proportion of air and blood suited to [them].
It is thus more probable that the common cause for the pleural adhesion is
some degree of inflammation connected with the disease we have seen here.

William Cullen, Clinical lectures, Edinburgh, 1772–1773, MSS Collection, Royal
College of Physicians, Edinburgh

In the next place, we have occasion to observe one of the most frequent causes of phthisis in this country: the numerous tubercles in the lungs. I have had occasion to say this before that these tubercles are of different kinds. The most frequent is the scrofulous type and we cannot doubt it in a person who evidently had laboured under scrofula before and from the nature of such scrofulous tumors. From what happened in this case you should understand how slow the progress of the disease may be, so that practitioners should be very attentive in discerning the first beginning of such cases. The disease should not be allowed to gain ground without taking measures to prevent it, or you should at least save yourselves by a proper diagnosis.

It has been supposed that an open ulcer is necessary for the disease to be a *phthisis confirmata*. But from this case we can observe that a phthisis may proceed to its fatal conclusion without purulent spitting appearing. Our judgment is confirmed by the dissection, as we did not observe any communication between the tubercles and the bronchia, nor any matter that could have issued from the tubercles. I am going to make some application from the fact that there was no open ulcer. I would say that the common symptoms and the fatal outcome of a phthisis, whether it has an open ulcer with vomica or not, depends rather upon the absorption of this material. If we are right in judging that there was no open ulcer here, we find the hectic fever suffered by the patient to have been produced by such an absorption alone while the debility and emaciation proceeded as in similar cases with open ulcers. Therefore, we must not, as physicians have frequently done when consulted for a cough and fever approaching a hectic type, examine the sputum and if it is not purulent, declare that the lungs are not yet tainted. That is a fallacious judgment and is to be guarded against.

Now these remarks from the dissection are based on the appearances of both lungs, but especially from the condition of the right one which we have the opportunity of examining more particularly. I have to say that it appeared that the increase in tubercles had so straightened the air vessels as to make them disappear. No room for the entrance of air into the right lung was found, although the organ still appeared pretty full of blood.

Now I am doubtful in admitting another conclusion, yet I think that from the firm consistence of the left lobe and its red colour, a true effusion of blood must have occurred there. At least in so many peripneumonic cases we take it as a certain mark of such effusion that it cannot be refused here. From the circumstances of that lobe and the whole disease, we are clearly led to perceive the cause for such effusions. Indeed, I must suppose that it happened a little before death, and I think that it has been the more immediate cause of this patient's death.

Diseases and patients presented during the clinical lectures of Dr. William Cullen November 1772–April 1773 (double rotation)

Nov. 28, 1772	Introductory lecture	
Dec. 1	Skin eruption	Anne Jackson
	Hematemesis	Elizabeth Ramsay
4	Jaundice	Margaret Bain
	Typhus	Margaret Blair
	Lepra ichtyosis	Amelia Fiar
8	Fever	Janet Crookshanks
	Catarrh	Christian Ross
	Rheumatism	Isabel Donaldson
11	Lumbago	Andrew Moffat
	Catarrh	John Beaton and William McKay
	Rheumatism	Alexander Sutherland
	Jaundice	James Burns
16	Intermittent fever	Alexander Black
	Smallpox	Archibald Alison
	Dysentery	Alexander Nicol and Neil Gordon
18	Epilepsy	John McFarlane
	Catarrh	Matthew Hiphant
23	Catarrh	John Crookshanks
24	Catarrh	John Crookshanks and John Baptist
	Anasarca	William Bruce
	(Christmas recess)	
Jan. 5, 1773	Synochus	David Panton
	Intermittent fever	Hugh Kerr
	Treatment of fevers	
8	Amenorrhea	Janet Sutherland
12	Fevers	Isabel Donaldson and Janet Williamson
15	Fevers – different types	Anne Ross, Catherine Henderson, Catherine McFarlane, William McFarlane, and James Imrie
19	Fevers – discussion of critical days	
22	Treatment of fevers	
26	Fevers – different types	Isabel Baird, Janet Sutherland, and Elizabeth Ramsay
29	Catarrh	Margaret Bain and Isabel Barclay
Feb. 2	Dysentery	Alexander Nicol and Neil Gordon (repeat)

5	Phthisis	John Crookshanks, William Boyd, and Donald McDonald
9	Catarrh	John Cochrane and Andrew McFarlane
	Paralysis	John Muir
	Rheumatism	James Harvey
12	Dyspepsia	John Watt
17	Anasarca	James Millar
23	Anasarca	James Millar (cont.)
26	Hydrothorax	Margaret Mills
Mar. 2	Bladder stone	Isabel Barclay
	Rheumatism	George Home
5	Autopsy reports	George Home and John Crookshanks
9	Canceled	
12	Canceled	
16	Canceled	
19	Rheumatism (acute)	Elizabeth Sutherland
23	Rheumatism (acute)	Elizabeth Sutherland, Anne Alison, Janet Cameron, and Jean Smith
26	Rheumatism (chronic)	Alexander Sutherland
30	Treatment of chronic rheumatism	
Apr. 1	Treatment of chronic rheumatism – use of electricity	
2	Treatment of chronic rheumatism – water treatment at spas	
	Blisters	Alexander Sutherland, and Isabel Waters
5	Sciatica	Colin Reid and William Lothian
	Rheumatism (acute)	Jean Webster and John Henderson
6	Intermittent fevers	Hugh Kerr and David Watson
8	Intermittent fever	John Nicolson
	Fevers (synocha)	Archibald McCall, Donald Frazer, Donald Bain, William Bain, Catherine McFarlane, Elizabeth Wear, and Janet Bain
12	Fevers (synocha)	Anne Corbet and John Mason
14	Fevers (synochus)	Robert Bain
	Peripneumonitis	Grizel Cockburn and Colin Reid
16	Erysipelas	Alexander Hutton
	Fevers	James Heron and Helen Norman
19	Anasarca	Mary Taylor
	Measles	Catherine Henderson

21	Paralysis	Janet Grieve
	Menorrhagia	Isabel Reid
23	Worms	John Marshall
	Jaundice	Donald Grant
	Kidney injury	Robert Glen
	Closing comments	

Diseases and patients presented during the clinical lectures of Dr. James Gregory at the infirmary, November 1779–January 1780 (regular rotation)

Nov. 16, 1779	Tusis convulsiva (whooping cough)	Elizabeth Sutherland
19	Dropsy	James Niven and Janet Anderson
23	Fever	Peggy Couts
26	Amenorrhea	Isabel Mitchell
30	Angina	Janet McDonald
Dec. 7	Phthisis pulmonaris	John Matthews and William Simpson
10	Chorea St. Viti (St. Vitus' dance)	Janet Wilson
14	Paralysis	John Young and Robert McDonald
17	Hydrothorax	George Auchinleck
21	Lues venerea	Alexander Macaulay
	Scurvy	John White
	Cynanche tonsillaris (sore throat and tonsilitis)	William Aberdeen and Gabriel Weir
24	Menorrhagia	Mary Gunn
28	Fevers	Isabel McDonald and Helen Cooper
31	Fevers	John Oakley and Nelly Moncurr
Jan. 4, 1780	Fevers – causes of contagion	
7	Treatment of fevers	
11	Treatment of fevers – use of diaphoretics	
14	Treatment of fevers – use of opium	
18	Intermittent fevers	Jane Wright, John Ferguson, Elizabeth McDonald, Katherine Graham, Nelly Kirkpatrick, and David Monro
21	Erysipelas	Grizel Cumming and Euphem Ramsay
25	Rheumatism	Anna Hutton
	Variola	Elizabeth White

| 28 | Ophthalmia | Janet Sinclair, Gavin Kilgour, and Ebenezer Finlay |
| | Amaurosis | Peter Robb |

Diseases and patients presented during the clinical lectures of Dr. Andrew Duncan, Sr., at the infirmary, February–April 1795 (regular rotation)

Intermittent fever (tertiana)	Margaret Campbell
Intermittent fever (quartana)	Lilly Campbell
Ophthalmia	Jane Henderson, Bell Mowatt, and Eleanor Terry
Cynanche tonsillaris	Catherine Preston
Enteritis	Mary Lindsey
Nephritis	Christian Grant and Daniel Manson
Rheumatismus	Alexander Forbes, William Patterson, and Trotter Anderson
Rheumatismus (chronic)	John Mather and Christian MacDonald
Podagra atonica	William Brown
Erysipelas	Janet Ross and James Shewster
Phthisis	Daniel MacIntosh, Margaret Dewer, Daniel Robertson, and Barbara Taylor
Pertussis	Jane Henderson
Leucorrhea	Sarah Forbes and Elizabeth Jameson
Menorrhagia	Elizabeth Jameson
Catarrhus	Isabel Bain, Jane Layl, David MacKenzie, Catherine Cameron, Elizabeth Haddock, John Inglis, John MacGregor, and John Rose
Hydrothorax	Barbara Hope
Dysenteria	Margaret Miller
Apoplexia	Jane Duncan
Paralysis	Naysmith Lind, Isabel Strachan, John Crawford, William Forrest, and Robert Grant
Dyspepsia	Jane Fraser, James Plant, Margaret Burnet, and Bell Robinson
Hypochondriasis	John Menter and James Smyth
Epilepsia	James Glen
Colica pictonum	Andrew Taylor
Diabetes mellitus	Phyllis Veitch
Asthma	Ann Anderson
Atrophia	Christian Cameron
Anasarca	James Gib, Janet Clark, and Alexander Duff
Hydrothorax	Jane Berkeley and James Lauder
Hydrocephalus	Charles MacDonald

Syphilis	John Mackay
Lepra	Nelly Henderson
Tetanus	Janet Elder
Caligo	William Stewart
Cancer	James Pennycock
Herpes	Euphan Smith and David Hodge

Principal cases of surgery in the infirmary, November 1772, prepared by the surgeon Mr. James Rae

Men's Ward

A large gunshot wound of the hand and forearm
A gunshot wound of the thigh
A lacerated wound of the leg
A white swelling of the knee with erysipelas on the leg, etc.
A large edematous leg with gangrenous symptoms and ulcer
A testis with induration and partial suppurations
Another with haematocele
Two patients with injuries on the cranium
A fracture of the thighbone above the trochanter
A fracture of the forearm with wound and contusion
A fracture of the humerus and both bones of the forearm
A singular case where amputation of the leg was performed two years ago
A fractured leg
A fractured leg with wound and bad symptoms
Two patients for lithotomy
A large tumour on the hand to be extirpated

Women's ward

An aneurism of the ulnar artery from a wound
An amputation above the knee, case singular
A fracture of the forearm
A fractured leg
A diseased mamma
A paronychia of the thumb
Variety of tumours, ulcers, etc.

Drug usage at the infirmary: the example of Dr. Andrew Duncan, Sr.

J. Worth Estes, M.D.

The detailed clinical notes of Andrew Duncan, Sr., collated and copied by an anonymous student during Duncan's attendance on the teaching ward of the infirmary, exemplify day-to-day drug usage at the hospital in the late eighteenth century.[1] Internal evidence suggests that Duncan was assigned to the ward between Feb. 1 and Apr. 25, 1795, but the student recorder has included clinical data for a few patients already in the ward before that time. Although Francis Home had prescribed for patients in the teaching ward during the preceding three months, the responsible physicians will not be differentiated in the following discussion; if they did differ in their practices, the differences are not discernible.

These admission and progress notes describe 65 patients (30 men and 35 women), probably all those in the male and female teaching wards between February and April. The tabulations given here may be taken as representative of professional attempts to counteract a fairly random sample of symptoms. Altogether, the 65 patients were hospitalized for a total of 2,633 days, during which time they received 4,363 different drugs or non-drug treatments, an overall average of 1.7 treatments per day per patient.

As Table A.1 shows, 94 different drugs or drug preparations were administered to the 65 patients. The drug prescribed most often was opium, in several dosage forms and for several indications (for which see the glossary at the end of this appendix). The next most frequently administered drug was cantharides, as a blister, prescribed for almost half of the patients. Virtually all patients received cathartics at some time during hospitalization;

I am very much indebted to Suzanne Messer for her painstaking collations of all drug administrations to each patient, for constructing pulse rate graphs for all of Duncan's patients, and for some of the statistical analyses required for interpreting the raw data of the clinical notes. Ida Hay at the Arnold Arboretum in Boston and Professor Richard Evans Schultes at Harvard University helped identify some of the plant species and clarified their nomenclatures. Richard J. Wolfe at the Boston Medical Library brought several helpful items to my attention.

Table A.1. *Drug use in the teaching ward of the infirmary, early 1795*

Drug name	% patients treated (N = 65)	% all treatments administered (N = 4,363)
AERATA, AQUA	1.5	0.05
AETHIOPS NARCOTICUS	10.8	0.55
ALKALINA AERATA, AQUA	3.1	0.25
ALOE	35.4	4.16
ALUMEN	1.5	0.09
AMARUM, INFUSUM	9.2	1.01
AMMONIACUS, SAL	1.5	0.39
AMMONIAE, LINIMENTUM	12.3	1.19
AMMONIA PRAEPARATA	1.5	0.12
AMYGDALA, OL	1.5	0.25
ANGOSTURA, CORTEX	7.7	1.31
ANTIMONIUM CRUDUM	1.5	0.25
ANTIMONIUM TARTARISATUM (tartar emetic)	7.7	0.28
ARNICA MONTANA, FOLIA	4.6	1.29
AROMATIC TINCTURE or ELECTU-ARY (AQUA CARDIACA)	12.3	3.01
ARSENICI, SOLUTIO MINERALIS (Fowler's solution)	4.6	0.67
ASAFETIDA	3.1	1.10
BELLADONNA	1.5	0.92
CALCIS, AQUA (and LINIMENTUM AQUAE CALCIS)	12.3	1.82
CAMPECHE	1.5	0.18
CAMPHOR	16.9	3.43
CANCRORUM LAPILLAE	1.5	0.35
CANTHARIDES, as BLISTER	47.7	1.45
CANTHARIDES, as TINCTURE administered orally	6.2	2.37
CARBONAS LIGNI, PULVIS	9.2	2.25
CASSIA LIGNEA	16.9	2.78
CATECHU	4.6	0.69
CERUSSA ACETATA, as UNGUEN-TUM or COLLYRIUM	16.9	3.45
CICUTA	13.8	5.52
CINCHONA	33.8	7.02
COLOCYNTHIS	6.2	1.01
COLUMBA	4.6	0.23
CORNU CERVIS, SAL	1.5	0.18
CRETA	3.1	0.16

Table A.1. *(cont.)*

Drug name	% patients treated (N = 65)	% all treatments administered (N = 4,363)
CUPRUM AMMONIACUM	1.5	1.10
DIGITALIS	1.5	0.44
FARINA POULTICE or FRICTION	3.1	0.07
FERRI RUBIGO and FERRUM PRAE-CIPITATUM	3.1	0.32
FERRUM VITRIOLATUM	3.1	0.74
GARLIC	4.6	0.51
GLYCERRHIZA	33.8	5.50
GUAIAC	4.6	0.51
HYOSCYAMUS	4.6	0.46
IPECAC	21.5	0.90
JALAP	27.7	1.66
JAMAICA EXTRACT	12.3	2.58
JULAP, SALINE	4.6	0.16
JUNIPER, INFUSUM or SPIRITS OF	4.6	1.01
KALI SULPHURATUM	4.6	1.73
MAGNESIA ALBA	1.5	0.07
MAGNESIA USTA	3.1	0.12
MAGNESIA VITRIOLATA (Epsom salts)	3.1	0.23
MAGNOLIA	3.1	0.83
MERCURIAL PILLS	29.2	4.18
MERCURIAL UNGUENTS	7.7	4.10
MICA PANIO (breadcrumbs)	3.1	0.16
MUCILAGINOUS MIXTURE	12.3	1.66
MYRRH	1.5	0.41
NICOTIANA, as SNUFF	3.1	0.14
NICOTIANI, VIN	6.2	1.75
NITRITI, UNGUENTUM	1.5	0.02
OLEO MIXTURE	3.1	0.14
OPIUM ENEMA	1.5	0.03
OPIUM PILLS	38.5	3.64
OPIUM TINCTURES and INFUSIONS	84.6	8.58
OPIUM UNGUENTS and LINIMENTS	21.5	3.04
RHEUM (Rhubarb)	21.5	2.97
RICINUS	10.8	0.97
ROSES, CONSERVE OF	4.6	0.48
RUBIA	1.5	0.18
SACCHARUM ALBUM	1.5	0.37
SARSAPARILLA	1.5	0.07

Table A.1. *(cont.)*

Drug name	% patients treated (N = 65)	% all treatments administered (N = 4,363)
SCILLAE	6.2	0.97
SENNA	36.9	1.84
SODA PHOSPHORATA	13.8	0.51
SOYMIDA	12.3	2.58
SUCCINI, OL	1.5	0.30
SULFUR, FLOWERS OF	7.7	1.33
TAMARINDORUM CUM SENNA, INFUSUM	7.7	0.12
TARTARI, CRYSTALLI (= SODA TARTARISATA, or Rochelle salt)	35.4	4.05
TARTARI, LIXIVIA	12.3	1.11
TEREBINTH, UNGUENTS and LINIMENTS	7.7	1.06
TOLU, SYRUP OF	4.6	1.06
TOXICODENDRI, INFUSUM	1.5	0.21
UNGUENTUM SIMPLEX	1.5	0.09
VALERIAN	6.2	1.68
VEGETABLE ACID, POTUS	12.3	0.85
VITRIOLICUM, ACIDUM	15.4	1.54
VITRIOLICUM, LINIMENT or UNGUENT	3.1	0.21
VITRIOLICUS, AETHER	4.6	0.18
WINE, RED (including PORTER)	7.7	1.47
ZINCUM PRAECIPITATUM	1.5	0.78
ZINCUM VITRIOLATUM	1.5	0.58
ZINGIBER	3.1	0.30

Note: Because 28.1% of all prescriptions were for extemporaneous mixtures of two or more active raw drug ingredients, the sum of the percentages in the final column is greater than 100. See the glossary at the end of this appendix for a definition of each drug or preparation and its therapeutic applications.

the most common were aloes, glycerrhiza, senna, crystals of tartar (prescribed elsewhere as cream of tartar), and mercury. Cinchona, the Peruvian bark, was administered to about one-third of the patients.

Table A.2 shows the nondrug treatments administered to the 65 patients. About one-sixth were bled, by the lancet, scarification, wet cupping, or leeches. One-third were given enemas when cathartics had failed, and one-tenth were treated with electricity.

Table A.2. *Use of nondrug treatments in the teaching ward of the infirmary, winter 1795*

Treatment	% patients treated (N = 65)	% all treatments administered (N = 4,363)
Bleeding		
By lancet	3.1	0.07
By scarification	1.5	0.02
By wet cupping	4.6	0.07
With leeches	7.7	0.37
Total bleeding	16.9	0.53
Seton	1.5	0.02
Cold water on kidneys	1.5	0.64
Heat on stomach	1.5	0.55
Warm bath	1.5	0.12
Torcularia (tourniquets)	1.5	0.05
Electricity	10.8	4.74
Enemas		
Domestic	32.3	1.52
Opium	1.5	0.07

Note: The treatments listed here represent a total of 8.2% of all treatments administered to these 65 patients. See the glossary at the end of this appendix for descriptions of the treatments.

Duncan indicated his therapeutic plans for some of his patients, including his contingency plans if others failed and his reasons for each. The rationales for the treatments administered to other patients must be inferred from their progress notes and the descriptions of each drug given in the *Edinburgh New Dispensatory* and other contemporary texts. Because the physicians of the infirmary wrote or compiled so many of the standard reference volumes, the clinical notes have been considered in conjunction with them in order to ascertain the actual rationale for the use of each treatment in each of the 65 patients, as summarized in the glossary.

Study of the individual patient records shows that treatments were aimed at separate symptoms, physical and "laboratory" findings, and specific stages in the evolution of each patient's illness, including complications; treatments were also adjusted to take into account individual patients' responses to putative contagions, miasmas, or other causative factors, including drug side effects. Significant physical findings were based on observations of the skin, tongue, pulse, abdomen (by percussion, measurement, and deep palpation), and extremities (by assessing, e.g., fine tremor, muscle strength, and pitting edema). "Laboratory" observations included assessing the vol-

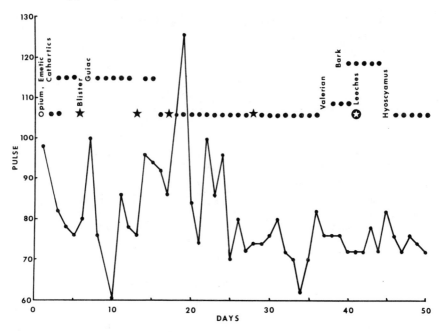

Figure A.1. Clinical course, as reflected by pulse rate and by the treatments prescribed by Duncan, of Alexander F., admitted to the infirmary with a diagnosis of rheumatismus. Closed circles indicate days on which treatments indicated to the left of each row were administered to the patient; closed stars indicate blister applications; and the open star indicates an application of leeches.

ume, color, sediment, and taste of urine and the volume, consistency, and color of stools; observing blood removed by the lancet or cupping for a buffy coat; and testing whether expectorated sputum sank in water. Food and drink intake were also compared with urine output when appropriate.

Pulse rates were especially useful to Duncan for assessing the responses of fever patients to his treatments. That is, fluctuations and stability in each patient's pulse appear to have helped him decide how best to adjust his prescriptions, and his patients' physiological balances, from one day to the next. Figures A.1 through A.4 illustrate how he used the pulse in determining therapeutic responses in four different kinds of fever.

Alexander F., aged 22, was admitted to the infirmary with a diagnosis of rheumatismus, which meant that he had pains in his head and chest, not necessarily joint pains. Duncan's first explicitly stated therapeutic objective was to inhibit the hyperactivity in the blood vessels of the patient's head and chest that was producing his symptoms. Figure A.1 shows that he began treating his patient with an opiate, to relieve his pain, and with an emetic, to strengthen his stomach so that it could remove the responsible contagious factors from the body by diverting them away from the diseased organs. He prescribed cathartics over the next four days because the patient became constipated, to prevent him from retaining the contagious matter. Duncan began his intended definitive treatment on day 6, when he applied a blister to the patient's sternum; his goal was first to divert the "morbid action" away from the thoracic organs; then, after a few hours, the cantharides would counteract the inflammatory process by relaxing the tense blood vessels that were responsible for it.

Tincture of guaiac was begun the next day, after the stools had become normal, in order to stimulate the stomach, urine, and sweat glands to remove the pain and, because guaiac was thought to be a tonic drug, to constrict the blood vessels. On the fourth day of guaiac treatment, Duncan increased its dose because the pulse rate had not yet stabilized, another blister was applied on the thirteenth day, between the shoulder blades. Guaiac was continued for two more days, although it provided little relief or inhibition of vascular hyperactivity. On day 17 another blister was applied, this time to the patient's head.

Despite these treatments, the patient's pains continued, so opiates were resumed and the guaiac was discontinued. On day 28 a fourth blister was applied, again to the head. By now the pulse was no longer fluctuating so wildly as it had been. On day 32 Duncan began an unsuccessful five-day trial of a new drug (not shown in Figure A.1), an extract of magnolia bark, which he thought should be an effective tonic. On day 37 he prescribed valerian, which he anticipated would potentiate the tonic effects of the magnolia extract, as well as calm the hyperexcited nervous system he thought was causing the patient's persistent headaches.

On day 39 Duncan replaced the experimental magnolia with Peruvian bark, the universally accepted astringent tonic. He and his colleagues also called it an antiseptic because they thought that it removed sepsis – inflammation – from the body. Although by then the pulse had more or less stabilized, the patient was not yet free from the typical symptoms of a continued fever, chiefly pain and evidence of vasoconstriction. Thus, on day 42, Duncan prescribed six leeches to be applied on the patient's temples overnight, for the removal of enough blood to relax the inflamed vessels in his head. On day 45 he made a trial of hyoscyamus, which he hypothesized should relieve the pain and relax the nervous system, much as he thought opium would do; this experiment, too, was unsuccessful.

Figure A.1 does not show the last fifteen days of the patient's hospitalization, but they included more cathartics, opiates, and two more doses of eight leeches each, applied to his head on days 60 and 62. He was discharged on day 65, apparently because his pulse was staying near normal, at around 75; this stabilization indicated to Duncan that the patient's system had been

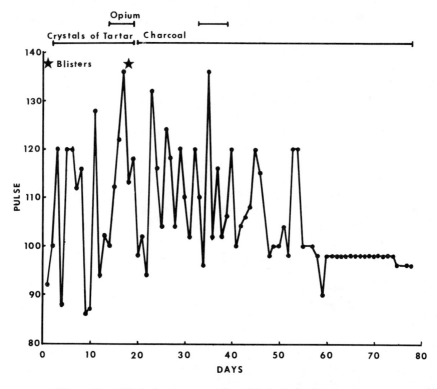

Figure A.2. Clinical course, as reflected by pulse rate and by the treatments prescribed by Duncan, of Daniel R., admitted to the infirmary with a diagnosis of phthisis catarrhalis. The duration of each treatment is indicated by the horizontal lines, and applications of blisters by closed stars.

adequately relaxed by his treatments, although the patient still had the pains that had precipitated his admission.

Figure A.2 outlines the clinical course of Daniel R., aged 34, who was admitted with a diagnosis of phthisis catarrhalis, characterized by retrosternal pain, cough, and copious expectoration. He was treated first with a blister to his sternum and then with crystals of tartar as a mild cooling cathartic expected to relieve the fluid accumulation and inflammatory activity in his chest. On day 14 opiates were begun, to help him sleep, and four days later another blister was applied on the lateral chest wall, to counter-irritate the disease in the chest cavity.

Two days later Duncan began treating the patient only with charcoal in water, in an explicit experimental attempt to absorb the septic material out of the body and into the intestinal canal. From days 33 to 39 he prescribed opiates again, but this time it was to reduce the number of stools. Finally,

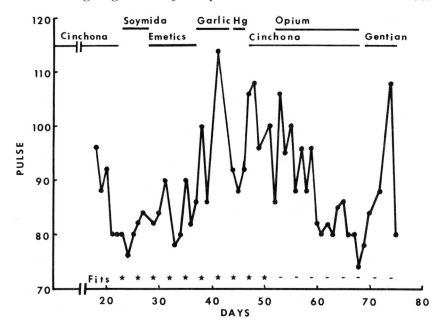

Figure A.3. Clinical course, as reflected by pulse rate, occurrence of "fits," and the treatments prescribed by Duncan, of Leslie C., admitted to the infirmary with a diagnosis of quartan fever. The duration of each treatment is indicated by the horizontal lines (Duncan's notes for the first two weeks are missing). The small stars across the bottom indicate days on which the patient had the characteristic attacks of this form of intermittent fever, or malaria, and the dashes to the right of the stars indicate days on which she did not suffer the expected attacks.

after about two months, the patient's pulse rate stabilized, although it was high, and he was discharged on day 79. Duncan reviewed this patient's hospital course and concluded that the charcoal had probably contributed to the recovery.

Leslie C. was a 22-year-old woman admitted with a quartan fever; she had shivering fits at 72-hour intervals at exactly 4:30 p.m., as indicated in Figure A.3. For the first three weeks she was treated with cinchona (Peruvian bark). However, it upset her stomach so badly that at the same time she was given preparations of gentian (infusum amarum) and cinnamon (tincture aromaticum), not shown in the figure, to settle her stomach. On one or two occasions during those first three weeks, tourniquets ("torcularia") were applied around her right arm and left thigh at the time the fits began, to calm her excited vascular system.

When the cinchona failed to cure her, Duncan tried a new drug, soymida bark, that had recently been introduced from India. As the stars at the bottom of Figure A.3 indicate, her fits continued to recur every fourth day. So, because the patient's pulse rate was still relatively high, and in order to strengthen her stomach's connections with the vascular system, he prescribed emetics, including ipecac and tartar emetic; at the same time he gave her arsenic, in Fowler's solution (not shown), to make her sweat out the disease. Nevertheless, the shivering fits continued to occur regularly, and her pulse remained hyperactive.

Duncan then tried garlic for a few days, because he thought it would enhance the activity and tone of the patient's whole body and thereby increase her production of sputum, urine, and sweat. Next he prescribed mercury, as a weak solution of corrosive sublimate (not shown), for a few more days, because he thought it had actions like those of garlic. Neither drug helped the patient, despite Duncan's opinion that "unquestionably they are capable of combatting the disease."

Finally, beginning on day 47 of the patient's hospitalization, he returned to prescribing cinchona, but this time he gave her doses eight times as large as those he had prescribed during the first three weeks. From day 50 on, the patient had no more attacks of her quartan fever; the clinical notes regularly indicate that she no longer suffered the expected fits every fourth day. She was given opiates for two weeks, for pain and to calm her blood vessels. Together, the two drugs were seen to lower her pulse rate. At the very end she was treated with gentian to stimulate her stomach (and her digestion), so Duncan was not surprised that her pulse rose somewhat on day 74; he discharged her as cured two days later.

James L. was a 50-year-old gardener admitted for hydrothorax as his principal sign of dropsy (see Figure A.4). Because the pulse was rapid in most cases of dropsy, this disease was regarded as a fever produced by weakness or laxity of the vessels, not as cardiac failure.[2] So the patient was first blistered on the sternum, to counterirritate the fluid-filled tissues of the chest and to promote an "artificial" evacuation of the fluid into the blister. For the next two days he was given jalap, as a potent cathartic and diuretic that would, Duncan anticipated, provide "natural" routes for evacuating more water from the chest. At the same time Duncan started prescribing digitalis, because it was a very potent diuretic. He had known Withering's studies of digitalis even before Withering published them ten years earlier.[3]

Duncan tripled the dose of digitalis on the second day, and the patient's symptoms had begun to diminish by the following day. His urine production was markedly elevated by day 5 and remained at over five pounds a day for the rest of his hospitalization. Soymida bark was added for the last five days, probably because, as a tonic, Duncan thought it would constrict the weakened blood vessels and thereby prevent fluid from reaccumulating in the chest.

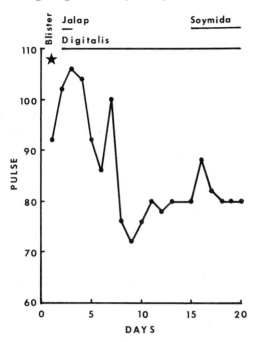

Figure A.4. Clinical course, as reflected by pulse rate and by the treatments prescribed by Duncan, of James L., admitted to the infirmary with a diagnosis of hydrothorax and dropsy. The horizontal lines indicate the duration of each treatment, and the star indicates a blistering.

Thus, by the time the patient was discharged, twenty-one days after his admission, Duncan had accomplished his original therapeutic goal: removing water from the chest with drugs that promoted the absorption of water from the tissues and that stimulated their evacuation from the body. About three and a half weeks later Duncan wrote that this cure was definitely attributable to the drugs he had prescribed. A number of other patients, he noted, probably would have recovered even without any treatment, because of the body's natural tendency to heal itself. However, he went on, he did not expect the cure in this case to be permanent. Duncan had seen the patient recently and found him still well, but, Duncan reported sadly, "I am afraid he pays too frequent visits to the Dram Shop"; that is, Duncan, like many of his contemporaries, thought that dropsy was associated with excessive alcohol intake.[4]

Phyllis V., age 42, was admitted to the infirmary with a diagnosis of diabetes mellitus, increased abdominal girth, and leucorrhea, although it is not clear from the clinical notes just how long she had been afflicted. She displayed the classic symptoms of polydipsia, polyphagia, and polyuria, as

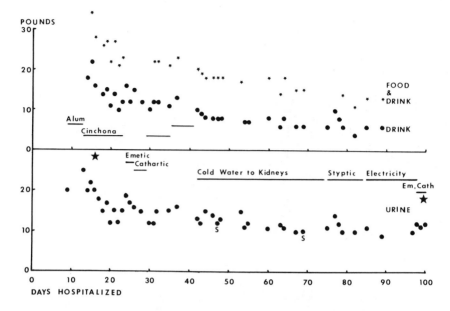

Figure A.5. Clinical course from day 10 to day 100, as reflected by the daily intake of food and drink and by the daily output of urine (both by weight) of Phyllis V., admitted to the infirmary with a diagnosis of diabetes mellitus. The large closed stars in the lower portion of the graph indicate blister applications; the letter *S* indicates days on which the patient's urine was tasted to determine if sugar was present (the test may have been performed on other days as well); and *Em* and *Cath* indicate, respectively, the administrations of emetics and cathartics.

shown graphically in Figure A.5, during the early days of her hospitalization. Duncan recorded her progress not by her pulse rates but by her food and drink intake and urine output, as shown in the upper and lower parts, respectively, of Figures A.5 and A.6. The data for the first ten days of her admission are missing.

The patient was first treated with alum, an astringent that Duncan expected would decrease both her leucorrhea and the fluid production responsible for her excessive urine output. She was then treated with cinchona, presumably for the same reason; there certainly were no signs or symptoms of fever at that time. She was blistered on day 15, to counterirritate the tissues that had become so weakened as to permit fluid to accumulate passively. By day 19 her abdominal girth had decreased by eight inches, and she lost another two inches over the next 24 hours as her urine output increased.

An emetic and a cathartic were added for a few days, to further strengthen

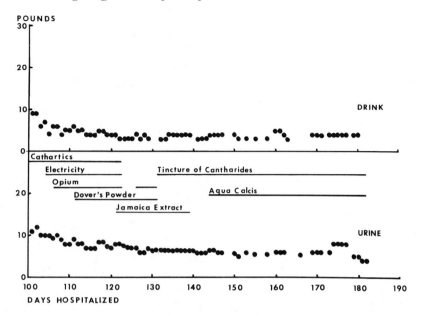

Figure A.6. Clinical course from day 101 to day 182 of Phyllis V.

the patient's stomach and relax her bowels, and Duncan resumed treating her with alum for a few days more when both intake and output remained relatively high. Then he treated her with cold water compresses applied over the kidneys for about a month. During this time her urine output decreased somewhat, but, as indicated in Figure A.5, she was still spilling excess sugar into her urine, as determined by tasting it.

Her urine output continued to be greater than the normal expected output of about three pounds a day, so Duncan prescribed a styptic of unspecified composition and then electricity to the area over the kidneys. Then, on day 98, the patient developed a pulmonary inflammation. As he did for other continued fever patients, Duncan treated this new complication with an emetic, a cathartic, and a blister applied between the shoulder blades.

For the next three weeks (see Figure A.6), he continued to give cathartics to keep the bowels open and help remove the factors responsible for the fever; a little later he added opium to treat her cough. He also prescribed Dover's powder as a diaphoretic to help remove the fever, because her pulse was ranging between 80 and 95, and the newly introduced Jamaica extract, an astringent that he thought would be an appropriate substitute for cinchona. The fever symptoms disappeared by day 130, about six weeks after they first appeared.

In the meantime Duncan had resumed electrical treatments to the kidneys, to constrict the patient's kidney fibers and thereby reduce her urine output; he was not disappointed with this treatment. After most of the fever symptoms had disappeared, he prescribed a very dilute solution of cantharides administered orally; he reasoned that the drug would "relieve the morbid action" of her blood vessels by stimulating them to achieve normal fluid balance. Finally, he prescribed aqua calcis, limewater, because the patient had a recurrence of her long-standing leucorrhea. He thought that the limewater, because of its astringent properties, would decrease the abnormal secretions of the uterus and perhaps even those that had produced the chief symptoms of her diabetes. During her last two months in the infirmary, the patient's urine output as well as her fluid intake stabilized at relatively low levels; she was discharged after a total hospitalization of six months because her average daily urine output remained at less than five pounds.

These five representative case reports illustrate Andrew Duncan's approach to adjusting his patients' humoral and tonic balances, their internal equilibria.[5] It is clear that his therapeutic decisions were made on the basis of his patients' symptoms as well as signs like pulse rates, urine and stool production, and even the amount of sugar in the urine. The student recorder of these 65 cases learned from Duncan that treatment must be empirical rather than dogmatic;[6] that is, physicians must base their treatments on their observations of their patients' responses to therapy.

Duncan prescribed seven drugs that were not officially accepted in the 1794 edition of the *Edinburgh New Dispensatory,* the edition published just before these 65 admissions: aethiops narcoticus, magnolia bark, Jamaica extract, soymida bark, carbonas ligni with kali sulphuratum, carbonas ligni alone, and toxicodendron. Duncan abandoned soymida and magnolia when they proved to be ineffective or not dependable. Carbonas ligni and toxicodendron had become official by the time the sixth (1811) edition of the *Dispensatory* appeared. His use of these drugs, together with his experience with and reading about digitalis, suggests that Duncan did indeed continue to prescribe drugs he found to be effective, and that he gave up prescribing drugs he found not effective in his own patients.

It is also clear from his clinical notes that Duncan adjusted the doses of the drugs he prescribed in accordance with his patients' responses to them. That is, he would increase the dose of a drug that he was certain would be beneficial if a patient did not respond to the first dose he prescribed. Similarly, he would almost always decrease the dose of a drug that produced too great an effect or an undesirable side effect (e.g., constipation in a patient given an opiate for pain), but only if he were certain that continued use of the drug would benefit his patient; otherwise, he would prescribe another drug with similar properties.

Because Duncan prescribed cathartics so often – like his contemporaries in America[7] – special patterns of their usage emerge from the records of his practical therapeutics. Although he prescribed strong or mild cathartics, as indicated, to adjust the tone of his patients' bowels or to speed evacuation of disturbing contagious matter, he also prescribed them if a patient produced no stool for what he took to be too long an interval, generally two days. In addition, he stopped prescribing cathartics for women when their menstrual periods began and resumed them afterward; he seems to have reasoned that the menstrual flow would achieve the same therapeutic evacuatory end.

Duncan concluded that 25 of the 65 patients admitted to his ward in the winter of 1795 (38.5%) had been completely cured and that 14 (21.5%) had been partially cured, for an overall partial or complete cure rate of 60.0%. He noted that he had not been able to cure another 12 (18.5%) and that 8 more could not have been cured (12.3%) despite all professional medical efforts. Another 4 of the patients (6.2%) died, and the final outcome of 2 cases is not known because of missing or torn pages in the clinical notes. He thought that 9 of the 39 partially or completely cured patients (23.1%, or 13.8% of all 65 patients) probably would have recovered without any treatment.

If the therapeutic methods of Andrew Duncan, Sr., were similar in all but the finest details to those of his English-speaking contemporaries, so were the outcomes of the illnesses he treated. For instance, among 10,000 patients treated at the Philadelphia Dispensary from 1786 to 1792, largely by physicians trained at Edinburgh, 14.2% were discharged as not cured and 4.5% died.[8] Mortality did, of course, vary with diagnosis; for instance, the incidence of death from serious diseases possibly of a cardiovascular nature was about five times the incidence of mortality from infectious diseases, which were far and away the most common illnesses of the time.[9] Duncan and other physicians of his generation could expect something like 95% of their nonsurgical patients to survive, regardless of the doctors' perception of, and reliance on, the influence of the healing power of nature. Although between one-sixth and one-third of the survivors might be regarded as incompletely cured, at least they had not died while in the hospital.

Many of the drugs prescribed by Duncan actually did cause vomiting, diarrhea, sweating, diuresis, blisters, and so on, before his patients recovered. He could, therefore, reasonably infer that he had good clinical evidence that most of the drugs he used (save for the few exceptions already noted among the drugs he tried experimentally) did benefit his patients. Duncan and his contemporaries – both physicians and their patients – had no clues that vomiting, catharsis, sweating, diuresis, purging, and blistering may not have contributed much to recovery from illness. In the absence of controlled trials, they lacked the information that could have led them to this conclusion.

Instead, Duncan and his colleagues at the Royal Infirmary of Edinburgh continued to prescribe those drugs which had, in the past, been associated with recovery from illness, and in accordance with their understanding of the body's reactions to the factors associated with the identifiable categories of disease. The specific reasons that led them to prescribe the drugs Duncan gave his patients in the infirmary's teaching ward in early 1795 are outlined next.

> Glossary of treatments prescribed by Dr. Duncan in the teaching ward of the infirmary, February–April 1795

In general, the main entries in this glossary are the drug, or treatment, names used in the majority of their mentions in Duncan's clinical notes; alternative names are employed in a minority of mentions in his notes or in the standard contemporary texts or references. All words capitalized in the texts of the definitions may be found as separate entries. See Tables A.1 and A.2 for the frequencies with which these treatments were prescribed. However, not all materials in this glossary are listed in table A.1, which includes only those drugs thought to have pharmacological effects and excludes materials used as flavoring, menstruums, vehicles, and so forth.

Each main entry begins with a modern identification, when possible, of the drug material, and for inorganic compounds of uncertain identity the method of preparation. Next is a synthesis of contemporary information about the treatment's presumed site(s) and mode(s) of action and the disease(s) or symptom(s) for which it had been found to be most effective. This information is expressed entirely within the framework of late eighteenth-century pathophysiological concepts, although more modern synonyms are used occasionally in order to avoid misunderstandings. Most of this information was collated from the following sources: *The Edinburgh New Dispensatory,* 4th ed. (Edinburgh: William Creech, 1794); *Pharmacopoeia Collegii Regii Medicorum Edinburgensis* (Edinburgh: Bell & Bradfute, 1792); J. Worth Estes, "Therapeutic practice in colonial New England," in *Medicine in Colonial Massachusetts, 1620–1820,* ed. by Philip Cash, Eric H. Christianson, and J. Worth Estes, Boston: Colonial Society of Massachusetts, 1980, pp. 289–383; and J. Worth Estes and LaVerne Kuhnke, "French observations of disease and drug use in late eighteenth-century Cairo," *J. Hist. Med.* 39 (1984): 121–152.

It should be noted that Andrew Duncan, Sr., was president of the Edinburgh College of Physicians when it published the *Pharmacopoeia Collegii Regii,* which can be taken as the "official" compilation of commonly accepted information about drugs. Some additional information, unavailable in these references and pertinent chiefly to the nonofficial remedies (that is, those not included in the *Pharmacopoeia Collegii Regii* or *Edinburgh New Dispensatory*), was collated from the clinical notes themselves or from other sources, including several mentioned by Duncan; these additional sources are cited in appropriate main entries. Although the *Edinburgh Dispensatory* provides the corresponding drug names and ingredients also specified in the *Pharmacopoeia of the Royal College of Physicians of London,* 6th ed. (London: Thomas Healde, 1793) – usually referred to as the London *Pharmacopoeia* – often they are not equivalent to Edinburgh specifications. Therefore, only the latter are used in this glossary.

The understanding of therapeutic action and of clinical efficacy apparent in Duncan's notes is also reflected in the works of two other physicians at the infirmary: Francis Home, *Clinical Experiments, Histories, and Dissections,* 3rd ed., London and Edinburgh: J. Murray & William Creech, 1783; and William Cullen, *First Lines of the Practice of Physic,* new ed., 4 vols., Edinburgh: C. Elliott; London: T. Kay, 1789. All editions chosen for use in this appendix are those published nearest to the date of the clinical notes analyzed or, in Cullen's case, the last edition he prepared before his death in 1790.

Asterisks indicate information that is explicit, or clearly implicit, in Duncan's clinical notes themselves. However, the total description of each treatment represents a fusion of information from all sources consulted. It should be remembered that even if a piece of information lacks an asterisk it may indeed have been included in Duncan's rationale for prescribing the treatment, but the necessary correlative clues are missing from his clinical notes.

Unless otherwise noted, all direct quotations are from Duncan's notes.

In general, the glossary is designed so that drugs of similar composition, insofar as Duncan was concerned, are grouped together, despite alphabetization. Note that the glossary does *not* alphabetize by words that indicate the nature of the preparation employed for administering the drugs: AETHER, AQUA, BALSAMUM, CONSERVE, CORTEX, ELECTUARIUM, FOLIA, GUM, INFUSUM, OL, PILL, PILULE, SAL, TINCTURA, UNGUENTUM, OR VIN.

AERATA, AQUA, or AQUA AERIS FIXI: Carbonic acid, prepared by dissolving chalk (calcium carbonate) in sulfuric acid and then saturating spring water with the evolving gas. Used chiefly as an antiemetic.★

AETHIOPS NARCOTICUS: Mercury dissolved in nitric acid and precipitated with KALI SULPHURATUM (potassium sulfate) to form mercuric sulfide. Nonofficial; recently introduced from Germany as a narcotic, to be used to induce sleep★ and/or allay pain,★ effects that Duncan ascribed to the sulfur content rather than the mercury. Side effects include confusion and vertigo. Because the new drug "keeps the belly open," it was thought to be superior to OPIUM, which regularly produces constipation. However, Duncan was not impressed by the clinical efficacy of aethiops narcoticus. Also see MERCURY.

ALKALINA AERATA, AQUA: Aerated alkaline solution prepared by saturating 2 oz. of LIXIVIUM (thought to be potassium carbonate) dissolved in one gal. water with fixed air (carbonic acid). Used as an antacid* and antiemetic* and to treat gout* and urinary tract stones.

ALLIUM: See GARLIC. However, in a few cases onion, *Allium cepa,* may have been meant.

ALOES: *Aloe perfoliata* or *A. barbadensis;* the best grade, known as socotrine, came from Socotrina Island in the Indian Ocean. Most often used as a cathartic;* also used to stimulate blood vessels* (especially of rectum and adjacent tissues), to warm the body, and to stimulate menstrual flow;* therefore, to regularize all discharges* in the treatment of, e.g., amenorrhea,* jaundice, worms, and some wounds.

ALOES CUM COLOCYNTHIDE, PILULULE: Potent cathartic* pill made with AL-OES, SCAMMONY, ANTIMONY SULFATE,* COLOCYNTHIS, oil of cloves, and GUM ARABIC; sometimes substituted for JALAP.

ALOETICAE, PILULULE, or ALOES PILL: Made from ALOES and GENTIAN extract, mixed with simple syrup. See ALOES for uses.

ALTHAEA: Gummy extract of *Althaea officinalis,* marshmallow. Used as a nonspecific binding agent* in several preparations; also as an emollient and for pulmonary inflammation, dysentery, kidney disease (including stones), and, externally, for "soft tumors."

ALUMEN: Alum, potassium aluminum sulfate. Used as an astringent,* in diabetes,* and to control bleeding.* Side effects: nausea and constipation.

AMARUM, INFUSUM (= infusum gentianae compositum): Water extract of GENTIAN root, dried orange peel, coriander seeds, and proof spirit. Used as a carminative* or stomachic,* that is, to enhance the appetite, and as a general tonic* to stimulate the vascular system.

AMMONIACUS, SAL: Ammonium chloride, prepared by sublimation of burned animal dung and sea salt or by mixing hydrochloric acid and "volatile ammonia" (ammonia). Given internally to produce diaphoresis,* diuresis, mild catharsis, and emesis; applied topically as an antiseptic gargle for tonsillitis* and perhaps for other swellings.

AMMONIAE, LINIMENTUM (= oleum ammoniatum or unguentum tussivum): Mixture of olive oil and a water solution of "caustic ammonium" (sodium hydroxide). Used as a gargle for tonsillitis* or sore throat* or to prevent suppuration* in the oral cavity; sometimes used as a warm tonic or as a diaphoretic, to treat inflammation, especially after BLEEDING.

AMMONIA PRAEPARATA (= diaphoretic salt): Ammonium acetate, originally extracted from ALOES (q.v.); introduced in 1610 as Spirits of Mindererus. Diaphoretic* and cathartic.*

AMYGDALA, OL: Oil of bitter almonds, from *Amygdala communis.* Used internally to relax solid organs and to diminish acrid humors in, e.g., cough,* hoarseness,* dysuria,* and other pains; applied externally to relax tense muscles. The *Edinburgh*

Dispensatory notes that it is poisonous to dogs but not to men.

ANGOSTURA, CORTEX: Bark of *Angostura* spp. Used to stimulate tone and vigor of stomach,★ to increase appetite, to decrease flatus and acidity in dyspepsia, and for diarrhea; a nonspecific aromatic bitter.

ANODYNE: Usually an opiate, used as an analgesic;★ see OPIUM.

ANODYNUM, BALSAMUM: see OPIATUM, LINIMENTUM.

ANTIMONIUM CRUDUM, PULVIS: Powdered antimony ore, chiefly the sulfide. Used (but rarely in this form) to stimulate diaphoresis,★ catharsis, emesis, and the circulation.★ ANTIMONIUM TARTARISATUM (tartar emetic) was probably the most frequently used antimony salt.

ANTIMONIUM TARTARISATUM (= tartar emetic): Antimony potassium tartrate. Used as a diaphoretic★ at lower doses and as an emetic★ at higher doses.

ANTIMONY SULFATE (SULPHATE): Used as a cathartic in ALOES CUM COLOCYN-THIDE (q.v.).

ARABIC, GUM: Extract of *Acacia senegal.* Used as a demulcent★ in, e.g., MUCILA-GINOUS MIXTURE (q.v.).

ARNICA MONTANA, FOLIA: Leaves of leopard's bane, *Arnica montana.* Used as a tonic for paralysis★ (although it was also thought to possess antispasmodic proper-ties) and for intermittent fevers and gangrene, though Duncan recognized that ex-perience had not validated these latter two applications.

AROMATICA, TINCTURA (= cinnamoni composita): According to official com-pendia, a tincture containing cinnamon *(Cinnamomum zeylanicum),* lesser cardamom seeds, angelica root, and long pepper *(Piper longum),* most of which are also the ingredients of CARDIACA, AQUA (q.v.). Used for languor,★ weak stomach,★ fla-tus,★ and other symptoms of gastric distress.

AROMATIC PILL (= electuarium aromaticum): Soft lozenge made of cinnamon *(cinnamomum zeylanicum),* lesser cardamom seeds, ginger (see ZINGIBER), and syrup of orange peel; the same ingredients are used in AQUA CARDIACA. Used to pro-mote digestion★ and as a tonic for weak viscera.★

ARSENICI, SOLUTIO MINERALIS (= Fowler's solution): Water solution of white arsenic (arsenic trioxide) and LIXIVIUM (thought to be potassium carbonate), with spirits of lavender added. Used as a diaphoretic for intermittent fevers;★ also taken internally or externally as a corrosive, for what was thought to be cancer.

ASAFETIDA: Extract of *Ferula assafoetida.* Used as a cathartic★ to promote release of all body fluids "in both sexes"; to raise the spirits in hysteric and nervous com-plaints, e.g., hypochondriasis;★ and for flatulent colic.★

AXUNGUENTUM PORCINUM: Hog fat, used chiefly as a pharmacologically inert emollient in topical ointments.

BARK: see CINCHONA.

BELLADONNA: Extract of deadly nightshade, *Atropa belladonna.* Used internally as a narcotic, diuretic, diaphoretic, and sialagogue (despite its now-recognized antimuscarinic effects), for treating melancholy, mania, and epilepsy and as an analgesic* in cancer. Applied topically to open superficial cancers.

BLEEDING: Used by Duncan to relieve symptoms of hyperactive blood vessels, e.g., flushing,* hemoptysis,* and pain,* chiefly in patients with inflammation,* fever,* apoplexy* (when accompanied by flushing), ophthalmia,* and gallstones.* For further details, see Chapter 4.

BLISTER: See CANTHARIS.

BREADCRUMBS: see MICA PANIO.

CALCINED MAGNESIA: see MAGNESIA USTA.

CALCIS, AQUA: Limewater. Used as an astringent* to decrease secretions, by constricting blood vessels,* in patients with diabetes,* leucorrhea,* foul skin ulcers,* diarrhea, and other conditions produced by laxity of solid tissue fibers; also administered orally or per rectum for gastrointestinal worms.

CALCIS, LINIMENTUM AQUAE: Equal parts of AQUA CALCIS and linseed (or olive) oil. Applied topically for skin conditions* (see CALCIS, AQUA), including scalds and burns, to decrease cutaneous inflammation.

CALOMEL (= hydrargyrus muriatus mitis or mercurius dulcis): Mercurous chloride. For actions and uses, see MERCURY.

CAMPECHE (= lignum campechense, haematoxylum, or logwood): Used as an astringent or styptic for leucorrhea,* diarrhea, etc.

CAMPHOR: Oil extracted from *Cinnamomum camphora.* Given internally to stimulate the *vis vitae,* especially to stimulate the nerves to the gastrointestinal tract in, e.g., hypochondriasis,* and to decrease spasm in, e.g., dysuria;* to enhance sleep and diaphoresis; and to inhibit suppuration in severe fevers. Applied externally as an unguent to inhibit inflammation,* spasm of cutaneous blood vessels,* and joint pains and to stimulate paralyzed muscles locally.

CANCRORUM LAPILLI PRAEPARATI: Purported to be powdered crab claws or crab's eyes; Duncan thought they were not. Used as absorbent* and antacid for leucorrhea,* heartburn, and diarrhea.

CANTHARIDIS, TINCTURA: Very dilute alcoholic solution of CANTHARIS (q.v.) administered by mouth, after further dilution, "to relieve morbid action" of spasmodic tissues of patients with diabetes,* leucorrhea, and gonorrhea, because of the drug's diuretic property.

CANTHARIDIS, UNGUENTUM (= epispastic unguent): Mixture of powdered CANTHARIS, water, and yellow resin, applied as a dressing to CANTHARIS-induced blisters (see next entry) to keep them running for up to five days.* Also used, after dilution, in a FRICTION or dressing with CAMPHOR dissolved in WINE, applied locally to stimulate paralyzed muscles.*

CANTHARIS or CANTHARIDES: Powdered "Spanish flies," *Lytta* (formerly *Cantharis*) *vesicatoria*. Applied externally as an "epispastic" or blistering plaster (composed of equal parts of powdered flies, melted suet, wax, and resin), it first operates as a general stimulant to remove fluid from the body "artifically," directly into the blister fluid and indirectly into urine or phlegm, and to "relieve torpor" by diverting "the impetus of the blood from the part affected to the part of application." These properties led Duncan to use it in the treatment of, e.g., dropsy,* hydrocephalus,* apoplexy,* paralysis,* catarrh,* fever,* cough,* dyspnea,* pain* (especially in the chest),* diabetes,* phthisis,* gonorrhea, and some skin and menstrual disorders. After a few hours, he inferred, the blister would begin to act as an antispasmodic* to reduce irritability, especially of the blood vessels, thereby changing the balance of the circulation; he therefore used it for treating severe fevers produced by inflammatory processes* and spasms of internal organs.

For the drug's internally administered form, see CANTHARIDIS, TINCTURA. When taken undiluted by mouth, cantharis produces severe dysuria, abdominal pain, hematuria, bloody stools, thirst, fetid breath, "madness," and death (the latter was presumably caused by cardiac arrhythmia produced by the drug's active principle, cantharidin). Its ability to irritate the lower urinary tract and thereby produce reflex stimulation of the sex organs presumably gave rise to the aphrodisiacal mythology of Spanish fly. For further details, see Chapter 4.

CARBONAS CALCIS, SAL: see CORNU CERVIS, SAL.

CARBONAS LIGNI, PULVIS: Powdered charcoal. Nonofficial until 1811. Used as an absorbent* and antiseptic* in rheumatism* and in phthisis (consumption) accompanied by hemoptysis.* Also see CHARCOAL AND KALI SULPHURATUM.

CARDIACA, AQUA: Water solution of cinnamon *(Cinnamomum zeylanicum)*, lesser cardamom seeds, ginger (see ZINGIBER), and syrup of orange peel, ingredients identical to those of the AROMATIC PILL and like those in TINCTURA AROMATICA. Used to promote digestion* and as a tonic* for lax viscera.* ("Cardiaca" = dyspepsia.)

CASSIA LIGNEA: Extract of *Cassia fistula*. Used as a mild cooling cathartic* to decrease the pulse,* as an emergency diuretic,* and to counteract the refrigerant effect of CRYSTALLI TARTARI produced by its antimony component.*

CATECHU: Extract of *Acacia catechu*. Mild astringent* used for treating diarrhea* (and to enhance OPIUM's constipating effect*), menorrhagia, catarrh, laxity of the viscera, etc., usually in extemporaneous prescriptions.

CATECHU, INFUSUM (= infusum Japonicum): Infusion of CATECHU (q.v.), cinnamon, and simple syrup. Used to treat diarrhea caused by laxity of the gastrointestinal tract and to potentiate tincture of OPIUM,* but also as a cathartic.*

CATHARTICUS AMARUS, SAL: see MAGNESIA VITRIOLATA.

CERUSSA ACETATA (= saccharum saturni): Lead acetate or sugar of lead, prepared by dissolving white lead (lead monoxide) in vinegar. Used as a cooling COLLYRIUM for ophthalmia;* as a styptic for treating skin cancers,* transudates, sweating, leucorrhea, etc.; and as CERUSSAE ACETATAE, UNGUENTUM (q.v.). An oral overdose produces colic, constipation, cramps, tremors, and nerve weakness.

CERUSSAE ACETATAE, UNGUENTUM: Ointment made with CERUSSA ACETATA and UNGUENTUM SIMPLEX. A cooling and dessicating ointment for treating skin sores★ and excoriations.★

CHALYBIS, SAL: see FERRUM VITRIOLATUM.

CHARCOAL: see CARBONAS LIGNI, PULVIS.

CHARCOAL AND KALI SULPHURATUM: Duncan notes that this nonofficial mixture of charcoal and potassium sulfate was recommended for the treatment of phthisis★ (consumption) by Garnet, on the basis of the following rationale: According to Dr. Thomas Beddoes, phthisis is caused by, or associated with, hyperoxygenation of the blood; therefore, Garnet reasoned, after the drug mixture enters the blood from the intestines, "the Chyle is impregnated with the sulphurated hydrogenous Gas, which unites with the Oxygen of the Blood & forms Water," thereby removing the excess oxygen from the blood. Duncan was not certain that Beddoes's theory was correct and would have preferred to treat his phthisis patients with air by inhalation; however, he judged that Garnet's recommended mixture would be safer to administer, and he did not doubt its efficacy a priori (although his clinical results disappointed him).

CICUTA: Powdered leaves of poison hemlock, *Conium maculatum.* Given internally, in small doses, as a potent tonic★ for diseases produced by obstructions, e.g., whooping cough, or for cachexia;★ also applied externally as a discutient to disperse solid tumors, especially cancer.★ Poisonous in larger doses.

CINCHONA (= bark, Peruvian bark, Cortex Peruvianus, or BARK VAN SWIE-TEN): Usually the powdered bark called pale or crown bark, from *Cinchona officinalis,* was meant. Sometimes "Cinchona Flavus" (yellow bark) or "Cinchona Rubra" (red bark) was specified. It is commonly believed that these definitely pigmented barks may have come from *C. calisaya* and *C. succirubra,* respectively. The technical and vernacular nomenclatures of *Cinchona* species, however, are not at all clear; the barks of other species may be yellow and red as well, so that it is not possible to ascertain precisely which species were used therapeutically merely from the reported or prescribed colors of the bark. At least both *C. calisaya* and *C. succirubra* are known to have been found in Peru, the chief source of the drug, in the late eighteenth century. Modern laboratory analyses show that the concentration of quinine varies not only in the bark from species to species but also in different parts of one tree, from year to year, and from one region to another. This complication means that, although the pale barks were prescribed more often than the colored varieties and were more often therapeutically effective, this information can provide no clues about which species was given. (For a review of the problems involved, see Leo Suppan, "Three centuries of cinchona," in *Proceedings of the Celebration of the Three Hundredth Anniversary of the First Recognized Use of Cinchona,* Oct. 31–Nov. 1, 1930, St. Louis: Missouri Botanical Garden, 1930, pp. 29–138.)

Used as a tonic★ (especially for patients weakened by a fever or by a cold); as an astringent★ (to constrict blood vessels and thus divert the "morbid action" away from the site of disease in, e.g., diabetes,★ anasarca,★ and podagra atonica★ [latent or long-remitting gout]); and as an antiseptic★ (i.e., to counteract suppuration or sepsis). Cinchona was regarded as especially suitable for patients with "periodical diseases," chiefly the intermittent fevers★ (i.e., the malarias) but also the spasmodic symptoms of chest disease, such as cough.★ It was prescribed also for some continued fevers, such as sore throat,★ dysentery,★ dropsy,★ and venereal diseases; in the latter case, it was prescribed as a gargle, with roses of conserve, (q.v.), to counteract the side effects of MERCURY in the oral cavity.★ Cinchona's side effects included vomiting (prevented by administering it in red WINE) and diarrhea (prevented by the concomitant administration of OPIUM).

Cinchona was not regarded as a specific for intermittent or other fevers. Cullen reasoned that, because its effects can be perceived very soon after it is taken into the stomach and before it can be absorbed into the blood, its tonic powers must be conveyed via nerves from the stomach to the rest of the body. Therefore, he went on, cinchona is not appropriate therapy for patients with phlogistic (inflammatory) disorders, because they would only worsen under such a stimulating influence, but it is appropriate for patients with debility induced by continued fevers, after remissions of phlogistic disorders have begun or after inflammatory symptoms have been removed (see Cullen, *First Lines,* vol. I, pp. 245–247). However, it is also likely that cinchona's well-known therapeutic success rate in the intermittent fevers led to its earliest trials in the continued fevers and that the results of those trials could only have facilitated the drug's widespread use for the majority of fevers.

CINNAMONI COMPOSITA: see AROMATICA, TINCTURA.

COLD WATER: Applied over the kidneys to stimulate them to excrete, as urine, fluid accumulated in the body★ in, e.g., diabetes.★

COLLYRIUM: Any medication to be applied topically to the eyes for inflammatory diseases such as ophthalmia.★

COLOCYNTHIS: Extract of *Citrullus colocynthus.* Very potent cathartic★ sometimes used instead of JALAP (q.v. for uses). May produce bloody stools, which cannot be prevented. Usually administered as pills of ALOES CUM COLOCYNTHIDE (q.v.).

COLOMBA, COLUMBA, or COLUMBO: Powdered root of *Swertia caroliniensis.* Used as an astringent★ "to brace the system,"★ and to stimulate the stomach, as well as to reduce its secretions,★ for patients with dyspepsia,★ dysentery,★ menorrhagia,★ and bilious symptoms;★ also used as an antiemetic.★ A less potent substitute for ANGOSTURA★ (q.v.).

CORNU CERVIS, SAL (= Sal Carbonas Calcis): Calcium carbonate. Used as an antacid.★

CORROSIVE SUBLIMATE: see HYDRARGYRUS MURIATUS CORROSIVUS.

CORTEX PERUVIANUS: see CINCHONA.

CRAB CLAWS or CRAB'S EYES: see CANCRORUM LAPILLI PRAEPARATI.

CREAM OF TARTAR or CREMOR TARTAR: see TARTARI, CRYSTALLI.

CRETA: Chalk, chiefly calcium carbonate. Used as an antacid in dyspepsia★ and as an absorbent.

CUCURBITA CUM FERRO: Wet cupping; see BLEEDING.

CUPRUM AMMONIACUM: Pill made from mixture of copper sulfate and ammonia. Used to inhibit "moving fibers" in epilepsy.★

DIAPHORETIC MIXTURE: see JULAP, SALINE.

DIET: Duncan clearly used diet as specific therapy. Overall, he upgraded the standard "low" diet that was given to all newly admitted patients to "milk" diets for 17% of the 65 patients and to "full" diets for another 14%, almost all within a week of their admissions. Another 31% were allowed "meat" or "a bit of meat," and a few more beef tea, after longer intervals, generally during convalescence. Duncan prescribed more nutritious or stronger diets for patients suffering from severe fevers, especially those with specific weaknesses (e.g., paralyses,★ hypochondriasis,★ diabetes,★ melancholia,★ hydrocephalus,★ hydrothorax,★ and anasarca★), skin diseases,★ blood loss (in, e.g., hemoptysis★), and conditions requiring strengthening of the gastrointestinal tract (e.g., dyspepsia★). He also prescribed stronger diets for patients convalescing from catarrhs★ and intermittent fevers.★ For further details, see Chapter 4.

DIGITALIS: Pills made from powdered leaves of foxglove, *Digitalis purpurea,* and GLYCERRHIZA (employed only as a vehicle for the active ingredient). Acts on kidneys as diuretic★ to remove fluid from chest in dropsy★ (hydrothorax★), especially when the pulse rate is high. Side effects include vomiting, slow pulse, vertigo, and change of vision. Apparently as a direct result of the early studies on which William Withering based his 1785 book, Duncan had included digitalis in his lectures and "sometimes employed it in his practice" (Withering, *An Account of the Foxglove and Some of Its Medical Uses,* Birmingham: M. Swinney, 1785, p. 8).

DOVER'S POWDER (= pulvis Doveri or pulvis ipecacuanhae compositus): Mixture of IPECAC and OPIUM introduced by Thomas Dover in 1740. Used as a diaphoretic,★ especially for treating rheumatism and dropsy, but also see IPECAC.

ELECTRICITY: Used chiefly to "relieve torpor" of the nerves in patients with prolonged paralysis★ of specific muscles and organs. It was also applied over the kidneys to stimulate their fibers to constrict, so as to reduce urine output in diabetes.★ For further details, see Chapter 4.

ENEMA, DOMESTIC: Salt and olive oil in warm water. Used to relieve prolonged constipation.★ OPIUM was sometimes added.

EPISPASTIC: see CANTHARIS.

EPSOM SALT: see MAGNESIA VITRIOLATA.

FARINA POULTICE or FRICTION: Poultice made from wheat flour. Used to counteract inflammation of skin;★ also used for nutritive value of gluten.

FERRI RUBIGO: Purified iron rust, often administered as FERRUM PRAECIPITATUM, TINCTURA (q.v.). Used to stimulate menstruation,★ especially in patients with chlorosis.

FERRUM [RUBRUM] PRAECIPITATUM, TINCTURA: Tincture of iron rust. Used as a tonic★ to stimulate menstrual flow in amenorrhea.★ sometimes given with ANGOSTURA for stomach pain and flatus.★ Also see FERRI RUBIGO.

FERRUM VITRIOLATUM (= sal chalybis): Ferrous sulfate. Used, because it contains iron, as a tonic* in diseases requiring strengthening of the weakened,* or perhaps merely recuperating,* body, for patients with, e.g., dyspepsia,* debility associated with epilepsy,* chlorosis, amenorrhea, melancholy, and worms; and, by stimulating the kidneys to diuresis, to prevent fluid accumulation in patients with, e.g., anasarca.*

FLORES SULPHURIS: see SULPHUR, FLOWERS OF.

FONTANA, AQUA. Spring water, used as a diluent for many drugs.

FONTICULUS: Literally, "little fountain"; professional jargon for CANTHARIDIS, UNGUENTUM (q.v.), or EPISPASTIC ointment; used to keep induced blisters running.

FOWLER'S SOLUTION: see ARSENICI, SOLUTIO MINERALIS.

FRICTION: A poultice designed to chafe and redden the skin, to stimulate its circulation.* Also see FARINA.

GARLIC or ALLIUM: Extract of garlic, *Allium sativum*. Administered orally as a tonic to stimulate the whole body, especially the peripheral blood vessels,* and as a carminative (to relieve flatus),* expectorant,* and diuretic,* for patients with catarrh, flatus, hysteria, dropsy, intermittent fevers, and other conditions attributable to "laxity of the solids." Applied externally to inflame the skin of patients with "cold tumors," as a diuretic, and for smallpox. Side effects include headache, flatus, fever, and piles; contraindicated for patients with ileus. The active principle is absorbed through the skin and exhaled through the lungs.

GENTIAN: Extract of gentian, *Gentiana lutea*. Used as a bitter stomachic* to stimulate the appetite and digestion and as a "curative" in many diseases; active ingredient of AMARUM, INFUSUM (q.v.).

GINGER: see ZINGIBER.

GLYCERRHIZA: Extract of licorice, *Glycerrhiza glabra*. Used to reduce thirst in, e.g., dropsy,* and as a gentle detergent to break up mucus in the pulmonary tree in chest diseases. Most often administered in drug mixtures as a vehicle for their active ingredients, but also as a gentle cathartic and, rarely, to enhance the effect of OPIUM.*

GUAIAC (GUIAC), GUIAIAC, or GUAIACUM: Resin of lignum vitae, *Guaiacum officinale*. Used to calm blood vessels;* as a diaphoretic,* diuretic, and cathartic; to "divert morbid action";* and as a warm stimulus to the stomach and viscera. Prescribed chiefly for patients with joint,* sciatic,* and other* pains and for those with paralyses; also for venereal disease patients, to potentiate the effects of MERCURIALS (q.v.).

HEAT: Applied to the abdomen as warm compresses* or sometimes as a bath heated to 84°F,* to relax the stomach in order to prevent repeated vomiting.*

HEPAR SULPHURIS: see KALI SULPHURATUM.

HORDEI, AQUA: Barley water, from Latin name *Hordeum distichon*. Used for same indications as MICA PANIO (q.v.).

HYDRARGYROSI MURIATI MITIS, PILULAE (= Plummer's Pills): Pills made of CALOMEL (q.v.), ANTIMONY SULFATE, and CONSERVE OF ROSES. For uses and action, see MERCURY.

HYDRARGYRUS MURIATUS CORROSIVUS (= corrosive sublimate): Mercuric chloride. Usually applied topically to clean foul cutaneous ulcers and to destroy insects infesting the skin. Taken internally to facilitate excretion through feces, urine, and sweat in the treatment of venereal disease and other contagions, e.g., intermittent fevers.* Regarded as a very dangerous drug, it may have been administered in a then new and nonofficial formulation containing SAL AMMONIACUS, ALTHAEA, and honey, as well as alone. Also see MERCURY.

HYDRARGYRUS MURIATUS MITIS: see CALOMEL.

HYDRARGYRUS PRAECIPITATUS CINEREUS: Mercuric oxide; see MERCURY. Usually applied topically, as an ointment, to syphilitic chancres.*

HYOSCYAMUS: Extract of black henbane, *Hyoscyamus niger.* Administered (as a pill that also contained CAMPHOR, GLYCERRHIZA, and GUM ARABIC) as a sedative and narcotic for patients with pain* and wakefulness* and for nervous diseases, e.g., mania, epilepsy, melancholy, and hysteria; also for enlarged glands. As with OPIUM, "its influence is very much diminished by habit." Side effects include delirium, mydriasis, convulsions, diaphoresis, sedation, pustules, vomiting, diarrhea, and diuresis; unlike OPIUM, it produces analgesia but not constipation.

IPECAC or IPECACUANHA: Extract of *Cephaelis ipecacuanha.* Used as a mild, safe emetic,* diaphoretic,* and/or expectorant* in diseases requiring diversion of "morbid action" away from the site of the disease, e.g., severe catarrh,* pain* (in almost any site), headache,* anasarca* (by promoting absorption of tissue fluids), fever,* cough,* dysentery, menorrhagia, and most other "obstructions." Often administered in DOVER'S POWDER (q.v.).

IPECACUANHAE COMPOSITUS, PULVIS: see DOVER'S POWDER.

IRON: Used in several forms chiefly as tonic.* See FERRI RUBIGO, FERRUM PRAECIPITATUM, and FERRUM VITRIOLATUM.

JALAP or JALAPA: Powdered root of *Exogonium purga.* A safe, mild, and preferred cathartic* used to treat colic* and other obstructions of the gastrointestinal tract,* to potentiate IPECAC,* to counteract inflammation,* to divert blood from the head in ophthalmia* and apoplexy,* and to counteract melancholy; also used in dropsy and during inoculation for smallpox. Contraindicated for patients with upset stomach or bilious fevers. Also see JALAPPAE COMPOSITUS, PULVIS.

JALAPPAE COMPOSITUS, PULVIS: Powdered JALAP and TARTARI, CRYSTALLI (q.v.). Duncan regarded this as the "best cathartic," although he prescribed JALAP alone eight times more frequently. The crystals of tartar were thought to potentiate the jalap, while the jalap was thought to antagonize the refrigerant action of crystals of tartar, also a mild cathartic; the combination was thought able to "purge the whole system" of morbid matter.

JAMAICA EXTRACT: According to Duncan, this drug had appeared recently in the shops of Edinburgh, where it was sold as a dye and, mixed with VALERIAN (q.v.), as a secret remedy with astringent properties. He had been told that the drug was extracted from the bark of the sea grape, *Coccolobis uviflora*. Twenty years later the resin from this plant was the most widely exploited source of the material known as gum kino, which Duncan had said the Jamaica extract resembled. The original gum kino is now thought to have been derived from two African tree genera, *Butea* and *Pterocarpus;* its source was not generally known in 1795. Duncan proposed to give the new drug the official name "Gummi rubrum astringens Jamaicensis." He used it as an astringent★ for treating menorrhagia,★ leucorrhea,★ and diarrhea★ and as a substitute for CATECHU in the treatment of rheumatism.★

JAPONICUM, INFUSUM: see CATECHU, INFUSUM.

JULAP or JULEP, SALINE (= mixtura diaphoretica salina): Mixture of LIXIVIA (thought to be potassium carbonate), lemon juice, and black currant syrup. Used as a gentle diaphoretic★ and diuretic, often to stop vomiting in, e.g., catarrh★ and dyspepsia.★

JULEP, MUCILAGINOUS: see MUCILAGINOUS MIXTURE.

JUNIPER, SPIRITS OF: Alcohol solution of juniper oil, caraway seeds, and fennel. Used as a diuretic★ and cordial★; see JUNIPERIS, INFUSUM, for clinical indications.

JUNIPERIS, INFUSUM: Water solution of juniper (*Juniperus communis* or *J. sabina*) oil. Used as a mild diuretic★ and as a carminative or stomachic, for patients with a weak gastrointestinal tract, especially elderly patients or patients with tissue fluid accumulations in, e.g., anasarca.★

KALI SULPHURATUM (= kali vitriolatum, hepar sulphuris, vitriolatum sulphuratum lixivium, vitriolated tartar, or sal polychrestum): Potassium sulfate. Administered internally as a mild cathartic★ and diaphoretic★ with a long duration of action and as an absorbent★ of morbid materials from the blood into the gut or into the phlegm★ for eventual evacuation; hence it was used as an antidote to mineral poisons, e.g., MERCURIALS, presumably because many metals form insoluble precipitates with sulfur. Also combined with PULVIS CARBONAS LIGNI; see CHARCOAL AND KALI SULPHURATUM. Applied topically for "herpetic" and other skin diseases and as a bath for psora (itch) and tinea capitis.

KINO, GUM: see JAMAICA EXTRACT.

LAUDANUM LIQUIDUM: see OPIUM and THEBAICA, TINCTURA.

LEECHES: see BLEEDING.

LICORICE: see GLYCERRHIZA.

LINI, INFUSUM: Infusion of flax seed (linseed) from *Linum usitatissimum*. Used as a demulcent in catarrh. Duncan prescribed it chiefly as an accompaniment to all the CANTHARIS (q.v.) blisters he prescribed. The ground seeds were also used for making poultices (so were those of wheat; see FARINA).

LIXIVIA, LIXIVIUM, or LIXIVE (= potash, fixed vegetable alkali, pearl ash, kali impurum, cineres clavellati, or sal tartari): Thought to be potassium carbonate, prepared by burning plant material with close smothering heat, but more likely potassium hydroxide or potassium chloride, if purified at all. Used to contribute the diuretic★ component of several inorganic chemical mixtures or salts.

MAGNESIA ALBA: Thought to be magnesium carbonate, prepared by reacting magnesium sulfate with LIXIVIA, which was thought to be potassium carbonate. However, because LIXIVIA is more likely to have been potassium hydroxide or chloride, the drug was probably magnesium hydroxide or chloride. Used as a strong cathartic for patients with gastric acidity and as a raw material for preparing the more commonly prescribed MAGNESIA VITRIOLATA (q.v.).

MAGNESIA USTA (= calcined magnesia): Magnesium oxide, prepared by subjecting magnesium to high heat. Used for treating flatus★ and gastric acidity.★

MAGNESIA VITRIOLATA (= sal catharticus amarus or Epsom salts): Magnesium sulfate. Used as a mild cathartic,★ antiemetic,★ diuretic, and diaphoretic and as an undependable analgesic for patients with colic. Has few side effects.

MAGNOLIA: Extract of *Magnolia accuminata*. Nonofficial. Used in a tincture as a sedative★ and as an experimental tonic.★

MELLI OPTIMI: The best grade of honey. Used in mixtures designed to soothe the throat★ and sometimes in unguents for topical application.

MERCURIUS DULCIS: see CALOMEL.

MERCURY, MERCURIALS (= hydrargyrus): Administered in several forms (including CALOMEL, HYDRARGYROSI MURIATI MITIS, HYDRARGYRUS MURIATUS CORROSIVUS, and HYDRARGYRUS PRAECIPITATUS CINEREUS) as a cathartic★ and/or diaphoretic★ to stimulate excretions and the circulation, especially when they had become obstructed, by promoting absorption from sites of disease. Thus Duncan used mercurials in the general treatment of intermittent fevers,★ rheumatism,★ amenorrhea,★ hydrocephalus,★ and several skin diseases,★ but as a "specific" for syphilis,★ because in the latter case mercury prevented the "virus" from acting or, less likely in Duncan's opinion, because mercury expelled the "virus" from the body or destroyed it.

MICA PANIO: Breadcrumbs, taken internally in water for treating a weak gastrointestinal tract, bilious vomiting, cholera morbus, and other fevers; applied externally as a plaster to stimulate suppuration.★

MUCILAGINOUS MIXTURE (= mucilago gummi arabici or mucilaginous julep): Powdered ARABIC, GUM (q.v.), administered in warm water or with CONSERVE OF ROSES or with ALTHAEA, to relieve "tickling cough."★

MYRRH: Resin extracted from *Commiphora abyssinica*. Used as a diaphoretic,★ expectorant,★ and tonic, because it could "remove the morbid state of the inflamed surfaces" in, e.g., phthisis catarrhalis.★

NARCOTICUS AETHOPICUS: see AETHIOPS NARCOTICUS.

NICOTIANA, VIN, or VINUM NICOTIANAE: Tobacco, *Nicotiana tabacum,* steeped in white wine. Administered as a quick-acting diuretic,★ for cough,★ and occasionally as an expectorant★ or mild laxative; given, rarely, per rectum for severe constipation, but regarded as too dangerous for routine use in this way. Also see SNUFF.

NITRITI or NITRI, SAL: Potassium nitrate (= saltpeter, niter, kali nitratum, or lixivium nitratum). Used most often in NITRITI, UNGUENTUM (q.v.), but also occasionally given internally as a cooling cathartic.*

NITRITI, UNGUENTUM: Ointment made with SAL NITRI (potassium nitrate). Applied topically as an antiseptic wound ointment.*

OLEO MIXTURE (= emulsio oleosa volatilis): A gargle mixture made with OL AMYGDALA, ALTHAEA, GUM ARABIC, and sometimes with volatile alkali (ammonia), the latter to minimize the side effects of amygdala oil. For patients with cough,* tonsillitis,* etc.

OPIATUM, LINIMENTUM (= balsamum anodynum, unguentum thebaicum, or unguentum opiatum): The official preparation contained OPIUM, CAMPHOR, WINE, oil of rosemary, and soap. Most often used for intestinal pain,* headache,* sprains,* and other joint pains.*

OPIUM: Dried exudate of seed pods of opium poppy, *Papaver somniferum*. Because it was thought to decrease the irritability of most tissues and organs, it was prescribed as a sedative,* analgesic,* remedy for persistent cough,* and antidiarrheal* and to relax the common bile duct when obstructed with stone.* It was sometimes given with CALOMEL* to reduce active inflammatory processes, especially those producing pain and fever, such as wounds, by diverting the "morbid action," or to minimize the effects of cathartics like SENNA.* When taken internally, opium was observed to induce serenity and drowsiness, slowing of the pulse, venous dilation, and diaphoresis and to reduce bowel discharge by inhibiting intestinal muscle activity; this last effect was generally regarded as detrimental to the success of therapeutic regimens. Larger doses were noted to induce confusion, vertigo, and deep sleep; even larger doses produced tremors, delirium, convulsions, stupor, dyspnea, and death during a fit of apoplexy. When Duncan noted that opium should "not . . . be used too freely," he may have been warning against the possibility of addicting the patient, but he may also have been concerned with avoiding excessive constipation or other side effects.

Preparations for internal administration included opium pills (prepared at the infirmary with soap and simple syrup), THEBAIC PILLS, and PACIFIC PILLS (these were probably equivalent names); tincture of opium, THEBAICA TINCTURA, and laudanum liquidum, which were certainly similar if not identical preparations; THEBAICUM INFUSION with or without CATECHU; and ANODYNE, a common name reflecting opium's analgesic property but implying no specific preparation. (For the relative potencies of these common solid and liquid preparations, see J. Worth Estes, "John Jones' *Mysteries of Opium Reveal'd* [1701]: key to historical opiates," *J. His. Med.* 34 (1979): 200–209.)

Opium was also applied topically to decrease sensibility (especially sensitivity to pain) in patients with e.g., chest pains,* rheumatic pains,* toothache, skin ulcers, ophthalmia, and gonorrhea. The several externally applied preparations probably had similar if not identical ingredients, chiefly opium and a menstruum: LINIMENTUM OPIATUM, balsamum anodynum, unguentum thebaicum, and unguentum opiatum. OPIUM ENEMAS were regarded as the most potent inhibitors of gastrointestinal activity, for treating both vomiting and diarrhea; they also produced analgesia and sedation.

OPIUM ENEMA: OPIUM added to ENEMA, DOMESTIC (q.v.).

PACIFIC PILL: same as THEBAIC PILL, but with pimento added.

PEPPERMINT WATER: Infusion of leaves of *Mentha piperita*. Used alone or, more commonly, as a diluent for other drugs, to warm the stomach* and to relieve cold* or flatulent colic.* (In Table A.1 the frequency of peppermint water use among Duncan's prescriptions is not included because he seems not to have prescribed it for any specific therapeutic purpose.)

PERUVIAN BARK: see CINCHONA.

PLUMMER'S PILLS: see HYDRARGYROSI MURIATI MITIS.

PORTER: Strong dark beer; alcohol content about 6.8%. Used therapeutically in same way as WINE, RED (q.v.).

RHEI or RHEUM: Extract of officinal or Chinese rhubarb, *Rheum officinalis* or *R. palmatum*. Used as a mild cathartic* and astringent* (i.e., as a tonic for the gut musculature) in patients with urinary obstruction,* menorrhagia,* constipation,* and continued vomiting,* as well as in many other conditions requiring catharsis; also used as an antiemetic in the presence of gallstones.* Principal side effect is abdominal pain, caused by excessive stimulation of intestinal activity.*

RICINI, OL, or RICINUS: Oil of castor bean, *Ricinus communis*. Used as a mild cathartic* for patients with colic, worms, bladder stones, gonorrhea, and many other conditions.

ROSES, CONSERVE OF (= rosa pallida or infusum or tinctura rosarum): Jelly made of dried damask roses (the *Edinburgh Dispensatory* specified *Rosa centifolia*, but *R. damascena* seems more likely), sugar, and VITRIOLIC ACID (sulfuric acid); instructions for preparing it specified that it should not be mixed in a lead vessel, because the lead would contaminate the drug and harm the patient. Used as a gargle* because it is an astringent* and detergent* that breaks up mucus* in patients with catarrh,* and to minimize the side effects of CALOMEL* and BLEEDING. Much of this drug's effect was thought to be attributable to its VITRIOLIC ACID component. Some regarded the drug as a tonic, for stimulating the spirits, and as an analgesic with mild laxative properties.

RUBIA: Extract of madder, *Rubia tinctorum*. Used for its detergent and mild cathartic properties, in combinations with other drugs, for treating diseases characterized by obstructions, e.g., amenorrhea,* jaundice, and dropsy.

SABIN, SAVIN, or SAVINE: Oil of berries of *Juniperus sabina*. See JUNIPERUS, INFUSUM.

SACCHARUM ALBUM: White sugar. Used as a sweetener or for its nutritive value.

SALINA, MIXTURA DIAPHORETICA: see JULAP, SALINE.

SARSAPARILLA: Usually the powdered root of *Smilax aristolochiaefolia* from South America, but sometimes *Aralia hispida* or *A. nudicaulis* from North America. Used chiefly as a flavoring, but rarely as a diaphoretic.

SATURNI, SACCHARUM: see CERUSSA ACETATA.

SCAMMONY: Dried root of Syrian bindweed, *Convolvulus scammonia*. Cathartic.★

SCARIFICATION: see BLEEDING.

SCILLAE, or SCILLITICAE, PILULULE (= squills): Dried powdered bulb of sea onion, *Urginea* (or *scilla*) *maritima,* mixed with gum ammoniac, GLYCERRHIZA, lesser cardamom seeds, and simple syrup. Used chiefly as the strongest and most dependable diuretic★ but occasionally as a diaphoretic or sialagogue, for patients with tissue fluid accumulations in, e.g., dropsy,★ anasarca,★ severe catarrh,★ and nephritis.

SENNA: Leaves of *Cassia acutifolia* or *C. angustifolia.* Used as a mild cathartic★ to reduce obstructions of the gut,★ urine,★ or common bile duct,★ in many kinds of disease, and for OPIUM-induced constipation. Side effects include abdominal pain★ and a bad taste in the mouth.

SETON: A thread or other fibrous material passed through subcutaneous tissue to form an issue, for the same reasons as those which motivated raising of blisters with CANTHARIS (q.v.). Used in one patient with epilepsy★ (apparent grand mal seizures) to procure issues from his neck; no clinical benefit was detected.

SNUFF: Finely pulverized tobacco, *Nicotiana tabacum,* drawn into the nostrils by inhalation. Used to make a patient sneeze,★ to facilitate release of phlegm.

SOCOTRINE ALOES: see ALOES.

SODA PHOSPHORATA: Sodium phosphate. Used as a cooling, pleasant cathartic★ in several inflammatory diseases,★ e.g., erysipelas,★ and in dysentery.★

SODA TARTARISATA: see TARTARI, CRYSTALLI.

SOYMIDA: Powdered bark of the rohun tree, *Soymida febrifuga,* which had recently been introduced from India to British medicine by Duncan; nonofficial in 1795. Used as an astringent★ and gentle tonic★ for diseases resulting from atony or laxity of the gut★ and blood vessels,★ e.g., dyspepsia,★ anasarca,★ diarrhea, and dysentery, but also to reduce irritability of the system;★ also used, because of its tonic property, as a substitute for CINCHONA (q.v.). Principal side effect is vertigo. (For the presumed pharmacology of this drug, which never gained acceptance in Western medicine, see Edward John Waring, *Pharmacopoeia of India,* London: India Office, 1868, pp. 55, 444. For botanical descriptions and illustrations of different kinds, see Robert Bentley and Henry Trimen, *Medicinal Plants,* 4 vols., London, J. & A. Churchill, 1880, vol. 1, article 63; and *The Wealth of India: Raw Materials,* 12 vols., New Delhi: Publications & Information Directorate, 1972, vol. 9, pp. 471–472.)

SQUILLS: see SCILLAE.

SUCCINI, OL: Oil of amber. Used as a tonic and antispasmodic in, e.g., paralysis, leucorrhea, gonorrhea, and hysteria; efficacy regarded as doubtful. Also applied topically in FRICTIONS (q.v.) for paralysis.★

SULFUR, FLOWERS OF (= flores sulphuris): Sublimated sulfur in olive oil. Used as a cooling cathartic★ and diaphoretic,★ to antagonize the side effects of MERCURY and ANTIMONIUM preparations, for skin disease (internally and externally), cough,★ catarrh,★ and dyspnea,★ the latter because the drug was "supposed to have some peculiar Effect in the Lungs & to have a particular Power in relieving Dyspnea" by diverting morbid matter from the lungs to the feces.

SULFURIC ETHER or AETHER: see VITRIOLICUS, AETHER.

TAMARINDORUM CUM SENNA, INFUSUM: Water extract of tamarinds, *Tamarindus indica,* SENNA (q.v.), TARTARI, CRYSTALLI (q.v.), coriander seeds, and brown sugar, mixed in a nonleaden vessel to avoid causing lead poisoning. Used as a mild cooling cathartic★ for fevers,★ melancholy,★ "delicate stomachs,"★ and other acute diseases.

TARTAR EMETIC: see ANTIMONIUM TARTARISATUM.

TARTARI, CRYSTALLI (= crystals of tartar, soda tartarisata, or Rochelle salt): Sodium potassium tartrate, extracted from the acid-saturated dregs of wine casks; the powdered form of these crystals was called cream of tartar or cremor tartar. Used as a mild, cooling, and brisk cathartic★ or mild diuretic,★ to decrease "the morbid state of inflamed surfaces" and "to diminish the Impetus of the Blood" by inhibiting hyperactive blood vessels;★ the net result of these actions was decreased expectoration★ and decreased sweating,★ for treating chest diseases,★ anasarca,★ and colica pictonum (lead colic),★ all of which were thought to be especially benefited by the evacuation of fluid via the stool. The drug was also used as a COLLYRIUM for ophthalmia;★ Duncan noted that the "Pulvis ophthalmicus" of Dr. Ballander was crystals of tartar mixed with white sugar. It was often combined with other cathartics, e.g., SENNA, JALAP, and ANTIMONIUM TARTARISATUM, to enhance their activity.

TARTARI, LIXIVIA: Potassium tartrate or "soluble tartar." Used as a cathartic★ especially suitable for mental patients.★

TARTARI, SAL: see LIXIVIA.

TEREBINTHA VENETA, OL: Volatile oil(s) of pine, *Pinus* spp.; turpentine. Given internally, but seldom, as a diuretic★ and gentle cathartic, because it strengthens weak vessels in, e.g., paralysis,★ chronic rheumatism,★ and leucorrhea. Most often applied externally, for the same reasons, as unguents and liniments for, e.g., rheumatic pains★ or paralysis or to potentiate CANTHARIS★ (q.v.).

THEBAICA, TINCTURA (= tincture of opium or laudanum liquidum): Made by letting 2 oz. OPIUM (q.v.) stand in 2 pints distilled spirits for 4 days and then straining and evaporating until 1 dram of tincture contains 3½ grains of pure opium.

THEBAIC PILL (= Pilulule or sometimes Pacific, Starkey's, or Matthews' Pills): Made with OPIUM (q.v.) evaporated from an alcoholic solution (e.g., from TINCTURA THEBAICA) and mixed with GLYCERRHIZA, soap, and sometimes pimento, to "correct" the opium by preventing its "bad effects"; a 10-grain pill should contain 1 grain of opium when dispensed.

THEBAICUM, INFUSUM: A water solution of OPIUM, often with CATECHU added. Probably because the active drug principles of opium are less soluble in water than in alcohol, this preparation was administered less often than TINCTURA THEBAICA.

TOLU, SYRUP OF, or SYRUPUS TOLUTANUS: Resin from *Myroxylon balsa*- Used for treating hoarseness,★ it seems to have been regarded as a tonic.

TORCULARIA: Tourniquets. Applied to one arm and the opposite thigh in one patient with a quartan intermittent fever just before the expected beginning of a paroxysm; this may well have been a therapeutic experiment because the treatment is not mentioned in standard texts of the time.

TOXICODENDRI, INFUSUM: Water extract of poison ivy, *Rhus toxicodendron* (Duncan called it "pubescent poison oak"). Dr. John Alderson of Hull, who had promoted this nonofficial remedy recently (in his *Essay on the Rhus Toxicodendron, or Sumach, with Cases Shewing It's* [sic] *Efficacy in the Cure of Paralytic Affections,* 2nd ed., Hull: 1794), specifically avoided discussing the drug's site and mode of action, but it is clear that he thought it stimulated nerve action in a manner analogous to poison ivy's irritating effect on the skin; perhaps he saw an analogy with CANTHARIS (q.v.). Duncan was unable to obtain the leaves specified by Alderson, presumably because it was winter, so he tried an infusion of poison ivy bark; it had no discernible clinical effect on his paralyzed patient. (The drug had become official by 1811.)

TURPENTINE: see TEREBINTHA VENETA.

UNGUENTUM SIMPLEX: Simple ointment made of five parts olive oil and two parts white wax. Used as a dressing for various skin conditions★ and for wounds.

VALERIAN or VALERIANA SYLVESTRIS: Water extract of root of valerian, *Valeriana officinalis.* Used as a tonic★ and antispasmodic for diseases caused by nervous debility, e.g., epilepsy★ and melancholy,★ to facilitate sleep, and to potentiate the tonic effects of CINCHONA★ (q.v.).

VAN SWIETEN, BARK: A preparation of CINCHONA (q.v.), introduced by Gerhard van Swieten of Vienna in the mid-eighteenth century.

VEGETABLE ACID, POTUS: A drink of what was thought to be potassium carbonate (derived from LIXIVIA, q.v.), prepared as an infusion of ashes or cinders of burned vegetable matter; it is more likely to have been very dilute potassium hydroxide or lye. Although sometimes "vegetable acid" was prepared by dissolving CRYSTALLI TARTARI in flour and water, it seems probable that Duncan meant the former recipe. Used to decrease thirst★ and to stimulate weak gastric muscle fibers in dyspepsia.

VEGETABLE ALKALI, FIXED: see LIXIVIA.

VITRIOLATED TARTAR: see KALI SULPHURATUM.

VITRIOLATUM SULPHURATUM LIXIVIA: see KALI SULPHURATUM.

VITRIOLIC ACID or ACIDUM VITRIOLICUM DILUTUM: 1 part sulfuric acid at specific gravity 1.85 and 7 parts water (1 and 9 parts, respectively, in the London *Pharmacopoeia*). Regarded as "subservient in effect to other preparations" with which it might be mixed in extemporaneous prescriptions. Used, because it increases both acidity and muscle tone, for weak stomachs (e.g., in dyspepsia★), venereal diseases,★

weeping skin sores,★ gall★ or bladder stones, and typhus fevers. It also has astringent, antiseptic, and antifermentation properties that make it useful when the gut is hyperactive, e.g., to antagonize OPIUM-induced constipation. Applied externally, as unguentum or linimentum vitriolicum, mixed with 8 parts of oil, as a rubefacient to stimulate blood vessels in itch,★ local palsy, and rheumatism and to counteract MERCURY's effect on the gums.

VITRIOLICUM, LINIMENTUM or UNGUENTUM: see VITRIOLIC ACID.

VITRIOLICUS, AETHER (= sulfuric ether): Ether, prepared by distilling equal parts of sulfuric acid and wine. Used as an antispasmodic, internally for violent headache,★ whooping cough, asthma, and other spasmodic affections, and topically for toothache. Also used to dissolve elastic gums. The vitriolic component was regarded as more important pharmacologically than the etheric component.

WARM BATH: Water heated to 85°F, prescribed to stimulate paralyzed muscles.★

WINE, RED: Because it was thought to be astringent, wine was used as a tonic for the gastrointestinal system, especially the stomach, and for the spirits,★ to strengthen and warm the body by stimulating the circulation★ and to increase the pulse rate and sweating.

ZINCUM PRAECIPITATUM: Zinc precipitated from ZINCUM VITRIOLATUM (zinc sulfate) with volatile alkali (ammonia). Used as an antispasmodic in, e.g., epilepsy.★

ZINCUM VITRIOLATUM: Zinc sulfate. Used, rarely, as an antispasmodic for treating epilepsy or, with CINCHONA, for treating intermittent fevers. Most often used externally as an astringent, for, e.g., ophthalmia.★

ZINGIBER: Ginger, *Zinziber officinale.* Used for "cold colic" and weak gastrointestinal tract action, usually in mixtures,★ e.g., CARDIACA, AQUA; AROMATICA, TINCTURA; and AROMATIC PILL (all q.v.).

Notes

Abbreviations used in the notes:

MB   Minute Books, MSS Collection, Medical Archives, University of Edinburgh

RCP   Royal College of Physicians

RCS   Royal College of Surgeons

RIE   Royal Infirmary of Edinburgh

INTRODUCTION

1 W. Bauer, "The responsibility of the university hospital in the synthesis of medicine, science, and learning," *New England J. Med.* 265 (1961): 1292–1298.

2 For an overview see John H. Woodward, *To Do the Sick No Harm: A Study of the British Voluntary Hospital System to 1875,* London: Routledge & Kegan Paul, 1974.

3 Numerous publications deal with the Scottish Enlightenment. For recent summaries see H. Trevor-Roper, "The Scottish Enlightenment," *Studies on Voltaire* 58 (1967): 1635–1658; and N. Phillipson, "Towards a definition of the Scottish Enlightenment," in *City and Society in the Eighteenth Century,* ed. by P. Fritz, Toronto: Hakkert, 1973, pp. 125–147.

4 Anand C. Chitnis, "Universities: medicine and science," in his *Scottish Enlightenment,* London: Croom Helm, 1976, chap. 6, pp. 124–194. Also useful and informative is J. B. Morrell, "The University of Edinburgh in the late eighteenth century: its scientific eminence and academic structure," *Isis* 62 (1971): 158–171. More details can be obtained from the classic book by Alexander Bower, *The History of the University of Edinburgh,* 2 vols., Edinburgh: Oliphant, Waugh & Innes, 1817.

5 Alexander Monro primus began publication of his *Medical Essays and Observations* in 1732, two years after the establishment of the Edinburgh infirmary. Many of the articles contained case reports taken from the hospital's register. The stress on practical medicine is also explained in J. R. R. Christie, "The rise and fall of Scottish science," in *The Emergence of Science in Western Europe,* ed. by M. Crosland, New York: Science History Publications, 1976, pp. 111–126.

6 See, for example, Neil Campbell and R. Martin Smellie, *The Royal Society of Edinburgh (1783–1983),* Edinburgh: The Royal Society, 1983; and for earlier institutions R. L. Emerson, "The social composition of enlightened Scotland: the Select Society of Edinburgh, 1754–1764," *Studies on Voltaire* 114 (1973): 291–329; and Emerson, "The Philosophical Society of Edinburgh, 1737–1747," *Brit. J. Hist. Sci.* 12 (1979): 154–191.

7 See A. Logan Turner, *Story of a Great Hospital: The Royal Infirmary of Edinburgh, 1729–1929,* Edinburgh: Oliver & Boyd, 1937, especially chap. 9, pp. 130–155.

8 See A. C. Chitnis, "Provost Drummond and the origins of Edinburgh medicine," in *The Origins and Nature of the Scottish Enlightenment,* ed. by R. H. Campbell and A. S. Skinner, Edinburgh: J. Donald, 1982, pp. 86–114.

9 See, for example, Edward Foster, *An Essay on Hospitals, or Succinct Directions for the*

Situation, Construction, and Administration of Country Hospitals, Dublin: W. G. Jones, 1768.

10 See, for example, statements made by the famous hospital and prison reformer John Howard in *Appendix to the State of the Prisons in England and Wales, Containing a Further Account of Foreign Prisons and Hospitals,* Warrington, England: W. Eyres, 1784, p. 151.

11 Logan Turner's *Story* belongs in this category. It was based on lists of officials and medical staff members, architectural plans, and a cursory examination of some Minute Books.

12 The remark appears in Brian Abel-Smith, *The Hospitals, 1800–1948: A Study in Social Administration in England and Wales,* Cambridge, MA: Harvard University Press, 1964, p. 1, and is attributed to John Simon, author of an 1848 work entitled *On the Aims and Philosophic Method of Pathological Research.*

13 The most explicit and earliest statement on this subject can be found in T. McKeown and R. G. Brown, "Medical evidence related to English population changes in eighteenth century," *Popul. Stud.* 9 (1955–1956): 125: "Indeed, the chief indictment of hospital work at this period is not that it did no good, but that it positively did harm." McKeown and Brown's conclusions were promptly echoed by several historians, among them K. F. Helleiner, who characterized eighteenth-century hospitals as "gateways to death": See K. F. Helleiner, "The vital revolution reconsidered," reprinted from the *Canadian Journal of Economics and Political Science,* in *Population and History,* ed. by D. V. Glass and D. E. C. Eversley, London: Arnold, 1965, p. 84.

14 Michel Foucault writes in chap. 1, p. 18, of *The Birth of the Clinic: An Archeology of Medical Perception,* trans. from French by A. M. Sheridan Smith, New York: Vintage Books, 1975: "The hospital creates disease by means of the enclosed, pestilential domain that it constitutes." Such blanket allegations did not go unchallenged. Studying the records of York County Hospital, E. M. Sigsworth discovered that over 90% of the patients admitted between 1740 and 1783 were discharged "cured" or "relieved," a far cry from the "gateway to death" image regardless of the precise meaning then attached to so-called cures: E. M. Sigsworth, "Gateways to death? Medicine, hospitals, and mortality, 1700–1850," in *Science and Society, 1600–1900,* ed. by P. Mathias, Cambridge University Press, 1972, pp. 97–110. In his recent book, McKeown took notice of Sigsworth's work but went on to explain that the cheerful statistics could not be taken seriously, since not even modern-day hospitals can expect to exhibit such success stories. See Thomas McKeown, *The Modern Rise of Population,* New York: Academic Press, 1976, pp. 13–14.

15 See a book review by Lawrence Stone entitled "Madness," *New York Review of Books* 29 (Dec. 16, 1982): 28. See also Phyllis Deane, *The First Industrial Revolution,* Cambridge University Press, 1965. On p. 29 she writes: "Hospitals and dispensaries were more likely to spread disease than to check it. People who went to hospital in the eighteenth century normally died there, generally from some disease other than that with which they were admitted."

16 Abel-Smith, *The Hospitals,* pp. ix–x.

CHAPTER 1 *The sick poor and voluntary hospitals*

1 These comments were made during a sermon to raise funds for the Edinburgh infirmary. See Ninian Niving, *Jesus Christ in the Poor, or the Royal Infirmary of Edinburgh Recommended to the Charity of Well-disposed Christians,* Edinburgh: Sands, Brymer, Murray & Cochran, 1739, pp. 17–18.

2 Cases of "Peggy" and Andrew Carmichael, in James Gregory, Clinical notes and lectures, Edinburgh, 1779–1780, MSS Collection, Royal College of Physicians [hereafter cited as RCP], Edinburgh.

3 The cases of Mary and Pat Carmichael are contained in *ibid.,* together with the clinical history of Margaret Clunie.

4 John C. Lettsom, *On the Improvement of Medicine in London on the Basis of Public Good,* 2nd ed., London: J. Phillips, 1775, p. 19.
5 Anonymous, *Remarks on the Situation of the Poor in the Metropolis, as Contributing to the Progress of Contagious Diseases,* London: R. Noble, 1801, pp. 708.
6 See, for example, the cases of Sophia Martin, in James Gregory, Clinical cases of Dr. Gregory in the Royal Infirmary of Edinburgh, taken by Nathan Thomas, Edinburgh, 1785–1786, MSS Collection, University of Edinburgh; Janet Cameron, in Francis Home, Cases of patients under the care of Francis Home, Edinburgh, 1780–1781, MSS Collection, RCP, Edinburgh; and James Johnston, in James Gregory, Cases of patients under the care of James Gregory, M.D., Edinburgh, 1781–1782, MSS Collection, RCP, Edinburgh.
7 For fevers that followed "overheating by dancing" see the cases of David Naime, in John Gregory, Clinical cases of the Royal Infirmary of Edinburgh, Edinburgh, 1771–1772, MSS Collection, Medical Archives, University of Edinburgh; and Daniel Sutherland, in William Cullen, Clinical cases and reports taken at the Royal Infirmary of Edinburgh from Dr. Cullen, taken by Richard W. Hall, Edinburgh, 1772–1773, MSS Collection, National Library of Medicine, Bethesda, MD. This recreation was observed by visitors: "The lower class of people here are as fond of dancing as their betters; . . . and frequently, when the labors and the fatigues of the day are over, they refresh themselves by a dance." Edward Topham, *Letters from Edinburgh Written in Years 1774 and 1775,* 2 vols., Dublin: Watson, 1776, vol. 2, p. 73.
8 Case of Betty Haddock, in Andrew Duncan, Sr., Clinical reports and commentaries, Feb.–Apr. 1795, presented by Alexander Blackhall Morison, Edinburgh, 1795, MSS Collection, RCP, Edinburgh.
9 Case of Isabel McKay, in James Gregory, Cases of patients, 1781–1782.
10 William Cullen, Clinical lectures, Edinburgh, 1772–1773, MSS Collection, RCP, Edinburgh, p. 101.
11 Case of John Menter, in A. Duncan, Sr., Clinical reports and commentaries, 1795.
12 Cases of Margaret Milne, in W. Cullen, Clinical cases and reports, 1772–1773; and Nelly Carnegie, in Thomas C. Hope, Clinical casebook, Edinburgh, 1796–1797, MSS Collection, RCP, Edinburgh.
13 Case of Margaret Brown, in James Gregory, Clinical notes and lectures, 1779–1780.
14 Case of Rachel Parkinson, in James Gregory, Cases of patients, 1781–1782.
15 Case of Mary Craig, *ibid.*
16 Case of Alexander McLaughlan, *ibid.*
17 Case of William Littlefear, *ibid.*
18 See the case of Robert McKirday and family, in F. Home, Cases of patients, 1780–1781.
19 Case from William Brown, Casebooks, 5 vols., Edinburgh, 1790–1810, MSS Collection, Royal College of Surgeons [hereafter cited as RCS], Edinburgh, vol. 5, p. 7.
20 Most of these cases are contained in James Russell, Surgical cases, 8 vols., Edinburgh, 1784–1792, MSS Collection, RCP, Edinburgh.
21 Cases of Euphemia Ross, in James Gregory, Clinical cases, 1785–1786; and William Forrest, in A. Duncan, Sr., Clinical reports and commentaries, 1795.
22 Case of William Manson, in James Gregory, Cases of patients, 1781–1782.
23 Case of Christian Anderson, in F. Home, Cases of patients, 1780–1781.
24 Case of Jane Duncan, in A. Duncan, Sr., Clinical reports and commentaries, 1795.
25 Case of William Bell, in Daniel Rutherford, Clinical cases, Edinburgh, 1799, MSS Collection, RCP, Edinburgh.
26 Case of William Manson, in James Gregory, Cases of patients, 1781–1782.
27 John Sinclair, *Analysis of the Statistical Account of Scotland,* 2 parts, Edinburgh: A. Constable, 1825, reprinted, New York: Johnson Reprint Co., 1970, part 1, p. 137. See also Marjorie Plant, *The Domestic Life of Scotland in the Eighteenth Century,* Edinburgh: Edinburgh University Press, 1952, p. 223.
28 These conclusions were reached by analyzing the 808 complete clinical histories contained in student notebooks. To ascertain whether the current criteria of acute

(up to 10 days), subacute (10–30 days), and chronic (more than 30 days) correspond to the standards employed during the eighteenth century, sixty cases of rheumatism available from the notebooks and characterized by practitioners of that time as either acute or chronic were analyzed and matched against modern yardsticks. The results confirm an overwhelming agreement with current standards about what constituted a chronic ailment and significant agreement regarding acute cases, although a small number of those termed acute by eighteenth-century measures tend to fall within the present subacute category.

29 The following figures regarding treatment prior to admission were obtained from the sample described in the preceding note:

	Frequency	%
Yes	385	47.64
No	227	28.09
Unknown	196	24.25

30 Cases of Margaret Griffith, in James Gregory, Cases of patients, 1781–1782; and A. Bolatis, in D. Rutherford, Clinical cases, 1799.

31 Case of Isabel Donaldson, in William Cullen, Clinical cases and reports taken at the Royal Infirmary of Edinburgh from Dr. Cullen, taken by Richard W. Hall, Edinburgh, 1773–1774, MSS Collection, National Library of Medicine, Bethesda, MD. See also Sinclair, *Statistical Account,* part 1, p. 136.

32 Case of James Hay, in T. C. Hope, Clinical casebook, 1796–1797.

33 Case of James Pennywick, in A. Duncan, Sr., Clinical reports and commentaries, 1795.

34 Joseph Wilde, *The Hospital: A Poem in Three Books,* Norwich, England: Stevenson, Matchett & Stevenson, 1810, p. 24.

35 W. H. McMenemey, "The hospital movement of the eighteenth century and its development," in *The Evolution of Hospitals in Britain,* ed. by F. N. L. Poynter, London: Pitman Medical Publishing, 1964, pp. 43–71.

36 For more details about conditions and events before the eighteenth century see B. G. Gale, "The dissolution and revolution in London hospital facilities," *Med. Hist.* 11 (1967): 91–96.

37 G. Rosen, "A slaughter of innocents: aspects of child health in the eighteenth-century city," in *Studies in Eighteenth-Century Culture,* ed. by R. C. Rosbottom, Madison: University of Wisconsin Press, 1976, vol. 5, pp. 293–316. For a general panorama consult J. Brownlee, "The health of London in the eighteenth century," *Proc. Roy. Soc. Med.* 18 (1925): 73–85.

38 William Black, *Observations Medical and Political on the Smallpox,* 2nd ed. enlarged, London: J. Johnson, 1781, p. 155.

39 John Bellers, *Essay towards the Improvement of Physick,* London: Sowle, 1714, p. 6.

40 For an overview see A. Deutsch, "Historical interrelationships between medicine and social welfare," *Bull. Hist. Med.* 11 (1942): 485–502. Further details can be obtained from essays contained in George Rosen, *From Medical Police to Social Medicine,* New York: Science History Publications, 1974.

41 The concept of a "medicalization" of society appears in the writings of Michel Foucault and of various members of the "Annales" school of history in France. See, for example, Michel Foucault, "La politique de la santé au XVIIIᵉ siècle," in Foucault et al., *Les Machines à Guerir,* Paris L'Institut de l'Environment, 1976, pp. 11–21, translated into English as "The politics of health in the eighteenth century," in *Power/Knowledge: Selected Interviews and Other Writings, 1972–1977,* ed. by C. Gordon, New York: Pantheon, 1972, pp. 166–182.

42 The German efforts are summarized in G. Rosen, "Cameralism and the concept of medical police," *Bull. Hist. Med.* 27 (1952): 21–42; and E. Lesky, "Johann Peter Frank and social medicine," *Annales Cisalpines d'Hist. Sociale* 4 (1973): 137–144. For France see G. Rosen, "Mercantilism and health policy in eighteenth century French thought," *Med. Hist.* 3 (1959): 259–275.

43 G. Rosen, "Medical care and social policy in seventeenth-century England," *Bull.*

N.Y. *Acad. Med.* 29 (1953): 420–437; J. H. Cassedy, "Medicine and the rise of statistics," in *Medicine in Seventeenth-Century England,* ed. by A. G. Debus, Berkeley: University of California Press, 1974, pp. 283–312. For more details see E. S. Pearson, ed. *The History of Statistics in the 17th and 18th Centuries, Against the Changing Background of Intellectual, Scientific and Religious Thought, Lectures by Karl Pearson, 1921–1933,* London: Griffin, 1978, especially chaps. 1 and 2.

44 For a survey see Peter Gay, "Enlightenment: medicine and cure," in his *Enlightenment: An Interpretation,* 2 vols., New York: Knopf, 1966–1969, vol. 2, pp. 12–23. A recent essay also contains valuable information about the topic: W. F. Bynum, "Health, disease and medical care," in *The Ferment of Knowledge,* ed. by G. S. Rousseau and R. Porter, Cambridge University Press, 1980, pp. 211–253. Still in press is G. B. Risse, "Medicine in the Age of Enlightenment," in *Social History of the Biomedical Sciences,* ed. by M. Piatelli-Palmarini, Milan: Ricci.

45 For an explanation of the classical roots of the non-naturals see L. J. Rather, "The six things 'non-natural,' " *Clio Medica* 3 (1968): 337–347. Additional information can be gathered from P. H. Niebyl, "The non-naturals," *Bull. Hist. Med.* 45 (1971): 486–492; and C. R. Burns, "The non-naturals: a paradox in the Western concept of health," *J. Med. & Philos.* 3 (1976): 202–211.

46 W. Coleman, "Health and hygiene in the Encyclopédie: a medical doctrine for the bourgeoisie," *J. Hist. Med.* 29 (1974): 399–421.

47 [Arnulfe d'Aumont], "Santé," in *Encyclopédie ou Dictionnaire Raisonée des Sciences, des Arts et de Métiers,* ed. by D. Diderot, Paris: Briasson, 1751–1765, vol. 14, p. 629. Here and elsewhere, the translation is mine unless otherwise noted.

48 [Arnulfe d' Aumont], "Hygiène," in Diderot, *Encyclopédie,* vol. 8, p. 385. For more details about the evolution of this concept, see L. J. Jordanova, "Earth science and environmental medicine: the synthesis of the late Enlightenment," in *Images of the Earth,* ed. by R. S. Porter and L. J. Jordanova, Chalfont St. Giles, England: Science History Publications, 1979, pp. 119–146.

49 The eighteenth-century endeavors to popularize medicine have been repeatedly studied in some detail. For an overview see G. B. Risse, "Introduction," in *Medicine without Doctors,* ed. by G. B. Risse, R. L. Numbers, and J. Walzer Leavitt, New York: Science History Publications, 1977, pp. 1–8. For details on England, see C. J. Lawrence, "William Buchan: medicine laid open," *Med. Hist.* 19 (1975): 20–35; and C. E. Rosenberg, "Medical text and social context: explaining William Buchan's Domestic Medicine," *Bull. Hist. Med.* 57 (1983): 22–42.

50 Black, *Observations Medical and Political,* p. 103. These comments were made in reference to popular opposition to the practice of smallpox inoculation.

51 Wilde, *The Hospital,* pp. 27–28. Wilde's work, which will be quoted extensively, is a unique document since it represents the impressions and reactions of a hospitalized patient around 1800. For a brief analysis see W. B. Howie, "Consumer reaction: a patient's view of hospital life in 1809," *Brit. Med. J.* 3 (1973): 534–536.

52 Roy Porter, *English Society in the Eighteenth Century,* Harmondsworth, England: Penguin Books, 1982, p. 302.

53 For details see David Owen, *English Philanthropy, 1660–1960,* Cambridge, MA: Harvard University Press, 1965, especially chap. 2, "The philanthropy of eighteenth-century humanitarianism," pp. 36–61. Useful background reading for this topic is Karl de Schweinitz, *England's Road to Social Security,* Philadelphia: University of Pennsylvania Press, 1943.

54 John Cary, *An Essay toward Regulating the Trade and Employing the Poor of This Kingdom,* 2nd ed., London, 1719, pp. 150–162; as quoted in Schweinitz, *Road,* p. 53.

55 M. G. Jones, *The Charity School Movement: A Study of Eighteenth-Century Puritanism in Action,* Cambridge University Press, 1938, p. 12.

56 Nelson suggested that these good works could be implemented if "you dedicate and lay apart a proportion of your gains or income, when it is certain, for alms-deeds; which will make the work easy and delightful." See Robert Nelson, "Letter to George Hanger" (1708), reprinted in Charles F. Secretan, *Memoirs of the Life and Times of the Pious Robert Nelson,* London: J. Murray, 1860, pp. 195–196. For a bio-

graphical sketch of Nelson, see James C. Hadden, ed. *Dictionary of National Biography*, 22 vols., reprinted, London: Oxford University Press, 1937–1938, vol. 14, pp. 210–213.

57 Robert Nelson, *Address to Persons of Quality and Estate, to Which is Added a Representation of the Several Ways and Methods of Doing Good*, London, 1795. The reprinted Dublin edition of 1752 omits this latter part of the text. The quotation is taken from Secretan, *Memoirs*, pp. 147–148.

58 Bellers, *Essay*, pp. 1–3. For a biography of Bellers, see *Dictionary of National Biography*, vol. 2, pp. 190–192.

59 For details see G. Rosen, "An eighteenth-century plan for a national health service," *Bull. Hist. Med.* 16 (1944): 429–436.

60 Bellers, *Essay*, pp. 10–11.

61 *Ibid.*, p. 14.

62 J. G. Humble and Peter Hansell, *Westminster Hospital, 1716–1966*, London: Pitman Medical Publishing, 1966, pp. 6–7. For further details concerning this institution see John Langdon-Davies, *Westminster Hospital – Two Centuries of Voluntary Service, 1719–1948*, London: Murray, 1952.

63 For more information on Guy's Hospital, consult Hector C. Cameron, *Mr. Guy's Hospital, 1726–1948*, London: Longmans, Green, 1954. A brief chapter describing the history of the hospital was written by Sir William Hale Wright and concluded by Hujohn A. Ripman in *Guy's Hospital, 1725–1948*, ed. by H. A. Ripman, London: Adprint, 1951, pp. 7–56.

64 J. Bloomfield, *St. George's Hospital, 1733–1933*, London: Medici Society, 1933.

65 A recent account is A. E. Clark Kennedy, *The London: A Study in the Voluntary Hospital System*, 2 vols., London: Pitman Medical Publishing, 1962. The first volume covers the first hundred years, 1740–1840. An older work to be consulted is E. W. Morris, *A History of the London Hospital*, 3rd revised ed., London: Arnold, 1926.

66 Hilary St. George Saunders, *The Middlesex Hospital, 1745–1948*, London: M. Parrish, 1949. An earlier work, covering the first century of the hospital's existence and compiled from its records, is E. Wilson, *The History of the Middlesex Hospital*, London: Churchill, 1845.

67 Isaac Maddox, *A Sermon Preached before the Trustees of the Public Infirmary in James Street*, Westminster, 1739, pp. 9–10; as quoted in Owen, *English Philanthropy*, p. 43.

68 For Bristol consult George Munro-Smith, *A History of the Bristol Royal Infirmary*, Bristol: J. W. Arrowsmith, 1917. The hospital in Liverpool is described by G. McLoughlin, *A Short History of the First Liverpool Infirmary, 1749–1824*, London: Phillimore, 1978. Information about the County Hospital at York is contained in E. M. Sigsworth, "Gateways to death? Medicine, hospitals, and mortality, 1700–1850," in *Science and Society, 1600–1900*, ed. by P. Mathias, Cambridge University Press, 1972, pp. 97–110.

69 Brian Abel-Smith, *The Hospitals, 1800–1948: A Study in Social Administration in England and Wales*, Cambridge, MA: Harvard University Press, 1964, p. 1.

70 Francis Home, *Clinical Experiments, Histories, and Dissections*, 2nd corrected ed., London: Murray; Edinburgh: W. Creech, 1782, p. v.

71 Thomas Beddoes, "Considerations on infirmaries, and on the advantages of such an establishment for the county of Cornwall, September 1, 1791," in John E. Stock, *Memoirs of the Life of Thomas Beddoes, M.D.: With an Analytical Account of His Writings*, London: Murray, 1811, pp. xxv–xxviii.

72 John Aikin, *Thoughts on Hospitals*, London: J. Johnson, 1771, p. 19. For a biography of Aikin see *Dictionary of National Biography*, vol. 1, pp. 185–186.

73 Aikin, *Hospitals*, p. 8.

74 William Buchan, *Domestic Medicine, or a Treatise on the Prevention and Cure of Diseases by Regimen and Simple Medicines*, Edinburgh, 1769; enlarged ed., New York: R. Scott, 1812, p. 90.

75 Aikin, *Hospitals*, pp. 79–80.

76 William Blizard, *Suggestions for the Improvement of Hospitals and other Charitable Institutions*, London: Dilly-Poultry, 1796, p. 34.

77 For details see L. M. Zimmerman, "Surgeons and the rise of clinical teaching in England," *Bull. Hist. Med.* 37 (1963): 167–177.
78 Peter Mac Flogg'em, *Aesculapian Secrets Revealed*, London, 1813, p. 42.
79 John Pringle, *Observations on the Nature and Cure of Hospital and Jail Fevers*, London: Millar & Wilson, 1750. For more details on Pringle consult S. Selwyn, "Sir John Pringle: hospital reformer, moral philosopher and pioneer of antiseptics," *Med. Hist.* 10 (1966): 266–274.
80 Thomas Percival, "To Mr. Aikin," a letter to the author appended in Aikin, *Hospitals*, pp. 87–98.
81 Aikin, *Hospitals*, p. 21.
82 *Ibid.*, p. 52.
83 *Ibid.*, p. 54.
84 For an overview of the eighteenth- and early nineteenth-century dispensary movement see I. S. L. Loudon, "The origins and growth of the dispensary movement in England," *Bull. Hist. Med.* 55 (1981): 322–342.
85 [Veri Amicus], *A Letter to Dr. John Hope of the Royal Infirmary on the Management of Patients in That Hospital*, Edinburgh, 1782, pp. 11–12.
86 Blizard, *Suggestions*, p. 73.
87 Aikin, *Hospitals*, p. 55. For an overview see W. B. Howie, "Complaints and complaint-procedures in the eighteenth and early nineteenth century provincial hospitals in England," *Med. Hist.* 25 (1981): 345–362.
88 William Nolan, *An Essay on Humanity, or a View of Abuses in Hospitals*, London: J. Murray, 1786, p. 24.
89 Mac Flogg'em, *Secrets*, p. 43–44.
90 Nolan, *Essay*, p. 26.
91 Black, *Observations Medical and Political*, pp. 73–74.
92 Nolan, *Essay*, pp. 31–42.
93 John Howard, *Appendix to the State of the Prisons in England and Wales, Containing a Further Account of Foreign Prisons and Hospitals*, Warrington, England: W. Eyres, 1784, p. 151. Howard's biographies and published works on prison and hospital reform are listed in L. Baumgartner, "John Howard (1726–1790), hospital and prison reformer: a bibliography," *Bull. Hist. Med.* 7 (1939): 486–534, 595–626. A biographical sketch written by A. M. Muirhead is included in *ibid.* on pp. 489–503. The best biographical account is by John Aikin, *A View of the Character and Public Services of the Late John Howard*, London: J. Johnson, 1792.
94 P. M. Eaves Walton, "The early years in the Infirmary," in *The Early Years of the Edinburgh Medical School*, ed. by R. G. W. Anderson and A. D. C. Simpson, Edinburgh: Royal Scottish Museum, 1976, pp. 71–80. A detailed account of the personalities and civic interests involved can be found in Christopher J. Lawrence, "Medicine as culture: Edinburgh and the Scottish Enlightenment," Ph.D. diss., University College, London, 1984, especially chap. 3, pp. 103–109.
95 Edinburgh Infirmary, *An Account of the Rise and Establishment of the Infirmary or Hospital for Sick Poor, Erected at Edinburgh*, Edinburgh, ca. 1730, p. 2.
96 "List of the original subscribers and other donors to the Infirmary or Hospital for Sick Poor, erected at Edinburgh, preceding November 1730," in *ibid.*, pp. 19–30.
97 *Ibid.*, p. 6.
98 *Ibid.*, p. 9.
99 For more details concerning contemporary administrative arrangements see W. B. Howie, "The administration of an eighteenth-century provincial hospital: the Royal Salop Infirmary, 1747–1830," *Med. Hist.* 5 (1961): 34–55.
100 Quoted from the *Caledonian Mercury*, Aug. 1, 1727, and the minutes of the RCP, Aug. 5, 1729, in A. Logan Turner, *Story of a Great Hospital: The Royal Infirmary of Edinburgh, 1729–1929*, Edinburgh: Oliver & Boyd, 1937, pp. 44, 55.
101 Also from the *Caledonian Mercury*, July 24, 1729, quoted in Turner, *Story*, p. 50.
102 Edinburgh Infirmary, Minutes of Nov. 2, 1730, meeting, as quoted in *ibid.*, p. 59.
103 Turner, *Story*, pp. 68–70.
104 Niving, *Jesus Christ*, p. 3.

105   Edward Foster, *An Essay on Hospitals, or Succinct Directions for the Situation, Construction, and Administration of Country Hospitals,* Dublin: W. G. Jones, 1768, pp. 20–24. The U plan avoided the problems of insufficient ventilation that existed in other contemporary hospitals built with enclosed courtyards. According to one architectural analysis, it became nationally and internationally famous and was copied as an expression of "scientific functionalism and order." See Thomas A. Markus, "Buildings for the sad, the bad and the mad in urban Scotland, 1780–1830," in his *Order in Space and Society: Architectural Form and Its Context in the Scottish Enlightenment,* Edinburgh: Mainstream Publishing, 1982, pp. 34–36.

106   Hugh Arnot, *The History of Edinburgh,* Edinburgh: Longman & Cadell, 1779, p. 546.

107   Wilde, *The Hospital,* p. 4.

108   Arnot, *History of Edinburgh,* p. 548.

109   The plans drawn by Willam Adams are inserted in [John Stedman], *The History and Statutes of the Royal Infirmary of Edinburgh,* Edinburgh: Balfour & Smellie, 1778, n.p.

110   Royal Infirmary of Edinburgh [hereafter cited as RIE], Minute Book [hereafter cited as MB], MSS Collection, Medical Archives, University of Edinburgh, vol. 3, meeting of Dec. 29, 1755, p. 226.

111   William Maitland, *The History of Edinburgh,* Edinburgh, 1753, book 7, p. 457.

112   *Ibid.,* p. 458.

113   RIE, MB, vol. 3, meeting of Oct. 1, 1750, p. 63.

114   *Ibid.,* vol. 3, meeting of July 6, 1752, p. 136.

115   *Ibid.,* vol. 3, meeting of Apr. 5, 1756, p. 241.

116   *Ibid.,* vol. 4, meeting of Sept. 5, 1768, pp. 172–173.

117   *Ibid.,* vol. 4, meeting of Feb. 6, 1769, p. 188.

118   See "The Statutes of the Royal Infirmary of Edinburgh," in [Stedman], *History and Statutes,* pp. 47–89.

119   RIE, MB, vol. 3, meeting of Jan. 7, 1751, p. 71.

120   Finances are not a major focus of this book, and extensive documentation pertinent to the subject is lacking for the Royal Infirmary. For more details consult the financial history of another provincial British hospital, the Salop Infirmary. W. B. Howie, "Finance and supply in an eighteenth-century hospital, 1747–1830," *Med. Hist.* 7 (1963): 126–146.

121   See Turner, *Story,* pp. 42–43. Most of the information has been extracted from figures supplied by the treasurer's account book, one of the few surviving records. The data have been tentatively interpreted within the context of Edinburgh's hospital management. The stock of the Royal Infirmary was worth £5,000 in 1750 and increased to £36,000 in 1790. See William Creech, *Letters Addressed to Sir John Sinclair . . . ,* Edinburgh, 1793, reprinted, New York: AMS Press, 1982, p. 23.

122   The minutes of the Edinburgh Town Council record a meeting with the managers of the infirmary about the interest due, vol. 125, Minutes for Dec. 16, 1795, p. 102.

123   Turner, *Story,* p. 102.

124   The managers were first notified of Kerr's death in 1750, and details of his legacy became available the following year. According to the stipulations of the testament, one of the slaves, named Jimmy, was to be set free and provided with fifty square yards of land. RIE, vol. 3, meeting of Jan. 7, 1751, p. 78. One historian claims that Scotsmen at that time constituted one-fourth of all the landholders in Jamaica: R. B. Sheridan, "The wealth of Jamaica in the eighteenth century," *Econ. Hist. Rev.* 18 (1965): 292–334.

125   RIE, MB, vol. 4, meeting of Jan. 5, 1761, p. 25.

126   *Ibid.,* vol. 4, meeting of Feb. 28, 1774, pp. 305–306. In the process the managers had to settle a number of related matters, including the sale of a negro woman named Julie and freedom for her two children fathered by a British physician living in Kingston.

127   *Ibid.,* vol. 3, meeting of Mar. 7, 1750, p. 48.

128   *Ibid.,* vol. 3, meeting of Feb. 21, 1755, p. 200.

129   *Ibid.,* vol. 3, meeting of Aug. 4, 1755, p. 215.

130 "Petition from the managers of the Infirmary for collection in the Churches to maintain a ward for admitting sick servants ordered to be observed Sunday, 8 August 1773," in Minutes of Town Council, vol. 90, meeting of July 16, 1773. Yearly acts for the years 1761, 1762, 1764, 1766, 1768, 1769, 1770, and 1771 are also recorded in the minutes. The Edinburgh Room of the Edinburgh City Library also has a pamphlet printed for public distribution, dated Jan. 31, 1771, that requests donations for the servants' fund.

131 Treasurer's Accounts, 1769–1795, 1796–1804, MSS Collection, Medical Archives, University of Edinburgh. Occasionally information regarding these tickets also appears in the MB as part of the treasurer's report to the managers.

132 RIE, MB, vol. 6, meeting of Jan. 31, 1791, pp. 79–80.

133 *Ibid.*, vol. 6, meetings of Apr. 7, 1791, p. 88, Mar. 9, 1795, p. 214, and Nov. 2, 1795, p. 232.

134 Also taken from the Treasurer's Accounts, 1769–1795, 1796–1804.

135 According to the regulations, contributors who had subscribed 1 guinea toward the construction of this facility were entitled to use it free of charge for the first year. All others were required to pay a fee of 4s. per visit for bath and massage. A cold bath alone cost 1s. and a hot one twice this amount. The fees were obtained from the "Regulations ordered for the bagnio and the hot and cold baths," as reproduced in RIE, MB, vol. 3, meeting of Apr. 5, 1756, p. 241. The revenues were listed in the Treasurer's Accounts.

136 This problem of lower apothecary costs needs further study. In the absence of documents for the 1776–1788 period, we are left with a number of possibilities. One is the significance of the infirmary's own medicinal herbarium, located in the adjacent College Garden. Perhaps it supplied the apothecary shop with the staple herbs needed to compound the most popular remedies. Another factor was the strict adherence to items contained in the in-house dispensatory, containing economical formulas specifically prepared by the hospital apothecary. The more important question concerns the prescribing habits of attending physicians. Did they order fewer drugs for their patients as time went on? If so, was this change a result of their new institutional experiences, especially therapeutic experiments?

137 Salaries are occasionally listed in the MB.

138 Several notes ordering wooden legs appeared in the MB for 1755 and 1756, but at least the practice of recording such orders seems to have been discontinued thereafter.

139 The water was piped from the city's reservoir at Castle Hill and stored in two systems located on the ground floor. A smaller pipe coming from Heriot Hospital led to storage in the western wing. The public bath had its own deep pump well. When the city experienced water shortages, so did the infirmary. See RIE, *Report of a Committee on the State of the Hospital*, Edinburgh, 1818, p. 87.

140 See especially RIE, MB, vol. 6, meetings of July 5, 1790, p. 56, Dec. 3, 1792, pp. 161–162, June 2, 1794, p. 201, and Apr. 13, 1795, p. 223.

141 *Ibid.*, vol. 6, meeting of Apr. 7, 1791, p. 89.

142 *Ibid.*, vol. 6, meeting of June 6, 1791, p. 101.

143 *Ibid.*, vol. 6, meeting of June 15, 1795, p. 228.

144 James Gregory, *Memorial to the Managers of the Royal Infirmary*, Edinburgh: Murray & Cochrane, 1800, p. 182: "It would be much better to admit only 150 patients at once, all of whom may be comfortably accommodated and properly taken care of than to receive into the hospital all that desired to be admitted, as used to be done in the Hôtel-Dieu at Paris."

145 RIE, *Annual Report for the Year 1801*, Edinburgh, 1802, p. 2.

146 *Ibid.*, p. 3. For the year 1800, however, this statement was misleading. Although over £260 are listed in the Treasurer's Account for that year as deriving from small subscriptions, the hospital experienced a staggering loss of £998. This sum represented close to 25% of the total revenues received during 1800 and had to be absorbed through the sale of capital.

147 Gregory, *Memorial*, p. 180.

148   The annual report for 1805, for example, listed only 71 more subscribers than were recorded for 1801, and 68 of them appeared in the half-guinea-per-year category.

149   Francis Clifton, *Tabular Observations, Recommended as the Plainest and Surest Way of Practicing and Improving Physick*, London: J. Brindley, 1731.

150   *Ibid.*, p. 21.

151   "Rules for the management of the Infirmary, or Hospital for Sick Poor, in the city of Edinburgh," in Edinburgh Infirmary, *Account of the Rise*, pp. 11–12. Since much of the information on which this book is based was obtained from surviving fragments of the infirmary's registration system, it seems necessary to explain its methods and documents in some detail.

152   The first such list, covering the 35 admissions between Aug. 6, 1729, and Aug. 4, 1730, omitted the age of patients, no doubt because, as will be seen later, this information was often inaccurate. A note attached to the document indicated that "besides these patients (who were all maintained in bed, board, and medicines in the hospital) several out-patients were attended by the physicians and surgeons." Although these patients remained outside the official statistics, there is evidence that medications dispensed to them were scrupulously accounted for.

153   Edinburgh Infirmary, *Account of the Rise*, p. 12.

154   Maitand, *History of Edinburgh*, book 7, p. 460. The information was taken verbatim from an anonymous pamphlet entitled *A Letter From a Gentleman in Edinburgh to His Friend in the Country*.

155   *Ibid.*, pp. 459–460.

156   *Ibid.*, p. 460. No portions of an Edinburgh ward journal seem to have survived.

157   *Ibid.*, p. 460. Surviving fragments of a ledger from a male ward primarily occupied by soldiers for the years 1773–1776 (Ward Journal, 1773–1776, MSS Collection, Medical Archives, University of Edinburgh) have been located and analyzed, and the findings will be discussed. The name *journal* officially given to this document seems incorrect on the basis of contemporary eighteenth-century evidence.

158   Edinburgh Infirmary, *Account of the Rise*, p. 13.

159   The information could usually be found under the section "Affairs in Scotland," in the Jan. issue or in the appendix.

160   RIE, MB, vol. 3, meetings of Nov. 5, 1753, p. 162, and Dec. 29, 1755, p. 226.

161   *Ibid.*, vol. 4, meeting of Jan. 4, 1762, p. 31.

162   *Ibid.*, vol. 4, meeting of Aug. 6, 1770, p. 227.

163   It is interesting to note that the missing persons were summarily placed in the "cured" category, either because of convenience or in a deliberate attempt to embellish the statistics.

164   See the surviving volumes of the General Register of Patients, MSS Collection, Medical Archives, University of Edinburgh. General Register volumes are available from 1770 with the exception of one folio listing patients admitted between Mar. 28, 1797, and July 27, 1799. Each volume contains about 500–600 pages.

165   RIE, MB, vol. 6, meeting of Nov. 9, 1789, p. 26.

166   Often, especially after 1780, the soldiers were listed with the regiment they belonged to – the First Royal, Royal Fusiliers, Third Regiment of Guards, First Regiment of Dragoons, etc. – or simply as "recruits."

167   In 1770 the clerks employed 231 different diagnostic entries, many of them combinations of two distinct symptoms. By 1790 only about 170 of them survived.

168   Other instances of clerical haste occurred. At times, the admission numbers and even complete entries were repeated, and diagnoses of specifically female ailments became attached to patients with male first names. Moreover, some of the discharge dates assigned by the clerks were earlier than those given for admission to the house, or the status of the patient was entered in the wrong column. Some erroneous calendar dates, such as Feb. 30 and Apr. 31, also occasionally appear. A more serious error in the patient count occurred in 1785, when the clerk responsible for inscribing a new page of the register unwittingly followed number 539 with 340 instead of 540, thereby omitting from the final tally 200 patients previously admitted. Finally, several patients taken in late in the year and listed as remaining in the hospital did

not appear on the lists of those still in the house early in the following year; their diagnoses and discharge dates were also missing.

169 It also seems strange that given this impressive system of medical registration, with all its drawbacks, the infirmary waited until 1818 to publish its first statistical analysis: Andrew Duncan, Jr., *Reports of the Practice on the Clinical Wards of the Royal Infirmary of Edinburgh*, Edinburgh: A. Constable, 1818. In advocating such hospital reports, the author stressed their importance to the public and the medical profession by noting that, among other things, they would reveal the health status of the community in which the infirmary was located. Such a statement is open to question, however, considering the selective admission policies of the voluntary hospital system. Nevertheless, an analysis of those patients who were admitted, their diseases, treatment, and the length as well as results of hospital therapy would have been helpful to the persons responsible for the administrative and medical affairs of the infirmary.

170 RIE, MB, vol. 4, meeting of July 2, 1774, pp. 315–316: "Regulations drawn by house physicians for better preservation of good order and harmony among the patients." One man insisted on smoking, but James Gregory ordered on his chart, "Let him give up the use of tobacco which he has been in the habit of using for seven years." Case of James Caldwell, in James Gregory, Clinical reports, Nov. 1, 1795–Feb. 1, 1796, Edinburgh, 1795–1796, MSS Collection, University of Edinburgh.

171 See cases of Peggy Maitland and Margaret Williamson, in D. Rutherford, Clinical cases, 1799; and John Dryborough, in James Gregory, Clinical reports, 1795–1796.

172 Cases of Margaret Tait, Agnes Hamilton, and Anne Thornburn, in D. Rutherford, Clinical cases, 1799; and John Bell, in James Gregory, Cases of patients, 1781–1782.

173 Cases of Peggy McKay, in John Gregory, Clinical cases, 1771–1772; Elizabeth Davidson, in F. Home, Cases of patients, 1780–1781; and Anne Hall, in T. C. Hope, Clinical casebook, 1796–1797. See letter written by Joseph Black as presiding officer of the infirmary's managers, dated Mar. 20, 1781, in Erskine–Murray correspondence, 1777–1790, MSS Collection, National Library of Scotland.

174 See letter written by Joseph Black as presiding officer of the infirmary's managers, dated Mar. 20, 1781, in the Erskine-Murrary Correspondence, 1777–1790, MSS Collection, National Library of Scotland, Edinburgh.

175 Wilde, *The Hospital*, p. 36. Wilde wrote most of his poem in darkness while hospitalized.

176 RIE, *Report of a Committee*, p. 61.

177 Case of Andrew McPherson, in W. Cullen, Clinical lectures, 1772–1773, pp. 125–126.

178 Cases of Simon Davis, in John Gregory, Clinical cases, 1771–1772; Pompey Graham, in W. Cullen, Clinical cases and reports, 1773–1774; and Anne McNicol, in F. Home, Cases of patients, 1780–1781. Speaking of cautherization, Cullen remarked, "We cannot find patients to submit to it and were we to employ it even in this house, we would drive many patients out of it and prevent others from coming in." W. Cullen, Clinical lectures, 1772–1773, p. 500.

179 [Amicus], *Letter*, p. 10.

180 RIE, *Report of a Committee*, pp. 60, 89. One patient was so addicted to liquor that "he could not live without it" and had his wife bring it to him "privately." Case of Robert Grant, in A. Duncan, Sr., Clinical reports and commentaries, 1795.

181 W. Cullen, Clinical lectures, 1772–1773, pp. 186–187.

182 RIE, MB, vol. 4, meeting of July 2, 1774, p. 316.

183 [Stedman], *History and Statutes*, p. 54.

184 Wilde, *The Hospital*, p. 57. For more detail see Howie, "Complaints."

185 Two important papers written by Nicholas T. Phillipson try to define and explain the Scottish Enlightenment: "Towards a definition of the Scottish Enlightenment," in *City and Society in the Eighteenth Century*, ed. by P. Fritz, Toronto: Hakkert, 1973, pp. 125–147; and "Culture and society in the 18th century province: the case of Edinburgh and the Scottish Enlightenment," in *The University in Society*, ed. by L.

Stone, vol. II, *Europe, Scotland and the United States from the 16th to the 20th Century*, Princeton, N.J.: Princeton University Press, 1975, pp. 407–448.

186 See R. L. Emerson, "The social composition of enlightened Scotland: the Select Society of Edinburgh, 1754–1764," *Studies on Voltaire* 114 (1973): 291–329; and Emerson, "The Philosophical Society of Edinburgh, 1737–1747," *Brit. J. Hist. Sci.* 12 (1979): 154–191.

187 This issue has been recently raised on the basis of modern epidemiological criteria and articulated in some of Thomas McKeown's work. The problem has been studied in detail by S. Cherry: See Cherry, "The role of a provincial hospital: the Norfolk and Norwich Hospital, 1771–1880," *Popul. Stud.* 26 (1972): 291–306; and more recently, Cherry, "The hospitals and population growth: the voluntary general hospitals, mortality and local populations in the English provinces in the eighteenth and nineteenth centuries," 2 parts, *Popul. Stud.* 34 (1980): 59–75, 251–265. Cherry's studies seem to support his contention that hospitals "appear to have exerted a reducing or containing effect on mortality in their local areas." "The hospitals," p. 265.

CHAPTER 2 *Hospital staff and the admission of patients*

1 Peter Mac Flogg'em, *Aesculapian Secrets Revealed*, London, 1813, p. 72.

2 RIE, MB, vol. 3, meeting of Jan. 7, 1751, p. 71.

3 A. Logan Turner, *Story of a Great Hospital: The Royal Infirmary of Edinburgh, 1729–1929*, Edinburgh: Oliver & Boyd, 1937, pp. 118–119.

4 *Ibid.*, pp. 120–121.

5 [John Stedman], *The History and Statutes of the Royal Infirmary of Edinburgh*, Edinburgh: Balfour & Smellie, 1778, p. 20.

6 *Ibid.*, p. 84.

7 James Gregory, *Memorial to the Managers of the Royal Infirmary*, Edinburgh: Murray & Cochrane, 1800, p. 195.

8 *Ibid.*, p. 62.

9 [Stedman], *History and Statutes*, pp. 62–63.

10 RIE, MB, vol. 4, meeting of Feb. 3, 1766, pp. 112–117; *ibid.*, vol. 6, meeting of Oct. 1, 1792, pp. 149–157.

11 See separate Medical Matriculation Records, University of Edinburgh, 2 vols., Edinburgh, 1783–1795, MSS Collection, University of Edinburgh.

12 [Stedman], *History and Statutes*, p. 87. Whether such appeals were successful in curbing prescribing habits is still unknown, although, as mentioned before, drug-related expenses diminished toward the end of the century.

13 *Ibid.*, p. 63.

14 RIE, MB, vol. 3, meeting of Oct. 4, 1756, p. 264.

15 *Ibid.*, vol. 6, meeting of Apr. 6, 1789, p. 21.

16 Turner, *Story*, app. 2, p. 367.

17 For more details consult Clarendon H. Creswell, "The early association of the Incorporation of Surgeons with the Royal Infirmary," in his *Royal College of Surgeons of Edinburgh*, Edinburgh: Oliver & Boyd, 1926, chap. 13, pp. 208–233.

18 RIE, MB, vol. 4, meeting of July 7, 1766, pp. 129–132.

19 *Ibid.*, vol. 4, meetings of Mar. 18, 1769, pp. 160–161, and Mar. 6, 1769, pp. 189, 194–195.

20 [Stedman], *History and Statutes*, p. 63.

21 *Ibid.*, p. 64.

22 *Ibid.*

23 Edward Foster, *An Essay on Hospitals, or Succinct Directions for the Situation, Construction, and Administration of Country Hospitals*, Dublin: W. G. Jones, 1768, p. 61.

24 Gregory, *Memorial*, p. 104.

25 RIE, MB, vol. 6, meeting of Feb. 3, 1794, p. 193.

26 Pamphlet collection, RCP, Edinburgh.

27 Gregory, *Memorial*, p. 193.

28 James Gregory, *Additional Memorial to the Managers of the Royal Infirmary*, Edinburgh: Murray & Cochrane, 1803, p. 154.

29 RIE, MB, vol. 4, meeting of Nov. 24, 1800, p. 394. For other details about the surgical rotation see Benjamin Bell, *Observations on the Mode of Attendance of the Surgeons of Edinburgh on the Royal Infirmary*, Edinburgh: Neill, 1800.

30 See Turner, *Story*, p. 145. The quotation was taken from the minutes of the infirmary, meeting of May 14, 1802. More information is available in James Arnot, *Remarks on the Present Mode of Chirurgical Attendance in the Royal Infirmary of Edinburgh*, Edinburgh: Neill, 1800; and Andrew Wardrop, *An Address to Members of the Royal College of Surgeons*, Edinburgh: Shaw, 1800.

31 Gregory, *Memorial*, p. 41.

32 [Stedman], *History and Statutes*, p. 65.

33 For a brief summary see "Clinical teaching in the Royal Infirmary in the eighteenth century," in Turner, *Story*, chap. 9, pp. 130–142.

34 For a biographical sketch of John Gregory see John D. Comrie, *History of Scottish Medicine*, 2 vols., London: Bailliere, Tindall & Cox, 1932, vol. 1 pp. 309–311. Further biographical information on John Gregory can be obtained from *Medical Commentaries* 1 (1773): 210–215; and John Ramsay, *Scotland and Scotsmen in the Eighteenth Century*, 2 vols., Edinburgh: W. Blackwood, 1888, vol. 1, pp. 477–482. For William Cullen see John Thomson, *An Account of the Life, Lectures, and Writings of William Cullen, M.D.*, 2 vols., Edinburgh: W. Blackwood & Sons, 1859. A brief sketch can be found in J. D. Comrie, "An eighteenth-century consultant," *Edinb. Med. J.* 32 (1925): 17–30.

35 Biographical details concerning James Gregory are in Robert Chambers, *A Biographical Dictionary of Eminent Scotsmen*, continued by Thomas Thomson, 3 vols., reprint of 1870 ed., New York: G. Olms, 1971, pp. 177–179. Other sources are Robert Christison, *Life of Sir Robert Christison*, 2 vols., Edinburgh: 1885, vol. 1, pp. 338–339; and Henry Cockburn, *Memorials of His Time*, ed. and with an introduction by K. F. C. Miller, Chicago: University of Chicago Press, 1974, pp. 96–97.

36 For Francis Home, see J. F. Enders, "Francis Home and his experimental approach to medicine," *Bull. Hist. Med.* 38 (1964): 101–112. More information on Home can be found in *Dictionary of National Biography*, ed. by James C. Hadden, 22 vols., reprinted, London: Oxford University Press, 1937–1938, vol. 9, pp. 1122–1123.

37 For biographical information about Duncan, see *Dictionary of National Biography*, vol. 6, pp. 161–162; personality sketches in Cockburn, *Memorials*, p. 273; Christison, *Life*, vol. 1, p. 75; and Comrie, *History*, vol. 2, pp. 479–482.

38 Thomas C. Hope is also mentioned in Comrie, *History*, vol. 2, pp. 482–485. He became the sole professor of chemistry at the University of Edinburgh in 1799. For biographical information consult R. H. Cragg, "Thomas Charles Hope (1766–1844)," *Med. Hist.* 11 (1967): 186–189.

39 Little is known about the medical activities of Daniel Rutherford. See *Dictionary of National Biography*, vol. 17, pp. 494–495; and the article by E. L. Scott in *Dictionary of Scientific Biography*, ed. by C. C. Gillispie, 16 vols., New York: Scribner, 1970–1980, vol. 12, pp. 24–25.

40 [Stedman], *History and Statutes*, pp. 65–66.

41 "Regulations respecting the clerks, dressers and students attending the Royal Infirmary of Edinburgh," in RIE, MB, vol. 6, meeting of Oct. 1, 1792, p. 153.

42 *Ibid.*, vol. 4, meeting of Aug. 8, 1775, p. 346.

43 *Ibid.*, vol. 4, meeting of Feb. 3, 1766, pp. 112–114.

44 The Minute Books contain several entries indicating that departing clerks received a £10 or £15 bonus.

45 RIE, MB, vol. 6, meeting of Oct. 1, 1792, p. 150: Each month the physician's first clerk had to lay before the authorities "an account of the patients then in the hospital, specifying what number are medical ordinary, what chirurgical, what servants, what soldiers, what sailors, what supernumeraries, what patients have been more than three months in the hospital."

46 *Ibid.*, vol. 4, meeting of Feb. 3, 1766, p. 115; *ibid.*, vol. 6, meeting of Oct. 1, 1792, pp. 151–153.

47 *Ibid.*, vol. 4, meeting of June 13, 1775, p. 342. Charges of receiving "putrid food" were renewed in the early 1800s. See RIE, *Report of a Committee on the State of the Hospital*, Edinburgh, 1818, p. 58.

48 The request was refused "as a dangerous precedent and as inconsistent with the regulations of the hospital." RIE, MB, vol. 6, meeting of Aug. 5, 1793, p. 178.

49 Turner, *Story*, p. 110.

50 Foster, *Essay on Hospitals*, p. 64.

51 *Ibid.*, p. 65.

52 RIE, MB, vol. 3, meeting of Dec. 1, 1754, pp. 195–196.

53 *Ibid.*, vol. 3, meeting of Feb. 3, 1755, p. 199.

54 [Stedman], *History and Statutes*, pp. 70–71.

55 *Ibid.*, p. 70.

56 RIE, MB, vol. 4, meeting of Feb. 3, 1766, p. 117.

57 *Ibid.*, vol. 4, pp. 116–117.

58 *Ibid.*, vol. 6, meeting of July 5, 1790, p. 56.

59 *Ibid.*, vol. 6, meeting of Apr. 13, 1795, p. 223.

60 The most detailed regulations regarding dressers appeared in 1792: *ibid.*, vol. 6, meeting of Oct. 1, 1792, pp. 154–157.

61 [Stedman], *History and Statutes*, p. 73.

62 RIE, MB, vol. 6, meeting of Mar. 4, 1793, p. 170.

63 *Ibid.*, vol. 6, meeting of Feb. 3, 1800, p. 346.

64 *The Students of Medicine in the University of Edinburgh Inform the Managers of the Royal Infirmary*, a pamphlet in possession of the Royal Medical Society of Edinburgh, p. 13.

65 Marjorie Plant, *The Domestic Life of Scotland in the Eighteenth Century*, Edinburgh: Edinburgh University Press, 1952, p. 161.

66 Foster, *Essay on Hospitals*, pp. 67–68.

67 See, for example, the cases of John Oakley, suffering from a fever, in James Gregory, Clinical notes and lectures, Edinburgh, 1779–1780, MSS Collection, Royal College of Physicians, Edinburgh; and Thomas Ashurst, a soldier with a bowel problem, in John Hope, Cases of patients in the Royal Infirmary under the care of John Hope, M.D., Edinburgh, 1781, MSS Collection, University of Edinburgh. The teaching ward usually had both a day and a night nurse, whom Andrew Duncan, Sr., characterized as "attentive and humane." See RIE, *Report of a Committee*, p. 68.

68 [Stedman], *History and Statutes*, p. 81.

69 RIE, MB, vol. 4, meeting of July 4, 1768, p. 168.

70 *Ibid.*, vol. 6, meeting of Dec. 3, 1792, p. 162.

71 Plant, *Domestic Life*, p. 162.

72 RIE, MB, vol. 4, meeting of July 4, 1768, p. 168. The issue of nurses' taking money from patients to "ensure kind offices" was also brought out in later investigations. See RIE, *Report of a Committee*, p. 17.

73 [Stedman], *History and Statutes*, p. 79.

74 *Ibid.*, pp. 79–80.

75 Foster, *Essay on Hospitals*, p. 68.

76 Gregory, *Memorial*, p. 331. The fact that some nurses were frequently intoxicated – but apparently never before noon – emerged from several statements from a senior attending surgeon: RIE, *Report of a Committee*, p. 16.

77 [Veri Amicus], *A Letter to Dr. John Hope of the Royal Infirmary on the Management of Patients in That Hospital*, Edinburgh, 1782, pp. 11–12.

78 RIE, MB, vol. 6, meeting of Nov. 3, 1794, pp. 204–205.

79 *Ibid.*, vol. 6, meeting of Jan. 3, 1799, p. 340. See also RIE, *Report of a Committee*, pp. 5–15.

80 William Cullen, Clinical lectures, Edinburgh, 1772–1773, MSS Collection, RCP, Edinburgh, p. 25.

81 [Stedman], *History and Statutes,* p. 89. Other instances of abusive behavior were reported in the early 1800s. In one instance one of the day nurses in the soldiers' ward lifted a poker from the fireplace and threatened to strike the patients. See RIE, *Report of a Committee,* p. 61.

82 W. Cullen, Clinical lectures, 1772–1773, p. 504.

83 Joseph Wilde, *The Hospital: A Poem in Three Books,* Norwich, England: Stevenson, Matchelt, & Stevenson, 1810, p. 58. Wilde's disappointment and dismay were evident, and he seriously entertained the thought of reporting the abuses to the authorities.

84 Edinburgh Infirmary, "Rules for the management of the Infirmary, or Hospital for Sick Poor, in the city of Edinburgh," in *An Account of the Rise and Establishment of the Infirmary, or Hospital for Sick Poor, Erected at Edinburgh,* Edinburgh, ca. 1730, pp. 12–13.

85 Foster, *Essay on Hospitals,* pp. 69–70.

86 Edinburgh Infirmary, *Account of the Rise,* p. 13.

87 [Stedman], *History and Statutes,* p. 60.

88 *Ibid.,* pp. 59–60.

89 Turner, *Story,* pp. 109–110. See also RIE, *Report of a Committee,* pp. 3–6.

90 [Stedman], *History and Statutes,* p. 61.

91 *Ibid.,* p. 62.

92 *Ibid.,* p. 61.

93 Turner, *Story,* pp. 113–114.

94 [Stedman], *History and Statutes,* p. 62.

95 RIE, *Report of a Committee,* pp. 2–19.

96 [Stedman], *History and Statutes,* pp. 81–82.

97 RIE, MB, vol. 3, meeting of Apr. 5, 1756, p. 241.

98 William Nolan, *An Essay on Humanity, or a View of Abuses in Hospitals,* London: J. Murray, 1786, p. 30.

99 *Ibid.,* p. 29.

100 [Stedman], *History and Statutes,* p. 23. See also Turner, *Story,* p. 115.

101 RIE, MB, vol. 6, meeting of Dec. 1, 1794, p. 207.

102 Wilde, *The Hospital,* pp. 5–6.

103 RIE, MB, vol. 4, meeting of Nov. 7, 1768, p. 175.

104 [Stedman], *History and Statutes,* p. 88.

105 RIE, MB, vol. 4, meeting of Mar. 14, 1774, pp. 308–309.

106 A collection of issues of this newspaper is available in the Edinburgh Room of the Edinburgh City Library.

107 See W. B. Howie, "The administration of an eighteenth-century provincial hospital: the Royal Salop Infirmary, 1747–1830," *Med. Hist.* 5 (1961): 49.

108 [Stedman], *History and Statutes,* p. 10.

109 For details about the various possible modes of transportation consult H. W. Hart, "The conveyance of patients to and from hospital, 1720–1850," *Med. Hist.* 22 (1978): 397–407.

110 Cases of Janet Cameron, in W. Cullen, Clinical lectures, 1772–1773, p. 434; and Hannah Cameron, in William Cullen, Clinical lectures, delivered for John Gregory, Feb.–Apr. 1772, Edinburgh, 1772, MSS Collection, RCP, Edinburgh, p. 136.

111 Cases of Kenneth Stewart and James Imlach, in J. Hope, Cases of patients, 1781.

112 This case was extracted from James Russel, Surgical cases, 8 vols., Edinburgh, 1784–1792, MSS Collection, RCP, Edinburgh vol. 6, pp. 112–117.

113 In one of his lectures, Cullen said of two individuals received into the teaching unit, "I would have refused to practice upon them had they not been particularly recommended." Cullen, Clinical lectures, Feb.–Apr. 1772, p. 338.

114 [Stedman], *History and Statutes,* p. 88.

115 W. Cullen, Clinical lectures, 1772–1773, p. 60.

116 RIE, MB, vol. 4, meeting of May 7, 1764, p. 77.

117 *Ibid.,* vol. 6, meeting of Aug. 3, 1798, p. 307.

118 Gregory, *Memorial,* p. 182.

119 Turner, *Story*, p. 93.
120 [Stedman], *History and Statutes*, pp. 87–88.
121 RIE, MB, vol. 6, meeting of Aug. 3, 1798, p. 306.
122 [Stedman], *History and Statutes*, p. 76.
123 *Ibid.*, pp. 88–89.
124 *Ibid.*, p. 76.
125 Gregory, *Additional Memorial*, p. 477.
126 Wilde, *The Hospital*, p. 16.
127 RIE, MB, vol. 4, meeting of Sept. 6, 1773, p. 291.
128 Wilde, *The Hospital*, p. 16.
129 RIE, MB, vol. 6, meeting of June 4, 1792, p. 137.
130 This information was obtained from the General Register for the years 1777–1787, when the document listed by wards all patients remaining as of Jan. 1.
131 RIE, MB, vol. 3, meeting of Jan. 1, 1750, p. 38.
132 *Ibid.*, vol. 6, meeting of July 5, 1790, p. 56.
133 W. Cullen, Clinical lectures, 1772–1773, p. 29.
134 Turner, *Story*, p. 94.
135 RIE, MB, vol. 3, meetings of Feb. 21, 1755, p. 200, and June 8, 1756, p. 244.
136 See Cyril N. Parkinson, *Britannia Rules: The Classic Age of Naval History, 1793–1815*, London: Weidenfeld & Nicolson, 1977, pp. 40–41.
137 RIE, MB, vol. 3, meeting of Aug. 2, 1756, pp. 257–258.
138 *Ibid.*, vol. 3, meeting of Aug. 2, 1756, pp. 258–261.
139 *Ibid.*, vol. 3, meeting of Dec. 4, 1759, p. 341.
140 *Ibid.*, vol. 3, meeting of Dec. 21, 1759, pp. 342–344.
141 *Ibid.*, vol. 6, meeting of Oct. 1, 1798, p. 313.
142 The infirmary statistics published in *Scots Magazine* counted soldiers separately only for the years 1762–1778. An approximate idea of the proportion of soldiers admitted can be gathered from counting those who remained in the hospital on Jan. 1. The soldiers' ward is identified as such between 1777 and 1786, and so a total count of those hospitalized in it is possible for those years.
143 See, for example, the cases of Thomas Eagle and William Frazer, in James Gregory, Cases of patients under the care of James Gregory, M.D., Edinburgh, 1781–1782, MSS Collection, RCP, Edinburgh.
144 Cases of Henry Drinkwater and Isaac Day, in *ibid.*
145 For example, the case of George Drury, in *ibid.*
146 Case of Robert Wishart, in Daniel Rutherford, Clinical cases, Edinburgh, 1799, MSS Collection, RCP, Edinburgh.
147 Case of Anne McIntosh, in Thomas C. Hope, Clinical casebook, Edinburgh, 1796–1797, MSS Collection, RCP, Edinburgh.
148 Case of James McDonald, in William Cullen, Clinical cases and reports taken at the Royal Infirmary of Edinburgh from Dr. Cullen, taken by Richard W. Hall, Edinburgh, 1773–1774, MSS Collection, National Library of Medicine, Bethesda, MD: Gilbert Anderson, in J. Hope, Cases of patients, 1781; and William Brown, Casebooks, 5 vols., Edinburgh, 1790–1810, MSS Collection, RCS, Edinburgh, vol. 5, p. 79.
149 After signing a treaty with Russia on June 22, 1799, British forces prepared a joint expeditionary army against Napoleon. The goal was the invasion of Holland, and on August 13, 1799, the allied contingent left England under the protection of the North Sea Squadron. Following capture of the Dutch Fleet, the 40,000 troops under the command of the duke of York landed on the Continent, only to be repulsed two months later and forced to return. (For details, see G. J. Marcus, *The Age of Nelson: The Royal Navy, 1793–1815*, New York: Viking Press, 1971.)
      As a result, the city of Edinburgh received a considerable number of Russian soldiers, many of them sick, who came ashore from ships landing at Leith. A Russian military band even gave concerts in Edinburgh Assembly Rooms, and the sick were brought to the infirmary for admission and treatment. *Scots Magazine* 61 (Nov. 1799): 791, 856. Indeed for the period Nov. 19, 1799–May 7, 1800, the General Register of Patients contains the names of 236 Russian soldiers who came into the

house in about four separate groups. Because of Russia's secession from the alliance in Apr. 1800, no further Russian soldiers appeared on the admission lists after May 7. Those still remaining in the house were all evacuated before or on June 9, 1800. Their care was paid for by the commissioner of sick and wounded seamen, who remitted to the infirmary £204 in 1799 and £251 in 1800.

Many of the Russian soldiers were despearately ill. A statistical study of the 236 cases reveals that almost half of them (47.4%) suffered from fevers; also significant were scurvy (18.6%), diarrhea (10.1%), and several surgical problems. As will be seen later, these men were in poor physical condition after the brief campaign in Holland, and a fifth of them died in the infirmary, a fivefold increase in the average mortality reported to hospital subscribers. See Marcus, *Age of Nelson*, p. 151.

150 John C. Lettsom, *On the Improvement of Medicine in London on the Basis of Public Good*, 2nd ed., London: J. Phillips, 1775, p. 28.

151 Plant, *Domestic Life*, pp. 161–162.

152 Henry G. Graham, *The Social Life of Scotland in the Eighteenth Century*, London: A. & C. Black, 1909, pp. 60–61.

153 *Ibid.*, p. 87.

154 One maid, a young woman named Bell Mowatt, was a domestic servant of James Gregory, a hospital manager and university professor periodically in charge of the teaching ward. This patient, suffering from an inflammation of her eyes after extended "nightwatching," was admitted to the teaching ward in Feb. 1795 while Andrew Duncan, Sr., was in charge. See Andrew Duncan, Sr., Clinical reports and commentaries, February–April 1795, presented by Alexander Blackhall Morison, Edinburgh, 1795, MSS Collection, Royal College of Physicians, Edinburgh. A cookmaid with irregular menstrual bleeding actually received in 1773 a personal visit from William Cullen in the house of her employers, no doubt arranged by them. Several days later she was sent to the hospital and admitted to Cullen's teaching ward for more extensive treatment. See Cullen, Clinical lectures, 1772–1773, pp. 625–626.

155 Case of Gilbert McIntosh, in D. Rutherford, Clinical cases, 1799.

156 Case of Janet Sutherland, in James Gregory, Clinical notes and lectures, 1779–1780.

157 Case of Margaret Burton, in W. Cullen, Clinical cases and reports, 1773–1774.

158 RIE, MB, vol. 3, meeting of Aug. 4, 1755, p. 215.

159 Appeal for funds made in behalf of Lord Provost, Magistrates and Council, Edinburgh, Jan. 31, 1771, no pagination.

160 *Ibid.*

161 RIE, MB, vol. 3, meetings of Nov. 26, 1755, p. 225, and Apr. 5, 1756, p. 243.

162 Lettsom, *Improvement of Medicine*, p. 29.

163 Appeal for funds, 1771.

164 RIE, MB, vol. 3, meeting of Apr. 3, 1758, p. 312.

165 Christopher Lloyd and Jack L. S. Coulter, "The decline of the contract system," in their *Medicine and the Navy, 1200–1900*, vol. 3, *1714–1815*, Edinburgh: E. & S. Livingstone, 1961, chap. 14, pp. 187–195.

166 James Lind, *An Essay on the Most Effectual Means of Preserving the Health of Seamen in the Royal Navy*, London: J. Murray, 1779, reprinted in *The Health of Seamen: Selections from the Works of Dr. James Lind, Sir Gilbert Blane and Dr. Thomas Trotter*, edited by C. Lloyd, London: Navy Records Society, 1965, p. 77.

167 See discussion about the costs involved in the transport of seamen, RIE, MB, vol. 6, meeting of Apr. 7, 1791, p. 89.

168 *Ibid.*, vol. 6, meetings of Jan. 31, 1791, pp. 79–80, and Apr. 7, 1791, pp. 90–91.

169 *Ibid.*, vol. 6, meeting of Apr. 7, 1791, p. 91.

170 An example of the infirmary's interest in the subject was John Bell's *Discourse on the Nature and Cure of Wounds*, published in 1795. Not surprisingly, it was also Bell who in 1800 wrote a programmatic *Memorial Concerning the Present State of Military and Naval Surgery*, based on experience acquired in part before his expulsion from the infirmary. See Lloyd and Coulter, *Medicine and the Navy*, vol. 3, chap. 21, "Surgery," pp. 359–370.

171 RIE, MB, vol. 6, meeting of Mar. 9, 1795, p. 214. Operating in conjunction with

Admiral Duncan's North Sea Fleet was also a Russian squadron under the command of Vice-Admiral Peter Hanikoff. The foreign task force, nicknamed the "Curious Squad," joined the fleet in the summer of 1795, although the condition of its vessels and health of the crews made it more an encumbrance than an asset for the Royal Navy. Not surprisingly, the infirmary admitted from time to time some of the Russian seamen whose ships anchored at Leith. Their treatment was also paid for by the commissioner, but the men were omitted from the official hospital statistics. Between Feb. 20 and Sept. 1796, fifteen Russian sailors were allowed into the infirmary, over half of them suffering from scurvy. Marcus, *Age of Nelson,* p. 55.

172   *Ibid.,* meeting of Nov. 2, 1795, p. 232.
173   Thomas Trotter, *Medicina Nautica: An Essay on the Diseases of Seamen,* 2nd ed., 3 vols., London: Longman, Hurst, Rees & Orme, 1804, reprinted in Lloyd, *Health of Seamen,* p. 267.
174   *Ibid.,* pp. 108–109.
175   Gilbert Blane, "On the comparative health of the British Navy, from the year 1779 to the year 1814, with proposals for its farther improvement," originally published in *Transactions of the Medico-Chirugical Society* 6 (1815) and reprinted in Lloyd, *Health of Seamen,* pp. 197–198.
176   RIE, MB, vol. 3, meetings of Feb. 20, 1749, p. 3, and Dec. 3, 1750, p. 67.
177   [Stedman], *History and Statutes,* p. 11.
178   *Ibid.*
179   M. A. Waugh, "Attitudes of hospitals in London to venereal disease in the 18th and 19th centuries, *Brit. J. Vener. Dis.* 47 (1971): 146–150.
180   John Aikin, *Thoughts on Hospitals,* London: J. Johnson, 1771, p. 37.
181   [Stedman], *History and Statutes,* p. 86.
182   RIE, MB, vol. 3, meetings of July 7, 1755, p. 211, and Oct. 6, 1755, p. 218.
183   T. Champney, *Medical and Chirurgical Reform Proposed, from a Review of the Healing Art,* London: J. Johnson, 1797, p. 29.
184   RIE, MB, vol. 6, meeting of Aug. 5, 1793, p. 178. For details on the new hospital see *Laws, Orders and Regulations of the Edinburgh General Lying-In Hospital,* Edinburgh, 1793.
185   The letter is available in the Scottish Record Office.
186   RIE, MB, vol. 6, meeting of Apr. 6, 1789, p. 15.
187   For a brief summary concerning lunacy in Scotland and the institutional response see Comrie, *History,* vol. 2, pp. 464–467. Details about the Montrose Asylum can be found in a paper by K. M. G. Keddie, "Straightjackets and seclusion: Montrose Asylum, 1781–1834." A summary of this work was published in *Med. Hist.* 26 (1982): 202.
188   RIE, MB, vol. 6, meetings of Apr. 4, 1791, p. 84, and Nov. 7, 1791, p. 117.
189   RIE, *Report of a Committee,* p. 9.
190   Wilde, *The Hospital,* p. 18.
191   Case of Saunders Balmands, in D. Rutherford, Clinical cases, 1799. For more details about the importance of a clinical history, see Stanley J. Reiser, "Examination of the patient in the seventeenth and eighteenth centuries," in Reiser, *Medicine and the Reign of Technology,* Cambridge University Press, 1978, chap. 1, pp. 1–22.
192   Francis Home, Clinical lectures delivered in the year 1769, taken by John Goodsir, Edinburgh, 1769, MSS Collection, RCP, Edinburgh, preliminary lecture, p. 2.
193   *Ibid.,* p. 7.
194   See, for example, the cases of Fanny Kennedy, in James Gregory, Clinical cases of Dr. Gregory in the Royal Infirmary of Edinburgh, taken by Nathan Thomas, Edinburgh, 1785–1786, MSS Collection, University of Edinburgh; and Elizabeth Watson, in T. C. Hope, Clinical casebook, 1796–1797.
195   "Our patient may be inaccurate in speaking of some pain in her breast when perhaps it was in her belly," Cullen observed in a clinical lecture. See W. Cullen, Clinical lectures, 1772–1773, p. 376.
196   Cases of Andrew Carmichael, in James Gregory, Clinical notes and lectures, 1779–1780; and Janet Shanks, in John Gregory, Clinical cases of the Royal Infirmary of

Edinburgh, Edinburgh, 1771–1772, MSS Collection, Medical Archives, University of Edinburgh.

197 Such an incomplete history was blamed for the death of a patient with fluid in the chest. Not only did the attending physicians have no clue about the chest disorder, but they likewise were not aware that the patient had been bled prior to admission. See W. Cullen, Clinical lectures, Feb.–Apr. 1772, p. 300.

198 W. Cullen, Clinical lectures, 1772–1773, p. 120.

199 Case of Alexander Gillen, in D. Rutherford, Clinical cases, 1799.

200 Case of John Black, in James Gregory, Cases of patients, 1781–1782.

201 W. Cullen, Clinical lectures, 1772–1773, p. 651.

202 *Ibid.*, p. 506.

203 *Ibid.*, p. 213.

204 F. Home, Clinical lectures, 1769, p. 7.

205 Case of Ann Webster, in J. Hope, Cases of patients, 1781.

206 For an overview see Lester S. King, *Medical Thinking: A Historical Preface,* Princeton, N.J.: Princeton University Press, 1982, chap. 10, pp. 207–211. More details are contained in King's "Some problems of causality in eighteenth century medicine," *Bull. Hist. Med.* 38 (1963): 15–24.

207 [Stedman], *History and Statutes,* pp. 83–84.

208 F. Home, Clinical lectures, 1769, p. 8.

209 W. Cullen, Clinical lectures, 1772–1773, p. 103.

210 See, for example, cases of Jean McKenzie and Mary Boulsby, in Francis Home, Cases of patients under the care of Francis Home, Edinburgh 1780–1781, MSS Collection, RCP, Edinburgh.

211 Case of Christian Cameron, in A. Duncan, Sr., Clinical reports and commentaries, 1795.

212 Case of Christy Howard, in T. C. Hope, Clinical casebook, 1796–1797.

213 Case of James Hay, in *ibid.*

214 Case of Catherine Duff, in James Gregory, Clinical reports, Nov. 1, 1795–Feb. 1, 1796, Edinburgh, 1795–1796, MSS Collection, University of Edinburgh.

215 Case of Thomas Bell, in J. Hope, Cases of patients, 1781.

216 W. Cullen, Clinical lectures, 1772–1773, p. 277. The use of a watch is described in John Floyer, *The Physician's Pulse Watch,* 2 vols., London: S. Smith & B. Walford, 1707–1710.

217 Case of Nelly Kirkpatrick, in James Gregory, Clinical notes and lectures, 1779–1780.

218 William Fordyce, *A New Inquiry into the Causes, Symptoms and Cure of Putrid and Inflammatory Fevers,* 4th ed., London: T. Cadell, 1777, p. 45.

219 Case of Mary Blaikie, in James Gregory, Clinical reports, 1795–1796.

220 William Falconer, *Observations Respecting the Pulse, Especially in Feverish Complaints,* London: T. Cadell & W. Davies, 1796.

221 Case of William Johnston, in W. Cullen, Clinical cases and reports, 1773–1774.

222 George Fordyce, *A Dissertation on Simple Fever,* London: J. Johnson, 1794, p. 9. An earlier work suggesting clinical thermometry was George Martine, *Essays Medical and Philosophical,* London: A. Millar, 1740. For an overview see W. F. Bynum, "Cullen and the study of fevers in Britain, 1760–1820," *Med. Hist.,* supplement no. 1 (1981): 135–147.

223 W. Cullen, Clinical lectures, Feb.–Apr. 1772, pp. 122–123.

224 Cases of Elizabeth Davidson, in F. Home, Cases of patients, 1780–1781; and Mary Tennant, in Francis Home, Clinical cases from the Royal Infirmary and reports with notes as delivered by Francis Home, by Robert Dunlop, Edinburgh, 1786–1787, MSS Collection, Edinburgh Room, Edinburgh City Library.

225 Case of Mary Cockburn, in D. Rutherford, Clinical cases, 1799.

226 Case of Colin Lennox, in John Gregory, Clinical cases, 1771–1772. See also case of James Cairns, in F. Home, Cases of patients, 1780–1781.

227 Case of Charles Crawford, in D. Rutherford, Clinical cases, 1799.

228 Case of Barbara Millar, in James Gregory, Clinical reports, 1795–1796.

229 See cases of Hector McKenzie and Donald Murray, in W. Cullen, Clinical cases and reports, 1773–1774; see also W. Cullen, Clinical lectures, 1772–1773, p. 110.
230 Case of Alexander Cunningham, in T. C. Hope, Clinical casebook, 1796–1797. Some of these procedures to detect sugar were based on the work of Matthew Dobson, "Experiments and observations on the urine of diabetes," *Med. Obs. & Inquiries* (London) 5 (1776): 298–316.
231 George Fordyce, *A Third Dissertation on Fever*, London: J. Johnson, 1798, part 1, p. 92.
232 For a useful summary of eighteenth-century disease classifications consult Lester S. King, "Nosology," in his *Medical World of the Eighteenth Century*, Chicago: University of Chicago Press, 1958, chap. 7, pp. 193–226.
233 Thomas Sydenham, *The Works of Thomas Sydenham, M.D.*, trans. from Latin by R. G. Latham, 2 vols., London: Sydenham Society, 1847, vol. 1, p. 13.
234 L. S. King, "Boissier de Sauvages and 18th century nosology," *Bull. Hist. Med.* 40 (1966): 43–51.
235 An English translation of this work first appeared in 1792: William Cullen, *Synopsis and Nosology*, Hartford, CT: N. Palten.
236 William Cullen, *Nosology, or Systematic Arrangement of Diseases*, trans. from Latin, Edinburgh: W. Creech, 1800, pp. xvi–xvii.
237 W. Cullen, Clinical lectures, Feb.–Apr. 1772, pp. 75–80.
238 William Cullen, "On nosology," introductory lecture reprinted in *The Works of William Cullen, M.D.*, ed. by John Thomson, 2 vols., Edinburgh: Blackwood, 1828, vol. 1, p. 447.
239 For a discussion of the "medicine of species" see Michel Foucault, *The Birth of the Clinic: An Archeology of Medical Perception*, trans. from French by A. M. Sheridan Smith, New York: Vintage Books, 1975, chap. 1, pp. 3–21. Foucault cites several French sources in his contention that the hospital environment itself could likewise distort a particular species of disease, but the Edinburgh sources remain silent about the issue.

CHAPTER 3 *Patients and their diseases*

1 John Sinclair, *Analysis of the Statistical Account of Scotland*, 2 parts, Edinburgh: A. Constable, 1825, reprinted, New York: Johnson Reprint Co, 1970, part 1, p. 110.
2 The data were obtained by taking all consecutive diagnostic entries recorded in every fourth page of the General Register for the years 1770, 1775, 1780, 1785, 1790, 1795, and 1800. A total of 3,047 diagnoses were thus collected, distributed among 278 categories.
3 Although it is tempting to diagnose each eighteenth-century disease entity retrospectively, using contemporary medical criteria, the practice has been consistently avoided. Insufficient historical data and important clinical transformations that have occurred as a result of changing biological and social relationships make this procedure at times hazardous guesswork. For a discussion of the problem, see Jean-Pierre Peter, "Disease and the sick at the end of the eighteenth century," trans. from French by E. Forster in *Biology of Man in History*, ed. by E. Forster and O. Ranum, Baltimore: Johns Hopkins University Press, 1975, pp. 81–124. The original article appeared in the *Annales E.S.C.* in 1968.
4 For specific rules governing the admissions of venereal patients one should consult the histories of individual voluntary hospitals of the period, notably those located in London. For an overview of the issues at the end of the period under discussion see T. J. Wyke, "Hospital facilities for, and diagnosis and treatment of, venereal disease in England, 1800–1870," *Brit. J. Vener. Dis.* 49 (1973): 78–85.
5 William Buchan, *Domestic Medicine, or a Treatise on the Prevention and Cure of Diseases by Regimen and Simple Medicines*, Edinburgh, 1769, enlarged ed., New York: R. Scott, 1812, p. 293.
6 This information about prostitution in Edinburgh is contained in William Creech, *Letters Addressed to Sir John Sinclair . . .* , Edinburgh, 1793, reprinted, New York:

AMS Press, 1982, p. 36. This source is also quoted in an article by N. Smith, "Sexual mores and attitudes in Enlightenment Scotland," in *Sexuality in Eighteenth-Century Britain,* ed. by Paul-Gabriel Bouce, Manchester, England: Manchester University Press, 1982, pp. 47–73.

7 Buchan, *Domestic Medicine,* p. 308.

8 Andrew Duncan, *Observations on the Operation and Use of Mercury in the Venereal Disease,* Edinburgh: Kincaid & Creech, 1772, p. i.

9 William Nisbet, *First Lines of the Theory and Practice in Venereal Diseases,* Edinburgh: C. Elliot, 1787, pp. 17, 308–309. Nisbet was a student of William Cullen and received a doctorate in medicine from the University of Edinburgh. He also became a fellow of the RCS, Edinburgh. His book is dedicated to Cullen.

10 William Cullen, *Synopsis and Nosology,* Hartford, CT: N. Palten, 1792, pp. 54–55.

11 William Cullen, "Of syphilis or the venereal disease," in his *First Lines of the Practice of Physic,* new ed., Edinburgh: C. Elliot, 1786, vol. 4, chap. 2, pp. 383–384.

12 Benjamin Bell, *A Treatise on Gonorrhea Virulenta and Lues Venerea,* 2 vols., Edinburgh: J. Watson, 1793, vol. 2, p. 6. There is a brief biographical sketch of Benjamin Bell written by J. Wilson: "Benjamin Bell (1749–1806), the first of the Edinburgh scientific surgeons," *Practitioner* 218 (1977): 886–892.

13 Bell, *Gonorrhea,* vol. 2, pp. 36–37.

14 Cullen, *First Lines,* vol. 4, chap. 2, p. 386; Francois X. Swediaur, *Practical Observations on the More Obstinate and Inveterate Venereal Complaints,* London: T. Johnson, 1784. For biographical details about Swediaur see M. Kelly, "Swediaur: the vicious anti-Hunter rheumato-venereologist," *Med. Hist.* 11 (1967): 170–174.

15 John Hunter, *A Treatise on the Venereal Disease,* London, 1786. For a brief history of gonorrhea see R. S. Morton, "Gonorrhea in earlier times," in his *Gonorrhea,* Philadelphia: W. B. Saunders, 1977, pp. 1–24.

16 Francis Balfour, *De Gonorrhea Virulenta,* Edinburgh: Balfour, Auld & Smellie, 1767. More information about contemporary concepts in venereology is available in John Howard, *Practical Observations on the Natural History and Cure of Venereal Disease,* 3 vols., London: Baldwin, Longman & Johnson, 1787–1794.

17 Bell, vol. 1, especially pp. 1–7.

18 The arguments of Hunter and Bell are reviewed in Solomon Sawrey, *An Inquiry into Some of the Effects of the Venereal Poison on the Human Body,* London: E. Rider, 1802. For more details consult K. M. Flegel, "Changing concepts of the nosology of gonorrhea and syphilis," *Bull. Hist. Med.* 48 (1974): 571–588.

19 For more details see R. S. Morton, "The sibbens of Scotland," *Med. Hist.* 11 (1967): 374–380. The author suggests that this ailment was a nonvenereal treponematosis eradicated in the middle of the nineteenth century. A possible relationship between yaws and venereal syphilis is postulated in C. J. Hackett, "On the origin of the human treponematoses," *WHO Bull.* 29 (1963): 7–41.

20 Thomas Pennant, "A Tour in Scotland 1769," in his *Works,* 9 vols., London: B. White, 1776, vol. 9, part 2, appendix, number 14, p. 447.

21 Benjamin Bell, "Of some peculiarities of form under which lues venerea has appeared in Scotland and Canada," in his *Gonorrhea,* vol. 2, section 7, pp. 438–439.

22 Such an association led James Hill, a Dumfries surgeon, to define sibbens as "a mongrel breed" between a "*pocky cock* with a *scabbed hen* producing a *yaw chick.*" See James Hill, *Cases in Surgery,* Edinburgh: J. Balfour, 1772, pp. 229–230.

23 *Ibid.,* pp. 260–261.

24 Three women were admitted together on Feb. 12, 1780, and released together on July 14. A group of five, two men and three women, came into the ordinary medical ward on Apr. 18, 1795. All were dismissed exactly a month later.

25 Bell, vol. 1, p. 34.

26 Cullen, *First Lines,* vol. 3, pp. 9–48. The best-known contemporary gynecologic textbook was Jean Astruc, *Traité des maladies des femmes,* 6 vols., Paris: P. G. Cavelier, 1761–1765.

27 Cullen, *Synopsis and Nosology,* p. 14.

28 William Nisbet, *The Clinical Guide, or a Concise View of the Leading Facts on the*

History, Nature, and Treatment of Such Local Diseases as Form the Object of Surgery, 2nd ed., Edinburgh: J. Watson, 1800, pp. 304–307.

29 *Ibid.,* p. 304. The problem of bladder stone formation is examined by E. L. Priens, "The riddle of urinary stone disease," *J.A.M.A.* 216 (1971): 503–507.

30 Buchan, *Domestic Medicine,* p. 97. A connection between diabetes and injury to the pancreas was suggested in an article by Thomas Cawley, "A singular case of diabetes, consisting entirely in the quality of the urine; with an inquiry into the different theories of that disease," *London Med. J.* 9 (1788): 286–308.

31 Cullen, *Synopsis and Nosology,* p. 41.

32 Buchan, *Domestic Medicine,* pp. 206–207.

33 George Fordyce, *A Dissertation on Simple Fever,* London: J. Johnson, 1794, p. 6.

34 Cullen, *Synopsis and Nosology,* p. 1.

35 William Cullen, "Of fevers," in his *First Lines,* vol. 1, pp. 65–85. For a useful overview see the article "Febris" in Bartholomew Parr, *The London Medical Dictionary,* 2 vols., Philadelphia: Mitchell, Ames & White, 1819, vol. 1, pp. 642–654.

36 For eighteenth-century explanations and classifications of fever consult Lester S. King, "Of fevers," in his *Medical World of the Eighteenth Century,* Chicago: University of Chicago Press, 1958, chap. 5, pp. 123–138. Cullen's quotation is from his *First Lines,* vol. 1, p. 111. A social context in which the Edinburgh neurophysiological doctrines seemingly flourished has been presented by C. Lawrence, "The nervous system and society in the Scottish Enlightenment," in *Natural Order: Historical Studies of Scientific Culture,* ed. by B. Barnes and S. Shapin, Beverly Hills, CA: Sage Foundation, 1979, pp. 19–40.

37 James Gregory, *Additional Memorial to the Managers of the Royal Infirmary,* Edinburgh: Murray & Cochrane, 1803, p. 351.

38 *Ibid.*

39 For a complete discussion consult L. J. Bruce-Chwatt, "Ague as malaria (An essay on the history of two medical terms)," *J. Trop. Med. & Hyg.* 79 (1976): 168–176. Another explanation is that the word derives from the Gothic *agis,* meaning trembling: see Henry A. Skinner, *The Origin of Medical Terms,* New York: Hafner, 1970, p. 12.

40 A recent study of mortality rates in Kent and Essex from the sixteenth to the nineteenth centuries postulates such a linkage: M. Dobson, " 'Marsh fever' – the geography of malaria in England," *J. Hist. Geography* 6 (1980): 357–389.

41 Cullen, *First Lines,* vol. 1, pp. 83–85.

42 Buchan, *Domestic Medicine,* p. 109.

43 William Cullen, Clinical lectures, delivered for John Gregory, Feb.–Apr. 1772, Edinburgh, 1772, MSS Collection, RCP, Edinburgh, pp. 281–282.

44 Cullen, *First Lines,* vol. 1, pp. 140–142.

45 For an overview, see L. J. Bruce-Chwatt and J. De Zulueta, *The Rise and Fall of Malaria in Europe,* Oxford: Oxford University Press, 1980, pp. 131–135.

46 For example, cases of Margaret and Leslie Campbell, in Andrew Duncan, Sr., Clinical reports and commentaries, Feb.–Apr. 1795, presented by Alexander Blackhall Morison, Edinburgh, 1795; John Stewart and Rachel Parkinson, in James Gregory, Cases of patients under the care of James Gregory, M.D., Edinburgh, 1781–1782, both in MSS Collection, RCP, Edinburgh.

47 Sinclair, *Statistical Account,* part 1, p. 135.

48 Sinclair lists about eight parishes. Abernyte, Arngask, Dron, St. Madois, Kilspindie, and Kinnaird were in Perthshire, located between Perth and Dundee. Another, Barrie, was in Forfarshire just north of Dundee. Two additional parishes can be located in Berwickshire: Eccles and Cummertrees.

49 William Cullen, Clinical lectures, Edinburgh, 1772–1773, MSS Collection, RCP, Edinburgh, pp. 546–547.

50 W. Cullen, Clinical lectures, Feb.–Apr. 1772, p. 281.

51 These statistics were published in Charles Creighton, *A History of Epidemics in Britain,* 2 vols., Cambridge University Press, 1894, vol. 2, p. 370.

52 William Black, *Observations Medical and Political on the Smallpox*, 2nd ed. enlarged, London: J. Johnson, 1781, p. 100.
53 Cullen, *First Lines*, vol. 2, pp. 126–145.
54 John Aikin, *Thoughts on Hospitals*, London: J. Johnson, 1771, p. 47.
55 W. Cullen, Clinical lectures, 1772–1773, p. 71.
56 Aikin, *Hospitals*, p. 48.
57 [John Stedman], *The History and Statutes of the Royal Infirmary of Edinburgh*, Edinburgh: Balfour & Smellie, 1778, p. 85.
58 William Cullen, *Nosology, or Systematic Arrangement of Diseases*, trans. from Latin, Edinburgh: W. Creech, 1800, pp. 38–42.
59 Benjamin Bell, "On inflammation" in his *System of Surgery*, 7th ed., 7 vols., Edinburgh: Bell, Bradfute & Dickson, 1801, vol. 1, pp. 17–18 [subsequent citations to the *System of Surgery* are to this edition unless otherwise indicated]. See also John Hunter, *A Treatise on the Blood, Inflammation, and Gun-shot Wounds*, London: G. Nicol, 1794.
60 Benjamin Bell, *A Treatise on the Theory and Management of Ulcers*, Edinburgh: C. Elliot, 1778. This work is also reprinted in his 7-vol. *System of Surgery*, the first edition of which was published between 1783 and 1788. Quotations and references to *Ulcers* are from the U.S. edition, Boston: Thomas & Andrews, 1791, p. 79.
61 These statistics are presented in I. S. L. Loudon, "Leg ulcers in the eighteenth and early nineteenth centuries," *J. Royal Coll. Gral. Practitioners* 31 (1981): 263.
62 C. Brown, "On the necessity of establishing an hospital for the treatment of ulcerated legs," *Med. & Phys. J.* 3 (1800): 135–136. This information is included in Loudon's article "Leg ulcers."
63 Bell, *Ulcers*, pp. 82–85.
64 *Ibid.*, p. 247.
65 *Ibid.*, p. 249.
66 *Ibid.*, pp. 248–250.
67 *Ibid.*, pp. 90–101.
68 See Loudon, "Leg ulcers," or the sequel to that article, "Leg ulcers in the eighteenth and early nineteenth centuries – treatment," *J. Royal Coll. Gral. Practitioners* 32 (1982): 301–309.
69 Bell, *Ulcers*, p. 115.
70 Bell, *System of Surgery*, vol. 1, pp. 50–57.
71 *Ibid.*, vol. 1, pp. 76–78.
72 *Ibid.*, vol. 1, pp. 312–314.
73 *Ibid.*, vol. 1, pp. 251–262.
74 Cullen, *Synopsis and Nosology*, p. 36.
75 [Sedman], *History and Statutes*, p. 88.
76 Aikin, *Hospitals*, p. 51.
77 A. J. Youngson, *The Making of Classical Edinburgh, 1750–1840*, Edinburgh: Edinburgh University Press, 1966, p. 36.
78 Cullen, *First Lines*, vol. 3, p. 83.
79 *Ibid.*, vol. 3, pp. 90–91.
80 Case of Janet Kidd, in Daniel Rutherford, Clinical cases, Edinburgh, 1799, MSS Collection, RCP, Edinburgh.
81 W. Cullen, Clinical lectures, 1772–1773, p. 97; case of Daniel Rose, in A. Duncan, Sr., Clinical reports and commentaries, 1795.
82 Cullen, *First Lines*, vol. 2, pp. 356–358.
83 *Ibid.*, vol. 2, p. 384.
84 Sinclair, *Statistical Account*, part 1, p. 138.
85 The Edinburgh Bill of Burials was printed monthly in *Scots Magazine;* a General Bill of Mortality for the entire year appeared in the same publication.
86 Cullen, *First Lines*, vol. 2, p. 386.
87 *Ibid.*, vol. 2, p. 390.
88 *Ibid.*, vol. 1, p. 362.

89 George Motherby, *A New Medical Dictionary or General Repository of Physic*, 3rd ed., London: J. Johnson, 1791, p. 79; Cullen, *Synopsis and Nosology*, p. 9. The best work on croup or diphtheria was written by one of the Edinburgh professors: Francis Home, *An Inquiry into the Nature, Cause, and Cure of the Croup*, Edinburgh: Kincaid & Bell, 1765.

90 Parr, *London Medical Dictionary*, vol. 1, pp. 587, pp. 146–147.

91 Cullen, *First Lines*, vol. 3, pp. 217–225.

92 *Ibid.*, vol. 4, pp. 9–16.

93 *Ibid.*, vol. 3, pp. 225–226.

94 Sinclair, *Statistical Account*, part 1, p. 142.

95 *Caledonian Gazetteer*, no. 1, Friday, May 31, 1776.

96 Frederick W. Watkeys, *Old Edinburgh*, 2 vols., Boston: L. Page, 1908, vol. 2, pp. 192–193.

97 Parr, *London Medical Dictionary*, vol. 1, p. 146; Cullen, *First Lines*, vol. 3, p. 225.

98 Sinclair, *Statistical Account*, part 1, p. 141.

99 Cullen, *First Lines*, vol. 3, p. 225.

100 Cullen, *Synopsis and Nosology*, pp. 40–41.

101 *Ibid.*, p. 38.

102 Anonymous, *The Edinburgh Practice of Physic and Surgery*, 5 vols., London: Kearsley, vol. 1, 1800, pp. 435–436. For more details see Thomas Percival, *Observations and Experiments on the Poison of Lead*, London: J. Johnson, 1774. For a recent review of the history of lead poisoning see T. Eisinger, "Lead and wine: Eberhard Gockel and the colica pictonum," *Med. Hist.* 26 (1982): 279–302.

103 Buchan, *Domestic Medicine*, p. 197. For the problems in Devon consult H. A. Waldron, "The Devonshire colic," *J. Hist. Med.* 25 (1970): 383–413.

104 Buchan, *Domestic Medicine*, p. 193.

105 *Edinburgh Practice of Physic*, vol. 1, p. 439.

106 Cullen, *First Lines*, vol. 1, pp. 437–439.

107 Motherby, *New Medical Dictionary*, p. 420.

108 Cullen, *Synopsis and Nosology*, pp. 56–57.

109 Cullen, *First Lines*, vol. 4, pp. 435–441.

110 W. Cullen, Clinical lectures, 1772–1773, p. 543.

111 W. Cullen, Clinical lectures, Feb.–Apr. 1772, pp. 32–33.

112 Sinclair, *Statistical Account*, part 1, pp. 132–134.

113 *Ibid.*, p. 134.

114 W. Cullen, Clinical lectures, 1772–1773, p. 411.

115 Cullen, *Synopsis and Nosology*, p. 15.

116 W. Cullen, Clinical lectures, 1772–1773, p. 420. For more details see Cullen, *First Lines*, vol. 2, pp. 9–37.

117 W. Cullen, Clinical lectures, 1772–1773, p. 440. For an overview consult W. S. C. Copeman, "Acute rheumatism and chorea," in his *Short History of the Gout and the Rheumatic Diseases*, Berkeley, CA: University of California Press, 1964, chap. 8, pp. 118–124.

118 Aikin, *Hospitals*, pp. 43–44.

119 W. Cullen, Clinical lectures, 1772–1773, pp. 411–412.

120 John Haygarth, *A Clinical History of Diseases*, London: Cadell & Davies, 1805, p. 30.

121 *Ibid.*, pp. 20–21.

122 Christopher Lloyd and Jack L. S. Coulter, *Medicine and the Navy, 1200–1900*, vol. 3, *1714–1815*, Edinburgh: E. & S. Livingstone, 1961, p. 348.

123 *Edinburgh Practice of Physic*, vol. 1, p. 251; Motherby, *New Medical Dictionary*, p. 642.

124 Cullen, *First Lines*, vol. 4, pp. 332–343.

125 Buchan, *Domestic Medicine*, p. 39.

126 Cullen, *First Lines*, vol. 4, p. 343.

127 *Ibid.*, vol. 3, p. 286. See also *Edinburgh Practice of Physic*, vol. 1, pp. 398–409.

128 Cullen, *First Lines*, vol. 3, p. 170.

129 *Ibid.*, vol. 3, pp. 170–171. The special type of leg paralysis that follows tuberculosis

of the spine was described by Percivall Pott, *Remarks on That Kind of Palsy of the Lower Limbs Which Is Frequently Found to Accompany a Curvature of the Spine*, London: J. Johnson, 1779.

130 Motherby, *New Medical Dictionary*, pp. 226–227. The first description of so-called migraine headaches was made by John Fothergill, "Remarks on that complaint known under the name of sick headache," *Med. Obs. & Inquiries* (London) 6 (1777–1784): 103–137.

131 W. Cullen, Clinical lectures, 1772–1773, pp. 85–86. This signal before the fit was frequent enough so that physicians attempted to intercept its ascent and thus prevent an epileptic attack.

132 Buchan, *Domestic Medicine*, pp. 262–263.

133 Motherby, *New Medical Dictionary*, p. 726.

134 *Ibid.*, p. 133.

135 Cullen, *Synopsis and Nosology*, p. 33.

136 *Edinburgh Practice of Physic*, vol. 1, pp. 180–182.

137 Cullen, *First Lines*, vol. 4, pp. 93–99. One of the influential works of the period was Robert Whytt, *Observations on the Nature, Causes and Cure of Those Disorders Which Have Been Commonly Called Nervous, Hypochondriac, or Hysteric*, Edinburgh: T. Becket & P. du Hondt, 1765.

138 Buchan, *Domestic Medicine*, p. 62; Cullen, *First Lines*, vol. 4, pp. 99–105.

139 Cullen, *First Lines*, vol. 3, p. 250. An important contemporary monograph on the subject was John Hill, *Hypochondriasis: A Practical Treatise on the Nature and Cure of That Disorder*, London, 1766, reprinted with an introduction by G. S. Rousseau, Los Angeles: Williams Andrews Clark Memorial Library, 1969. See E. Fischer-Homberger, "Hypochondriasis of the eighteenth century – neurosis of the present century," *Bull. Hist. Med.* 46 (1972): 391–401.

140 Buchan, *Domestic Medicine*, p. 53. The classic eighteenth-century monograph on hypochondriasis was George Cheyne, *The English Malady*, London: G. Strahan, 1733.

141 Motherby, *New Medical Dictionary*, p. 506; Cullen, *First Lines*, vol. 4, pp. 168–184. Background information is available in T. H. Jobe, "Medical theories of melancholia in the seventeenth and early eighteenth centuries," *Clio Medica* 11 (1976): 217–231; and S. W. Jackson, "Melancholia and mechanical explanations in eighteenth-century medicine," *J. Hist. Med.* 38 (1983): 298–319.

142 Buchan, *Domestic Medicine*, p. 95.

143 Cullen, *First Lines*, vol. 4, pp. 146–147. For details see William Battie, *A Treatise on Madness (1758) and Remarks by John Monro: A Psychiatric Controversy of the Eighteenth Century*, introduction by R. Hunter and I. Macalpine, London: Dawsons, 1962.

144 Cullen, *First Lines*, vol. 4, p. 123.

145 James Gregory, "Mania," a lecture delivered in 1788–1789, in MSS Collection, National Library of Medicine, Washington, D.C.

146 Bell, *System of Surgery*, vol. 6, pp. 406–412. See also one of the best contemporary works on the subject: Percivall Pott, *Some Few Remarks on Fractures and Dislocations*, London: L. Hawes, W. Clarke, R. Collins, 1765.

147 Bell, *System of Surgery*, vol. 1, pp. 186–188.

148 *Ibid.*, vol. 1, p. 327.

149 *Ibid.*, vol. 1 pp. 414–429. More details are in Percivall Pott, *Observations on the Nature and Consequences of Wounds and Contusions of the Head, etc.*, London: C. Hitch & L. Hawes, 1760.

150 Bell, *System of Surgery*, vol. 2, p. 203.

151 *Ibid.*, vol. 2, p. 211.

152 Cullen, *First Lines*, vol. 4, pp. 357–358. An attempt to classify skin diseases – he distinguished about 115 different entities – is contained in Joseph J. Plenk, *Doctrina de Morbis Cutaneis*, Vienna: R. Graeffer, 1776. An improvement, albeit incomplete, was Robert Willan, *On Cutaneous Diseases*, London: J. Johnson, [1796] 1808; only one volume was published.

153 Buchan, *Domestic Medicine*, p. 46.

154 W. Cullen, Clinical lectures, Feb.–Apr. 1772, pp. 203, 231–232.
155 Cullen, *First Lines*, vol. 2, pp. 222–229.
156 Buchan, *Domestic Medicine*, pp. 49, 171–173.
157 *Ibid.*, pp. 243–244.
158 *Edinburgh Practice of Physic*, vol. 1, pp. 512–522. The problem of scurvy and its impact on the mortality of ship crews has been extensively studied. In a series of articles under the title "Scurvy as an occupational disease," C. P. McCord summarizes the history of the disease throughout the centuries: *J. Occup. Med.* 13 (1971): 306–307, 348–351, 393–395, 441–447, 484–491, 543–548.
159 Much has been written about James Lind and his experimental method in the discovery of lemon juice as a cure for scurvy. See, for example, R. E. Hughes, "James Lind and the cure of scurvy: an experimental approach," *Med. Hist.* 19 (1975): 342–351; and C. Lloyd, "The introduction of lemon juice as a cure for scurvy," *Bull. Hist. Med.* 35 (1961): 123–132. Lind's original *Treatise of the Scurvy* was first published in Edinburgh during the year 1753 and is available in reprint: *Lind's Treatise on Scurvy*, ed. by C. P. Stewart and D. Guthrie, Edinburgh: Edinburgh University Press, 1953.
160 Cullen, *Synopsis and Nosology*, p. 80.
161 Motherby, *New Medical Dictionary*, p. 617.
162 Buchan, *Domestic Medicine*, p. 325.
163 Motherby, *New Medical Dictionary*, p. 415. See also Bell, *System of Surgery*, vol. 2, pp. 405–410.
164 Cullen, *Synopsis and Nosology*, p. 56.
165 *Edinburgh Practice of Physic*, vol. 1, pp. 525–526.
166 Buchan, *Domestic Medicine*, p. 325.
167 Cullen, *Synopsis and Nosology*, p. 80; Bell, *System of Surgery*, vol. 2, p. 428.
168 Cullen, *First Lines*, vol. 4, p. 249. Details are contained in Donald Monro, *An Essay on the Dropsy and Its Different Species*, 3rd ed., London: A. Millar, 1765.
169 Cullen, *First Lines*, vol. 4, pp. 253–267.
170 *Ibid.*, vol. 4, p. 321.
171 *Edinburgh Practice of Physic*, vol. 1, pp. 485–488. See also Cullen, *First Lines*, vol. 4, pp. 321–327.
172 Cullen, *First Lines*, vol. 4, pp. 308–317.
173 Motherby, *New Medical Dictionary*, pp. 442–423. For details see Robert Whytt, *Observations on the Dropsy of the Brain*, Edinburgh: J. Balfour, 1768.
174 W. Cullen, Clinical lectures, 1772–1773, p. 337.
175 Case of James Lauder, in A. Duncan, Sr., Clinical reports and commentaries, 1795; Cullen, Clinical lectures, Feb.–Apr. 1772, p. 325.
176 Bell, *System of Surgery*, vol. 6, p. 321. See also Cullen, *First Lines*, vol. 2, pp. 424–430.
177 Bell, *System of Surgery*, vol. 6, pp. 325–327; see also Cullen, *First Lines*, vol. 2, pp. 431–440.
178 Bell, *System of Surgery*, vol. 1, p. 111.
179 *Ibid.*, vol. 1, pp. 114–116.
180 Cullen, *Synopsis and Nosology*, p. 54.
181 Buchan, *Domestic Medicine*, p. 246.
182 Cullen, *First Lines*, vol. 4, p. 367.
183 *Ibid.*, vol. 4, pp. 359–371. For further details see William Nisbet, *An Inquiry into the History, Nature, Causes and Different Modes of Treatment of Scrophula and Cancer*, Edinburgh: Chapman, 1795.
184 Cullen, *Synopsis and Nosology*, p. 78.
185 Motherby, *New Medical Dictionary*, p. 658.
186 Cullen, *Synopsis and Nosology*, p. 78.
187 Bell, *System of Surgery*, vol. 2, pp. 375–381.
188 *Ibid.*, vol. 2, p. 375.
189 Motherby, *New Medical Dictionary*, pp. 188–192; John Pearson, *Practical Observations on Cancerous Complaints*, London: J. Johnson, 1793, pp. 89–95. A contemporary

monograph on the subject of breast cancer is George Bell, *Thoughts on the Cancer of the Breast*, Birmingham: J. Johnson, 1788. An overview of eighteenth-century ideas about breast cancer can be found in D. de Moulin, "Historical notes on breast cancer, with emphasis on the Netherlands: Pathophysiological concepts, diagnosis and therapy in the 18th century," *Netherlands J. Surg.* 33–34 (1981): 206–216.

190 Bell, *System of Surgery*, vol. 2, p. 368.

191 Motherby, *New Medical Dictionary*, pp. 678, 607.

192 Buchan, *Domestic Medicine*, pp. 176–177; Cullen, *First Lines*, vol. 1, p. 316. The terminology remained vague until the turn of the century. A more accurate pathology facilitated a better classification system: James Wardrop, *Essays on the Morbid Anatomy of the Human Eye*, 2 vols., Edinburgh: G. Ramsay, 1808–1818.

193 Cullen, *Synopsis and Nosology*, pp. 57–58; Motherby, *New Medical Dictionary*, p. 183.

194 Parr, *London Medical Dictionary*, vol. 1, p. 88–89; Motherby, *New Medical Dictionary*, p. 58.

195 W. Cullen, Clinical lectures, Feb.–Apr. 1772, p. 128.

196 W. Cullen, Clinical lectures, 1772–1773, p. 64. The trial by blisters is explained in ibid., p. 47.

197 Case of John Chaplain, in Francis Home, Cases of patients under the care of Francis Home, Edinburgh, 1780–1781, MSS Collection, RCP, Edinburgh. One of the widely accepted medical methods of smallpox inoculation at that time is described by Thomas Dimsdale, *The Present Method of Inoculating for the Smallpox*, London: W. Owen, 1767.

198 Bell, *System of Surgery*, vol. 4, pp. 180–256. For more details see also Percivall Pott, *Chirurgical Observations Relative to the Cataract, etc.*, London: L. Hawes, W. Clarke, R. Collins, 1775.

199 Bell, *System of Surgery*, vol. 5, p. 251. See also Percivall Pott's *Treatise on Ruptures*, originally published in 1756, 5th ed., London: L. Hawes, 1775.

200 Bell, *System of Surgery*, vol. 5, p. 270.

201 *Ibid.*, vol. 5, pp. 273–279.

202 *Ibid.*, vol. 5, p. 387. For more details on this topic, see Percivall Pott, *Practical Remarks on the Hydrocele*, 2nd ed., London: L. Hawes, 1767.

203 Bell, *System of Surgery*, vol. 4, pp. 447–473.

204 *Ibid.*, vol. 5 p. 9. The best contemporary work on dental diseases was John Hunter, *A Practical Treatise on the Diseases of the Teeth*, London: J. Johnson, 1778.

205 Bell, *System of Surgery*, vol. 7, p. 226.

206 *Ibid.*, vol. 7, p. 227.

207 *Ibid.*, vol. 7, pp. 228–229. For an overview also consult J. Watt, "The injuries of four centuries of naval warfare," *Ann. Roy. Coll. Surg. Engl.* 57 (1975): 3–24.

208 Bell, *System of Surgery*, vol. 7, p. 253.

209 Alexander Monro's mortality rate for amputations at the infirmary in the 1740s and early 1750s was reported as being 8%. See his "Remarks on the amputations of the larger extremities," in his *Medical Essays and Observations*, 4th ed., vol. 4 (1752), p. 276, quoted in O. H. Wangensteen, J. Smith, and S. D. Wangensteen, "Some highlights in the history of amputation reflecting lessons in wound healing," *Bull. Hist. Med.* 41 (1967): 106.

210 For a summary of the historical developments consult Owen H. Wangensteen and Sarah D. Wangensteen, "Lithotomy and lithotomists," in their *Rise of Surgery*, Folkestone, England: Dawson, 1978, chap. 4, pp. 65–92. For the prevalance of urinary stones in Norwich and eighteenth-century hospital statistics about lithotomy at the local hospital, see A. Batty Shaw, "The Norwich School of lithotomy," *Med. Hist.* 14 (1970): 221–259.

211 William Falconer, *An Account of the Efficacy of the Aqua Mephitica Alkaline*, 2nd ed., London, 1787; Robert Whytt, *An Essay on the Virtues of Lime-water in the Cure of the Stone*, 3rd ed., Edinburgh, 1761. See A. J. Viseltear, "Attempts to dissolve bladder stones by direct injection," *Bull. Hist. Med.* 43 (1969): 477–481.

212 Bell, *System of Surgery*, vol. 1, p. 111

213 *Ibid.*, vol. 1, pp. 184–185. The "lateral" lithotomy pioneered by William Cheselden

was described in his *Treatise on the High Operation for the Stone*, London: J. Osborn, 1723. Cheselden was a surgeon at St. Thomas Hospital, London.

214 Bell, *System of Surgery*, vol. 3, pp. 400–401.

215 Data for the Newcastle and Manchester infirmaries in the 1750s were taken from John Woodward, *To Do the Sick No Harm: A Study of the British Voluntary Hospital System to 1875*, London: Routledge & Kegan Paul, 1974, app. 5, pp. 160–162. Woodward's figures were obtained from annual hospital reports. The information for the Bristol Royal Infirmary comes from George Munro Smith, *A History of the Bristol Royal Infirmary*, Bristol: J. W. Arrowsmith, 1917, p. 89. It covers the period Jan. 1–Dec. 31, 1762, and deals only with medical cases.

CHAPTER 4 *Hospital care*

1 Francis Home, *Clinical Experiments, Histories, and Dissections*, 2nd corrected ed., London: Murray; Edinburgh: W. Creech, 1782, p. vi.

2 William Cullen, "Therapeutics," in Institutes of Medicine, lecture notes, Edinburgh, 1772, MSS Collection, National Library of Medicine, Washington, D.C., vol. 7, p. 6. For a useful outline of the logic governing traditional therapeutics see C. E. Rosenberg, "The therapeutic revolution: medicine, meaning, and social change in nineteenth-century America," *Perspect. Biol. Med.* 20 (1977): 485–506.

3 Francis Home, Clinical lectures delivered in the year 1769, taken by John Goodsir, Edinburgh, 1769, MSS Collection, RCP, Edinburgh, preliminary lecture, pp. 10, 24. For a historical review of the healing power of nature see Max Neuburger, *Die Lehre von der Heilkraft der Natur im Wandel der Zeiten*, Stuttgart: F. Enke, 1926.

4 William Cullen, Clinical lectures, Edinburgh, 1772–1773, MSS Collection, RCP, Edinburgh, pp. 359–360, 541.

5 John C. Lettsom, *Reflections on the General Treatment and Cure of Fevers*, London: Cornish, 1772, preface (no pagination). For an overview of eighteenth-century therapeutics see Lester S. King, "The practice of medicine," in his *Medical World of the Eighteenth Century*, Chicago: University of Chicago Press, 1958, chap. 10, pp. 297–325.

6 George Fordyce, *A Dissertation on Simple Fever*, London: J. Johnson, 1794, p. 37. See L. S. King, "Theory and practice in eighteenth century medicine," *Studies on Voltaire* 153 (1976): 1201–1218.

7 Fordyce, *Simple Fever*, p. 27.

8 W. Cullen, Clinical lectures, 1772–1773, pp. 199–200.

9 Cullen, "Therapeutics," pp. 8–17. See also Andrew Duncan, Sr., *Elements of Therapeutics*, 2 vols., 2nd ed., Edinburgh: Drummond, 1773, vol. 1, pp. 8–9.

10 George Fordyce, *A Third Dissertation on Fever*, London: J. Johnson, 1798, part 1, p. 223.

11 F. Home, Clinical lectures, 1769, p. 3.

12 Edward Topham, *Letters from Edinburgh Written in Years 1774 and 1775*, 2 vols., Dublin: Watson, 1776, vol. 2, p. 76.

13 George Fordyce, *A Second Dissertation on Fever*, London: J. Johnson, 1795, p. 154.

14 William Cullen, Clinical lectures delivered for John Gregory, Feb.–Apr. 1772, Edinburgh, 1772, MSS Collection, RCP, Edinburgh, p. 276.

15 W. Cullen, Clinical lectures, 1772–1773, p. 595.

16 RIE, *Report of a Committee on the State of the Hospital*, Edinburgh, 1818, p. 67.

17 William Cullen, *First Lines of the Practice of Physic*, new ed., 4 vols. Edinburgh: C. Elliot, 1786, vol. 3, pp. 217–226.

18 James Gregory, *Additional Memorial to the Managers of the Royal Infirmary*, Edinburgh: Murray & Cochrane, 1803, pp. 412–413.

19 Joseph Wilde, *The Hospital: A Poem in Three Books*, Norwich, England: Stevenson, Matchett & Stevenson, 1810, p. 8.

20 *Ibid.*, p. 9.

21 *Ibid.*, p. 7.

22 "It is impossible to know all the several circumstances and occurrences that happen to our patients in this house." W. Cullen, Clinical lectures, 1772–1773, p. 560.

23 Peter Mac Flogg'em, *Aesculapian Secrets Revealed*, London, 1813, p. 43.
24 Thomas Percival, *Medical Ethics, or a Code of Institutes and Precepts, Adapted to the Professional Conduct of Physicians and Surgeons*, Manchester: J. Johnson, 1808, new ed. with an introduction by C. R. Burns, Huntington, N.Y.: R. E. Krieger, 1975. For an overview see I. Waddington, "The development of medical ethics – a sociological perspective, *Med. Hist.* 19 (1975): 36–51; and Lester S. King, "The development of medical ethics," in his *Medical World*, chap. 8, pp. 227–261.
25 John Gregory, *Observations on the Duties and Offices of a Physician*, London: W. Strahan & T. Cadell, 1770, pp. 18–19. For an explanation of Gregory's thought see L. B. McCullough, "Historical perspectives on the ethical dimensions of the patient-physician relationship: the medical ethics of Dr. John Gregory," *Ethics in Science & Medicine* 5 (1978): 47–53. For an overview see G. B. Risse, "Patients and their healers: historical studies in health care," in *Who Decides? Conflicts of Rights in Health Care*, ed. by N. K. Bell, Clifton, N.J.: Humana Press, 1982, chap. 2, pp. 27–45.
26 Wilde, *The Hospital*, pp. 17, 38.
27 *Ibid.*, p. 61.
28 James Gregory, *Memorial to the Managers of the Royal Infirmary*, Edinburgh: Murray & Cochrane, 1800, p. 62.
29 W. Cullen, Clinical lectures, 1772–1773, pp. 101, 63.
30 RIE, *Report of a Committee*, p. 90.
31 W. Cullen, Clinical lectures, Feb.–Apr. 1772, pp. 118, 239.
32 W. Cullen, Clinical lectures, 1772–1773, p. 97. See also pp. 284, 397.
33 W. Cullen, Clinical lectures, Feb.–Apr. 1772, p. 247.
34 *Ibid.*, p. 27.
35 Gregory, *Additional Memorial*, p. 349. As Cullen lectured, in "hospitals that receive infectious diseases there is no management but to give each of the patients a proper well ventilated apartment." Clinical lectures, Feb.–Apr. 1772, p. 309.
36 Robert Jackson, *Memorial addressed to the managers of the Royal Infirmary of Edinburgh*, Edinburgh: Mundell & Son, 1800, pp. 5–8.
37 For example, case of Janet Seaton, in William Cullen, *Clinical Lectures Delivered in the Years 1765 and 1766*, London: Lee & Hurst, 1797, p. 277.
38 John Howard, *Appendix to the State of the Prisons in England and Wales, Containing a Further Account of Foreign Prisons and Hospitals*, Warrington, England: W. Eyres, 1784, p. 151. Howard recommended that the ceiling and walls of every ward be well scraped and then washed with limestone taken hot from the kiln and flaked in boiling water. The procedure was called "lime-white" and was guaranteed "to destroy vermin, purify the air, and prevent infection."
39 John Howard, *The State of the Prisons in England and Wales*, 4th ed., London: J. Johnson, C. Dilly & T. Cadell, 1792, p. 30.
40 Gregory, *Additional Memorial*, p. 344.
41 RIE, *Report of a Committee*, p. 4. In spite of such favorable pronouncements, infirmary practitioners reported instances where a catarrh, fever, or diarrheal complaint was blamed on the patient occupying the next bed. See cases of Christian Grant, in Andrew Duncan, Sr., Clinical reports and commentaries, Feb.–Apr. 1795, presented by Alexander Blackhall Morison, Edinburgh, 1795, MSS Collection, RCP, Edinburgh; Mary Sharp, in James Gregory, Clinical reports, Nov. 1, 1795–Feb. 1, 1796, Edinburgh, 1795–1796, MSS Collection, University of Edinburgh; and Jean Cormie, in Thomas C. Hope, Clinical casebook, Edinburgh, 1796–1797, MSS Collection, RCP, Edinburgh.
42 RIE, *Report of a Committee*, pp. 5–19.
43 *Ibid.*, p. 68.
44 *Ibid.*, p. 5. The fumigations of nitrous air were proposed by James C. Smyth, *Account of the Experiment . . . to Determine the Effect of the Nitrous Acid in Destroying Contagion*, London: J. Johnson, 1796. The implications were discussed in a book review published in the *Annals of Medicine* 1 (1796): 110. Among the prescriptions copied in student notebooks are several concerning clean clothing. "To have clean shirt from the house" or "clean linen to her person and bed" were included in the physician's orders in the cases of Kenneth Steward, in John Hope, Cases of patients

in the Royal Infirmary under the care of John Hope, M.C., Edinburgh, 1781, MSS Collection, University of Edinburgh; and Ann Shillinglaw, in James Gregory, Cases of patients under the care of James Gregory, M.D., Edinburgh, 1781–1782, MSS Collection, RCP, Edinburgh.

45 Jackson, *Memorial*, p. 8.
46 RIE, *Report of a Committee*, pp. 2–3.
47 *Ibid.*, pp. 3–12. Conditions improved in the early nineteenth century when a new washhouse was completed, with facilities for boiling clothes and sheets and for soaking the linens in bleach.
48 Gregory, *Additional Memorial*, pp. 349–350.
49 *Ibid.*, p. 353.
50 See, for example, *Pharmacopoeia Colegii Regalis Medicorum Londinensis*, London, 1788, trans. by J. Latham as *The New Pharmacopea of the Royal College of Physicians of London*, 5th ed., revised, London, 1791; and Peter Shaw, *Pharmacopoea Edinburgensis or the Dispensatory of the Royal College of Physicians in Edinburgh*, 5th ed., London, 1753. For their historical development consult D. L. Cowen, "The Edinburgh Pharmacopoeia," *Med. Hist.* 1 (1957): 123–139.
51 *Pharmacopoeia Pauperum in Usum Nosocomii Regii Edinburgensis*, 3rd ed., Edinburgh, 1758. This book was translated into English a few years earlier as *The Dispensatory for the Use of the Royal Hospital in Edinburgh*, London, 1753 [hereafter cited as RIE, *Dispensatory*]. An even earlier edition used in this study was appended to William Lewis, ed., *The Pharmacopoeia of the Royal College of Physicians at Edinburgh*, London: J. Nourse, 1748, and titled "The dispensatory for the use of the poor in the Royal Hospital at Edinburgh," pp. 338–362. Most of the prescriptions are also listed in the anonymous *Practice of the British and French Hospitals, viz the Edinburgh, Military and Naval Hospitals, L'Hôtel Dieu, La Charité and Les Invalides*, 2nd ed., London: R. Baldwin, 1775, pp. 1–39.
52 William Cullen, *A Treatise of the Materia Medica*, 2 vols., Edinburgh: J. Cruikshank & R. Campbell, 1789.
53 W. Cullen, Clinical lectures, 1772–1773, p. 619. Such a purely clinical awareness of the effects caused by drugs has been termed "protopharmacology" by Chauncey D. Leake. See J. W. Estes, "Making therapeutic decisions with protopharmacologic evidence," *Trans. & Stud. Coll. Phys.* (Philadelphia), 5th ser., 1 (1979): 116–137. For practice in an Edinburgh dispensary see L. S. King, "The practice of medicine in 1787," *Illinois Med. J.* 130 (1955): 130–134. Cullen was always optimistic about the benefits of medicine: "We are never to hold any disease incurable till remedies have been tried to no purpose. There is no good to be gotten from despair. Efforts are to be used as long as they can be with any probability or safety." W. Cullen, Clinical lectures, 1772–1773, p. 567.
54 Fordyce, *Third Dissertation on Fever*, part 1, p. 175.
55 W. Cullen, Clinical lectures, 1772–1773, p. 78.
56 *Ibid.*, p. 616.
57 Duncan, *Elements of Therapeutics*, vol. 1, p. 135.
58 W. Cullen, Clinical lectures, 1772–1773, pp. 38, 44, 267.
59 Home, *Clinical Experiments*, pp. 1–13.
60 Case of Eleanor Jersy, in A. Duncan, Sr., Clinical reports and commentaries, 1795.
61 Gregory, *Memorial*, p. 143.
62 *Ibid.*, pp. 139–141.
63 *Ibid.*, p. 142.
64 Duncan, *Elements of Therapeutics*, vol. 1, pp. 18–19; Cullen, *Materia Medica*, vol. 1, pp. 115–117.
65 Duncan, *Elements of Therapeutics*, vol. 1, pp. 52–57.
66 *Ibid.*, vol. 2, pp. 12–20; Bartholomew Parr, *The London Medical Dictionary*, 2 vols., Philadelphia: Mitchell, Ames & White, 1819, vol. 1, pp. 374–378. See also Cullen, *Materia Medica*, vol. 2, pp. 333–368.
67 W. Cullen, Clinical lectures, 1772–1773, p. 81.
68 *Ibid.*, p. 511. For more details see Daniel Lyson, *Essay upon the Effects of Camphire and Calomel in Continual Fevers*, London: E. Reeve, 1771.

69 Case of Mary Guthrie, in John Gregory, Clinical cases of the Royal Infirmary of Edinburgh, Edinburgh, 1771–1772, MSS Collection, Medical Archives, University of Edinburgh.

70 James Hamilton, *Observations on the Utility and Administration of Purgative Medicines in Several Diseases*, Philadelphia: B. Johnson, 1809, p. 21.

71 *Ibid.*, pp. 22–25.

72 Parr, *London Medical Dictionary*, vol. 1, pp. 129–130; Cullen, *Materia Medica*, vol. 2, pp. 148–218.

73 RIE, *Dispensatory*, pp. 349, 359; case of Elizabeth Kyle, in James Gregory, Cases of patients, 1781–1782.

74 G. B. Risse, "The Brownian system of medicine: its theoretical and practical implications," *Clio Medica* 5 (1970): 45–51. See also Parr, *London Medical Dictionary*, vol. 2, p. 311–315.

75 John Leigh, *An Experimental Inquiry into the Properties of Opium and Its Effects on Living Subjects*, London: C. Elliot, 1785. This work won the Harveian Prize of 1785. See also Samuel Crumpe, *An Inquiry into the Nature and Properties of Opium*, London: G. G. & J. Robertson, 1793, especially pp. 168–192. Crumpe was a student of James Gregory who followed Brown's ideas.

76 Martin Wall, *Clinical Observations on the Use of Opium in Low Fevers*, Oxford: D. Prince & J. Cooke, 1786; David Campbell, *Observations on the Typhus or Low Contagious Fever*, Lancaster: Walmsley, 1785, especially pp. 80–96. Consult J. C. Kramer, "Opium rampant: medical use, misuse, and abuse in Britain and the West in the 17th and 18th centuries," *Br. J. Addict.* 74 (1979): 377–389; and Virginia Berridge and Griffith Edwards, *Opium and the People: Opiate Use in Nineteenth-century England*, London: Allen Lane, 1982.

77 Cullen, *Materia Medica*, vol. 2, pp. 312–332.

78 Duncan, *Elements of Therapeutics*, vol. 2, p. 1.

79 Parr, *London Medical Dictionary*, vol. 1, pp. 600–604.

80 William Nisbet, "Classifications of the principal articles of the materia medica," in his *Clinical Guide, or a Concise View of the Leading Facts on the History, Nature, and Cure of Diseases; to Which Is Subjoined a Practical Pharmacopoeia*, Edinburgh: J. Watson, 1793, pp. 69–70. Useful for comparative purposes is the anonymous *London Practice of Physic*, 6th ed., London: G. & J. Robinson, R. Baldwin, J. Walker, & T. N. Longman, 1797.

81 W. Cullen, Clinical lectures, 1772–1773, pp. 181, 589.

82 There were numerous examples. See case of David MacKenzie, in A. Duncan, Sr., Clinical reports and commentaries, 1795.

83 Case of Fanny Craig, in J. Hope, Cases of patients, 1781; W. Cullen, Clinical lectures, 1772–1773, p. 52.

84 Parr, *London Medical Dictionary*, vol. 1, pp. 552–555; Duncan, *Elements of Therapeutics*, vol. 2, pp. 23–33.

85 Nisbet, *Clinical Guide . . . ; to Which Is Subjoined a Practical Pharmacopoeia*, pp. 76–77.

86 RIE, *Dispensatory*, pp. 340, 353, 357.

87 Cullen, *Materia Medica*, vol. 2, p. 308.

88 Nisbet, *Clinical Guide . . . ; to Which Is Subjoined a Practical Pharmacopoeia*, pp. 70–71.

89 RIE, *Dispensatory*, pp. 340–341, 354.

90 Cullen, *Materia Medica*, vol. 2, pp. 308–312; Parr, *London Medical Dictionary*, vol. 1, p. 634.

91 Cullen, *Materia Medica*, vol. 2, pp. 36–59.

92 *Ibid.*, vol. 2, p. 59.

93 For an account, see F. Guerra, "The introduction of cinchona in the treatment of malaria," parts 1 and 2, *J. Trop. Med. & Hyg.* 80 (1977): 112–118, 135–140.

94 Cullen, *Materia Medica*, vol. 2, pp. 59–77; W. Cullen, Clinical lectures, 1772–1773, p. 36.

95 William Saunders, *Observations on the Superior Efficacy of the Red Peruvian Bark in the Cure of Agues and Other Fevers*, London: J. Johnson, 1782. This publication was

quickly followed by Edward Rigby, *An Essay on the Use of the Red Peruvian Bark in the Cure of Intermittents*, London: J. Johnson, 1783. Other works that reported on the use of both preparations were Ralph Irving, *Experiments on the Red and Quill Peruvian Bark*, Edinburgh: Elliott, 1785; and Thomas Skeete, *Experiments and Observations on Quilled and Red Peruvian Bark*, London: Murray, 1786.

96 Duncan, *Elements of Therapeutics*, vol. 2, pp. 44–53.

97 Cullen, *Materia Medica*, vol. 2, pp. 266–269.

98 *Ibid.*, vol. 2, pp. 275–277.

99 RIE, *Dispensatory*, pp. 340, 342, 344, 354, 357, 360. See also Nisbet, *Clinical Guide . . . ; to Which Is Subjoined a Practical Pharmacopoeia*, pp. 75–76; and D. L. Cowen, "Squill in the 17th and 18th centuries," *Bull. N.Y. Acad. Med.* 50 (1974): 714–722.

100 William Withering, *An Account of the Foxglove and Some of Its Medical Uses*, Birmingham: M. Swinney, 1785.

101 Cullen, *Materia Medica*, vol. 2, p. 375. For more details about the digitalis story, see E. A. Ackerknecht, "Aspects of the history of therapeutics," *Bull. Hist. Med.* 35 (1962): 389–419. Ackerknecht's thesis, that digitalis became a panacea, has been challenged by J. W. Estes in his book *Hall Jackson and the Purple Foxglove: Medical Practice and Research in Revolutionary America, 1760–1820*, Hanover, NH: University Press of New England, 1979, especially chaps. 5–7.

102 The patient with palpitations who was treated with digitalis was Christy Howard, in T. C. Hope, Clinical casebook, 1796–1797. See also D. A. Rytand, "The pulse, digitalis, diuretics, and William Withering," *J. Chron. Dis.* 28 (1975): 1–5.

103 W. Cullen, Clinical lectures, 1772–1773, pp. 485–486. See also his chapter "Sialogoga" in *Materia Medica*, vol. 2, pp. 298–307.

104 Andrew Duncan, *Observations on the Operation and Use of Mercury in the Venereal Disease*, Edinburgh: Kincaid & Creech, 1772, pp. 111–115.

105 *Ibid.*, pp. 128–135, 169–172.

106 *Ibid.*, p. 150.

107 W. Cullen, Clinical lectures, 1772–1773, p. 607; William Nisbet, *First Lines of the Theory and Practice in Venereal Diseases*, Edinburgh: C. Elliot, 1787, p. 414.

108 Nisbet, *First Lines*, pp. 400–420. For a brief historical sketch, see O. Temkin, "Therapeutic trends and the treatment of syphilis before 1900," *Bull. Hist. Med.* 29 (1955): 309–316.

109 Cullen, *First Lines*, vol. 4, pp. 408, 410–411.

110 Cullen, *Materia Medica*, vol. 2, pp. 284–287; Parr, *London Medical Dictionary*, vol. 1, p. 353.

111 See Duncan, *Elements of Therapeutics*, vol. 2, pp. 90–101; and Nisbet, *Clinical Guide . . . ; to Which Is Subjoined a Practical Pharmacopoeia*, pp. 74–75.

112 RIE, *Dispensatory*, p. 341; Nisbet, *Clinical Guide . . . ; to Which Is Subjoined a Practical Pharmacopoeia*, p. 82; Duncan, *Elements of Therapeutics*, vol. 2, pp. 174–183.

113 Cases of Mary Guthrie, in John Gregory, Clinical cases, 1771–1772; and Isabel Waters and Janet Sutherland, in William Cullen, Clinical cases and reports taken at the Royal Infirmary of Edinburgh from Dr. Cullen, taken by Richard W. Hall, Edinburgh, 1772–1773, MSS Collection, National Library of Medicine, Bethesda, MD.

114 Duncan, *Elements of Therapeutics*, vol. 2, pp. 201–210.

115 Cullen, *Materia Medica*, vol. 2, pp. 238–266.

116 Duncan, *Elements of Therapeutics*, vol. 2, pp. 64–71.

117 Cullen, *Materia Medica*, vol. 2, pp. 294–297. Sneezing was regarded as a convenient device for giving the body a number of small shocks, useful in lethargic or paralyzed patients. Simple tobacco snuff was equally effective.

118 Case of Alexander Forbes, in A. Duncan, Sr., Clinical reports and commentaries, 1795. Also see Andrew Duncan, Sr., ed. *The Edinburgh New Dispensatory*, 2nd ed., Edinburgh: C. Elliott, 1789, p. 557.

119 Duncan, *Elements of Therapeutics*, vol. 1, p. 135.

120 W. Cullen, Clinical lectures, Feb.–Apr. 1772, p. 219. See also Cullen's Clinical lectures, 1772–1773, p. 300; and the case of Janet McMillan, in James Gregory, Clinical cases of Dr. Gregory in the Royal Infirmary of Edinburgh, taken by Nathan

Thomas, Edinburgh, 1785–1786, MSS Collection, University of Edinburgh. Cullen was aware that in incurable ailments, palliation acted like a placebo. See his discussion of a terminal case of phthisis in Clinical lectures, 1772–1773, p. 397.

121 Cases of Nelly Henderson, in A. Duncan, Sr., Clinical reports and commentaries, 1795; Thomas Hunt, in T. C. Hope, Clinical casebook, 1796–1797; and Janet Muirhead, in James Gregory, Clinical notes and lectures, Edinburgh, 1779–1780, MSS Collection, RCP, Edinburgh.

122 Cases of Margaret Bain and Elizabeth Clark, in W. Cullen, Clinical cases and reports, 1772–1773.

123 Case of Hugh Carr, in *ibid.*

124 W. Cullen, Clinical lectures, 1772–1773, p. 46; cases of Janet Elder and Margaret Burnet, in A. Duncan, Sr., Clinical reports and commentaries, 1795.

125 For background information see Peter H. Niebyl, "Venesection and the concept of the foreign body: a historical study in the therapeutic consequences of humoral and traumatic concepts of disease," Ph.D. diss., Yale University, 1969.

126 Cullen, *First Lines*, vol. 1, p. 194.

127 W. Cullen, Clinical lectures, 1772–1773, p. 519.

128 William Buchan, *Domestic Medicine, or a Treatise on the Prevention and Cure of Diseases by Regimen and Simple Medicines*, enlarged ed., New York: R. Scott, 1812, pp. 129–130.

129 Unpublished lecture by James Gregory on bloodletting in fevers, quoted in Crumpe, *Inquiry into Opium*, pp. 224–225.

130 See articles on phlebotomy in Parr, *London Medical Dictionary*, vol. 2, pp. 385–391; and George Motherby, *A New Medical Dictionary or General Repository of Physic*, 3rd ed., London: J. Johnson, 1791, p. 591.

131 Benjamin Bell, *A System of Surgery*, 7th ed., 7 vols., Edinburgh: Bell, Bradfute & Dickson, 1801, vol. 3, p. 76.

132 Cases of Richard Aldridge, in James Gregory, Cases of patients, 1781–1782; and Henry Drinkwater, in J. Hope, Cases of patients, 1781.

133 Bell, *System of Surgery*, vol. 3, pp. 78–80.

134 W. Cullen, Clinical lectures, 1772–1773, p. 177. See also case of Janet Williamson, in W. Cullen, Clinical cases and reports, 1772–1773.

135 In a case of pheumonia treated by James Gregory, the progress note read: "Sixteen ounces venesection ordered; blood obtained with much difficulty on two attempts last night but a few ounces in all." Case of Margaret Clatchy, in James Gregory, Clinical reports, 1795–1796; see also case of David Young, in Daniel Rutherford, Clinical cases, Edinburgh, 1799, MSS Collection, RCP, Edinburgh.

136 "When the blood trickles down the arm I have always observed that bleeding is attended with bad consequences. The faster the blood flows from the arm, the greater will be the benefit derived from it." Case of David Cambell, in D. Rutherford, Clinical cases, 1799.

137 Cases of Barbara Stuart and Anne Corbet, in W. Cullen, Clinical cases and reports, 1772–1773; and Agnes Taylor, in James Gregory, Clinical reports, 1795–1796.

138 W. Cullen, Clinical lectures, 1772–1773, p. 556. Also see case of Elizabeth Weir, in W. Cullen, Clinical cases and reports, 1772–1773.

139 Cases of Helen Thykston, in John Gregory, Clinical cases, 1771–1772; and Janet Ross, in James Gregory, Clinical notes and lectures, 1779–1780.

140 Bell, *System of Surgery*, vol. 3, pp. 98–101.

141 Case of Janet Ross, in James Gregory, Cases of patients, 1781–1782.

142 Cases of John Parks and Elizabeth McPherson, in William Cullen, Clinical cases and reports taken at the Royal Infirmary of Edinburgh from Dr. Cullen, taken by Richard W. Hall, Edinburgh, 1773–1774, MSS Collection, National Library of Medicine, Bethesda, MD.

143 Anonymous, "Observations with regard to the siziness of the blood," *Med. Museum* (London) 1 (1763): 153–156.

144 Parr, "Blood," in his *London Medical Dictionary*, vol. 1, pp. 256–260. For details, see William Hey, *Observations on Blood*, London: Wallis, 1779.

145 Case of Elizabeth Small, in W. Cullen, Clinical cases and reports, 1773–1774.
146 Anonymous, "Of bloodletting," *Med. Museum* (London) 3 (1764): 473–474.
147 William Heberden, "Query, read July 21, 1768," *Med. Trans. Royal College of Physicians* (London) 2 (1772): 499–505.
148 W. Cullen, Clinical lectures, 1772–1773, p. 556. Cullen made similar observations in other cases: See his Clinical lectures, Feb.–Apr. 1772, p. 178.
149 One nearly contemporary physician has pointed out that an increased sedimentation rate of red blood cells accompanying inflammatory states and anemia would produce a greater buffy coat over the blood clot. Thus each blood removal would actually accentuate the siziness and set the stage for more withdrawals. See O. H. Perry Pepper, "Benjamin Rush's theories on blood letting after one hundred and fifty years," *Trans. Coll. Phys. of Philadelphia* 14/15 (1946–1947): 121–126.
150 Case of George Kemp, in J. Hope, Cases of patients, 1781.
151 John Sinclair, *Analysis of the Statistical Account of Scotland,* 2 parts, Edinburgh: A. Constable, 1825, reprinted, New York: Johnson Reprint Co., 1970, part 1, p. 136.
152 Bell, *System of Surgery,* vol. 3, p. 119.
153 John Sherven, "Case of the puncture of a nerve in phlebotomy," in *Medical and Philosophical Commentaries,* (by a Society of Physicians in Edinburgh), reprinted, Philadelphia: T. Dobson, 1793–1797, vol. 2 (1793), pp. 391–402. Also see Parr, *London Medical Dictionary,* vol. 1, p. 391.
154 Cases of William Monson and Robert Donaldson, in William Brown, Casebooks, 5 vols., Edinburgh, 1790–1810, MSS Collection, RCS, Edinburgh, vol. 2, pp. 66–67, pp. 76–77.
155 Case of Janet Williamson, in W. Cullen, Clinical cases and reports, 1772–1773.
156 J. Hunter, "Observations on the inflammation of the internal coats of veins," in *Trans. Soc. Improvement Medical and Chirurgical Knowledge* 1 (1793): 18, reprinted in *The Works of John Hunter F.R.S.,* ed. by J. F. Palmer, 4 vols., London: Longman, Rees, Orme, Brown, Green, & Longman, 1837, vol. 3, pp. 584–585.
157 Case of Helen Cowper, admitted in June 1803, in Brown, Casebooks, vol. 2, p. 186.
158 For more details see William Brockbank, "Leeching," in his *Ancient Therapeutic Arts,* London: W. Heinemann, 1954, pp. 87–97; and Audrey Davis and Toby Appel, "Leeching," in their *Bloodletting Instruments in the National Museum of History and Technology,* Washington, D.C.: Smithsonian Institution, 1979, pp. 34–36.
159 Cases of Elizabeth Sutherland and Jane Webster, in W. Cullen, Clinical cases and reports, 1772–1773.
160 Case of Donald McDonald, in Francis Home, Cases of patients under the care of Francis Home, Edinburgh, 1780–1781, MSS Collection, RCP, Edinburgh.
161 Case of James Bain, in James Gregory, Cases of patients, 1781–1782.
162 For details see Audrey Davis and Toby Appel, "Cupping," in their *Bloodletting Instruments,* pp. 17–32; and Samuel Bayfield, *A Treatise on Practical Cupping,* London, 1823.
163 Parr, "Cucurbitula," in his *London Medical Dictionary,* vol. 1, pp. 518–519; Bell, *System of Surgery,* vol. 3, pp. 155–161.
164 W. Cullen, Clinical lectures, 1772–1773, pp. 494–495.
165 Cases of James Bain and Christy Smith, in James Gregory, Cases of patients, 1781–1782.
166 Parr, "Blisters," in his *London Medical Dictionary,* vol. 1, pp. 254–256; Motherby, *New Medical Dictionary,* p. 291. Additional details can be found in Bell, *System of Surgery,* vol. 1, p. 49.
167 John Robertson, *A Practical Treatise on the Powers of Cantharides,* Edinburgh: Mundell, Doig & Stevenson, 1806. See also Cullen, *Materia Medica,* vol. 2, pp. 380–382.
168 W. Cullen, Clinical lectures, 1772–1773, pp. 497, 502.
169 Bell, *System of Surgery,* vol. 7, pp. 363–371.
170 Thomas Fowler, *Medical Reports on the Effects of Bloodletting, Sudorifics, and Blistering in the Cure of the Acute and Chronic Rheumatism,* London: J. Johnson, 1795, p. 241.

171 Cases of Mary Dempster and Janet Anderson, in D. Rutherford, Clinical cases, 1799.

172 Cases of Elizabeth Young and Isabel Waters, in W. Cullen, Clinical cases and reports, 1772–1773.

173 Case of John Thom, in W. Cullen, Clinical cases and reports, 1773–1774; W. Cullen, Clinical lectures, 1772–1773, p. 500.

174 RIE, MB, vol. 4, meeting of Aug. 7, 1769, p. 205.

175 W. Cullen, Clinical lectures, 1772–1773, pp. 49–50.

176 Case of David Monro, in James Gregory, Clinical notes and lectures, 1779–1780.

177 Cases of Elizabeth Miller and Helen Thykston, in John Gregory, Clinical cases, 1771–1772; and Mary Johnston, in J. Hope, Cases of patients, 1781. See also Motherby, *New Medical Dictionary,* p. 579.

178 See, for example, the case of Elizabeth Reilly, in T. C. Hope, Clinical casebook, 1796–1797.

179 Cases of John MacGregor, in A. Duncan, Sr., Clinical reports and commentaries, 1795; and Anne McIntosh, in T. C. Hope, Clinical casebook, 1796–1797. Also see the cases of John Bell and Alexander Leech, in James Gregory, Cases of patients, 1781–1782.

180 Parr, *London Medical Dictionary,* vol. 1, p. 227; W. Cullen, Clinical lectures, 1772–1773, pp. 492–493.

181 Case of Christian Donn, in W. Cullen, Clinical cases and reports, 1772–1773. Also see the cases of Jane Rollo and Barbara Manners, in James Gregory, Clinical reports, 1795–1796.

182 W. Cullen, Clinical lectures, 1772–1773, p. 492.

183 Cases of Isabel MacDonald, in James Gregory, Clinical notes and lectures, 1779–1780; and Janet Frazer, in James Gregory, Clinical reports, 1795–1796. The most influential writer of the period favoring the use of cold water was a student of Cullen: See James Currie, *Medical Reports on the Effects of Water, Cold and Warm, as a Remedy in Fever and Febrile Diseases,* Liverpool: Cadell & Davies, 1797.

184 W. Cullen, Clinical lectures, 1772–1773, p. 164. According to Cullen, total immersion in hot water could not "be administered with any convenience and propriety" in hospitals if the patients were not ambulatory.

185 See cases of William Johnston, in W. Cullen, Clinical cases and reports, 1773–1774; and Janet Williamson, in W. Cullen, Clinical cases and reports, 1772–1773. For Cullen's ideas, see his Clinical lectures, 1772–1773, p. 165.

186 Cases of Neil McCallum, in John Gregory, Clinical cases, 1771–1772; and Isabel Waters and Elizabeth Sutherland, in W. Cullen, Clinical cases and reports, 1772–1773.

187 W. Cullen, Clinical lectures, 1772–1773, p. 473. See also case of Isabel Monro, in John Gregory, Clinical cases, 1771–1772; and Fowler, *Medical Reports,* p. 250.

188 Cases of Robert Bethune, in John Gregory, Clinical cases, 1771–1772; and John Turnbull, in W. Cullen, Clinical cases and reports, 1773–1774.

189 W. Cullen, Clinical lectures, 1772–1773, p. 474. See also case of Janet Grieve, in W. Cullen, Clinical cases and reports, 1772–1773.

190 W. Cullen, Clinical lectures, 1772–1773, p. 473.

191 For an overview see Sidney Licht, "History of electrotherapy," in his *Therapeutic Electricity and Ultraviolet Radiation,* Physical Medicine Library, vol. 4, New Haven, CT: E. Licht, 1967, chap. 1, pp. 1–16.

192 E. Snorrason, *C. G. Kratzenstein and His Studies on Electricity during the Eighteenth Century,* Copenhagen: Odensee University Press, 1974, pp. 27–50.

193 For a discussion of such eighteenth-century theories see R. W. Home, "Electricity and the nervous fluid," *J. Hist. Biol.* 3 (1970): 235–251.

194 Joseph Priestley, "Of medical electricity," in his *History and Present State of Electricity,* 2 vols., 3rd ed., London, 1775, pp. 472–489. More information, with extracts of Priestley's *History,* can be found in J. B. Becket, "Medical electricity," in his *Essay on Electricity,* Bristol: J. B. Becket, 1773, pp. 49–114.

195   See, for example, Francis Lowndes, "Medical electrician," in his *Observations on Medical Electricity*, London: D. Stuart, 1787. Lowndes pioneered a mild form of treatment dubbed "electric vibrations." For one of the more portable machines invented during that period, see *The Description and Use of Nairne's Patent Electrical Machine*, London: Nairne & Blunt, 1783.

196   William Cullen, "On electricity as applied to medicine," in his *Clinical Lectures, 1765 and 1766*, p. 243.

197   RIE, MB, vol. 3, meeting of Apr. 20, 1750, p. 53.

198   Patrick Brydone, "Case of cure of palsy through use of an electrical machine, communicated to Dr. Whytt," in *The Works of Robert Whytt*, Edinburgh: Balfour, 1768, pp. 483–486.

199   James Saunders, "An account of the effects of electricity in different diseases," *Med. & Philos. Commentaries* 2 (1774): 240–251.

200   Parr, *London Medical Dictionary*, vol. 1, pp. 595–596; W. Cullen, Clinical lectures, 1772–1773, pp. 475–479.

201   RIE, MB, vol. 4, meeting of July 1, 1771, p. 248.

202   Anonymous, "Nachrichten über die edinburgischen akadem-medicinischen Anstalten," *Neues Magazin für Aerzte* 3 (1781): part 5, p. 452.

203   Tiberius Cavallo, *An Essay on the Theory and Practice of Medical Electricity*, 2nd ed., London: Dilly, 1781, p. 5.

204   Case of Euphemia McKay, in James Gregory, Clinical cases, 1785–1786.

205   Cases of John Stewart and Janet Christy, in James Gregory, Cases of patients, 1781–1782. See T. Fowler, "A case of an obstinate quartan ague of five months continuance, cured by electricity," *Mem. Med. Soc. London* 3 (1792): 114–122.

206   Cullen, *Clinical Lectures, 1765 and 1766*, p. 247.

207   W. Cullen, Clinical lectures, 1772–1773, p. 479.

208   Case of Grizzle Parker, in D. Rutherford, Clinical cases, 1799.

209   J. Sims, "On the paracentesis," *Mem. Med. Soc. London* 3 (1792): 472–474; J. Andree, "Account of an elastic trochar . . . for tapping the hydrocele . . . abdomen," *London Med. J.* 1 (1781): 418–423.

210   Case of William Rait, in James Gregory, Clinical reports, 1795–1796. See also cases of Margaret Watson, in James Gregory, Clinical cases, 1785–1786; and Archibald Malcolm, in D. Rutherford, Clinical cases, 1799.

211   Sims, "On the paracentesis," p. 476.

212   Cases of Colin Lennox, in John Gregory, Clinical cases, 1771–1772; and Robert Jameson, in W. Cullen, Clinical cases and reports, 1773–1774.

213   W. Cullen, Clinical lectures, 1772–1773, p. 362.

214   Bell, System of Surgery, vol. 4, p. 38.

215   Case of Ann Robinson, in W. Cullen, Clinical cases and reports, 1773–1774.

216   Bell, *System of Surgery*, vol. 4, p. 40.

217   See, for example, the cases of Peggy Thurnburn, in James Gregory, Clinical reports, 1795–1796; and Janet Sinclair, in James Gregory, Clinical notes and lectures, 1779–1780.

218   Cases of Isabel Waters and Jane Smith, in W. Cullen, Clinical cases and reports, 1772–1773; and George Auchinlek, Peter Begbie, and Grizel Cumming, in James Gregory, Clinical notes and lectures, 1779–1780.

219   Cases of Euphemia McKay, in James Gregory, Clinical cases, 1785–1786; Bell Smeeton, in Francis Home, Clinical cases from the Royal infirmary and reports with notes as delivered by Francis Home, by Robert Dunlop, Edinburgh, 1786–1787, MSS Collection, Edinburgh Room, Edinburgh City Library; and John McFarlane, in W. Cullen, Clinical lectures, 1772–1773, p. 267.

220   Bell, *System of Surgery*, vol. 6, pp. 241–245.

221   Case of Isabel Barclay, in W. Cullen, Clinical cases and reports, 1772–1773.

222   Case of Catherine Campbell, in *ibid.*

223   Cases of Isabel Tough and Robert McAlpin, in T. C. Hope, Clinical casebook. 1796–1797; and Robert Jameson, in Cullen, Clinical cases and reports, 1772–1773.

224 Case of Peggy Maitland, in D. Rutherford, Clinical cases, 1799.
225 These activities are summarized in Francis Fuller, *Medicina Gymnastica*, 3rd ed., London: R. Knaplock, 1707. For sailing see Ebenezer Gilchrist, *The Use of Sea Voyages in Medicine*, 2nd ed., London: Millar, Wilson & Durham, 1757. Cullen believed that sailing had favorable effects in the treatment of phthisis, and he quoted Gilchrist's work: Clinical lectures, Feb.–Apr. 1772, pp. 176–177.
226 [John Stedman], *The History and Statutes of the Royal Infirmary of Edinburgh*, Edinburgh: Balfour & Smellie, 1778, p. 79.
227 RIE, MB, vol. 3, meeting of Feb. 5, 1750, p. 39. There is a discussion of lint scrapers in A. E. Clark-Kennedy, *London Pride: The Story of a Voluntary Hospital*, London: Hutchinson Benham, 1979, p. 34.
228 Cases of John Monro, in D. Rutherford, Clinical cases, 1799; Janet Stuart, in W. Cullen, Clinical cases and reports, 1772–1773; and John Bell, in James Gregory, Cases of patients, 1781–1782.
229 Installation of an exercise machine is mentioned in RIE, MB, vol. 3, meeting of Apr. 20, 1750, p. 52. See cases of Jane Fraser and Betty Jameson, in Duncan, Sr., Clinical reports and commentaries, 1795.
230 Case of Janet Anderson, in James Gregory, Clinical notes and lectures, 1779–1780. For more comments see also W. Cullen, Clinical lectures, 1772–1773, p. 321.
231 Cullen, "Therapeutics," p. 27.
232 Samuel Davidson, "Observations on dietetics," in his *History of Medicine*, Newcastle: S. Hodgson, 1791, pp. 103–150; George Pearson, *Arranged Catalogues of the Articles of Food, Drink, Seasoning and Medicine for the Use of Lectures on Therapeutics and Materia Medica*, London, 1801.
233 [Stedman], *History and Statutes*, pp. 77–79.
234 For a comparison of published hospital diets see W. B. Rabenn, "Hospital diets in eighteenth century England," *J. Amer. Dietetic Ass.* 30 (1954): 1216–1221.
235 RIE, *Report of a Committee*, p. 87.
236 RIE, MG, vol. 3, meetings of Oct. 1, 1753, p. 159, and Dec. 6, 1756, p. 267.
237 [Veri Amicus], *A Letter to Dr. John Hope of the Royal Infirmary on the Management of Patients in That Hospital*, Edinburgh, 1782, p. 6. Authorship of this pamphlet has been imputed to John Brown, the creator of a new system of medicine and a disciple of William Cullen.
238 *Ibid.*, p. 7.
239 *Ibid.*, p. 11. Similar criticisms were made by the reformer John Howard, who visited the infirmary on several occasions and noticed "the want of a dietary." John Howard, *An Account of the Principal Lazarettos in Europe*, 2nd ed., London: J. Johnson, C. Dilly, & T. Cadell, 1791, p. 77.
240 W. Cullen, Clinical lectures, 1772–1773, p. 188.
241 [Stedman], *History and Statutes*, p. 77; Marjorie Plant, *The Domestic Life of Scotland in the Eighteenth Century*, Edinburgh: Edinburgh University Press, 1952, p. 98.
242 W. Cullen, Clinical lectures, 1772–1773, pp. 293–294.
243 Cases of Ann Wright and Jean Bain hospitalized in the country ward, probably under the direction of Henry Cullen. See Dr. Cullen's notebook of clinical case histories, Edinburgh, 1784–1785, MSS Collection, University of Edinburgh. For details about sowans see Plant, *Domestic Life*, p. 98.
244 RIE, *Report of a Committee*, pp. 12–13, 67.
245 *Ibid.*, p. 91.
246 *Ibid.*, pp. 63–67.
247 Plant, *Domestic Life*, p. 108.
248 RIE, *Report of a Committee*, pp. 64, 91.
249 Plant, *Domestic Life*, p. 102. In 1781 a supply operation brought ships of the Jamaica fleet – representing about 20,000 men – into the port of Leith: William Creech, *Letters Addressed to Sir John Sinclair . . .* , Edinburgh, 1793, reprinted New York: AMS Press, 1982, p. 29.
250 [Stedman], *History and Statutes*, p. 79. See cases of Margaret Blair, in W. Cullen,

Clinical cases and reports, 1772–1773; Andrew Carmichael, in James Gregory, Clinical notes and lectures, 1779–1780; and David Cunningham, in James Gregory, Cases of patients, 1781–1782.

251 Tea drinking was forbidden in the hospital in spite of the fact that it was popular even among the lower classes. Physicians blamed the tea for weakening the stomach and thus the entire organic system. See the anonymous article "Of diet in general and the bad effects of tea-drinking," *Med. Museum* (London) 2 (1763): 49–57.

252 Rabenn, "Hospital diets," p. 1220; case of Elizabeth Weir, in W. Cullen, Clinical cases and reports, 1772–1773. Complaints about adulterated beer were frequent in hospitals and forced some of them to organize their own breweries. For complaints in Edinburgh see RIE, MB, vol. 4, meeting of Aug. 8, 1775, p. 346.

253 William Sandford, *A Few Practical remarks on the Medicinal Effects of Wine and Spirits,* Worcester: J. Tymbs, 1799, pp. iv–v. Sandford was a surgeon to the Worcester Infirmary.

254 William Cullen, "Wine and alcohol," in his *Materia Medica,* vol. 2, pp. 216–218.

255 Cases of John Davis and Isabel Donaldson, in W. Cullen, Clinical cases and reports, 1773–1774. See also case of John Black, in James Gregory, Cases of patients, 1781–1782.

256 Cases of Isabel MacDonald, in James Gregory, Clinical notes and lectures, 1779–1780; and Elizabeth Fraser, in John Gregory, clinical cases, 1771–1772.

257 Sandford, *Wine and Spirits,* p. v.

258 Case of Andrew Gray, in W. Cullen, Clinical cases and reports, 1773–1774.

259 RIE, MB, vol. 6, meeting of July 5, 1790, p. 56; see also *ibid.,* vol. 6, meeting of Dec. 3, 1792, pp. 161–162.

260 *Ibid.,* vol. 6, meeting of Apr. 13, 1795, p. 223.

261 Some of the background is described in S. E. Williams, "The use of beverage alcohol as medicine, 1790–1860," in *J. Stud. Alcohol* 41 (1980): 543–566.

262 Risse, "Brownian system," pp. 47–51.

263 Sandford, *Wine and Spirits,* pp. 85–86.

264 Cases of Peggy Maitland in D. Rutherford, Clinical cases, 1799; and Robert Hutchinson, in James Gregory, Clinical reports, 1795–1796.

265 [Stedman], *History and Statutes,* p. 86.

266 See cases of John MacGregor and John Mathews in A. Duncan, Sr., Clinical reports and commentaries, 1795. Other cases with similar extensions were those of Thomas Thompson, in T. C. Hope, Clinical casebook, 1796–1797; and Elizabeth Miller, in John Gregory, Clinical cases, 1771–1772.

267 "Whenever the weather and her state of health will permit, we shall dismiss her, for her best chance of recovery is form pure air and free exercise." Case of Mary Lindsey, in A. Duncan, Sr., Clinical reports and commentaries, 1795. Other relevant cases in the same notebook were those of Daniel MacIntosh and Nelly Henderson.

268 For example, see the case described by Cullen in his Clinical lectures, Feb.–Apr. 1772, p. 338.

269 See RIE, MB, vol. 4, meeting of Mar. 14, 1774, pp. 308–309.

270 RIE, *Report of a Committee,* p. 9.

271 W. Cullen, Clinical lectures, 1772–1773, p. 47.

272 [Stedman], *History and Statutes,* p. 86.

273 W. Cullen, Clinical lectures, Feb.–Apr. 1772, p. 128.

274 See the case of Isabel Donaldson, in W. Cullen, Clinical lectures, 1772–1773, p. 50.

275 [Stedman], *History and Statutes,* p. 86. See also the cases of Donald McDonald, in W. Cullen, Clinical cases and reports, 1773–1774; and Margaret Burnet, in A. Duncan, Sr., Clinical reports and commentaries, 1795.

276 Cases of Andrew Gibson and Mary Tennant, in F. Home, Cases of patients, 1780–1781, and in F. Home, Clinical cases, 1786–1787.

277 Case of Henry Drinkwater, in J. Hope, Cases of patients, 1781.

278 [Amicus], *Letter,* p. 15.

279 Anonymous, "Nachrichten," p. 446.

280 Cases of Grizzle Wilson and Peggy Coventry, in D. Rutherford, Clinical cases,

1799. "His paralytic limbs continue nearly in the same state as at admission but he is unwilling to remain any longer in the house." Quoted from case of Robert Grant, in A. Duncan, Sr., Clinical reports and commentaries, 1795. Similar situations occurred in the cases of Nanny Gray, in James Gregory, Clinical cases, 1785–1786; Johanna Drysdale, in D. Rutherford, Clinical cases, 1799; Jean Miller, in James Gregory, Cases of patients, 1781–1782; and Thomas Bell, in J. Hope, Cases of patients, 1781. See also the causes of Charles MacDonald, a five-year-old boy with hydrocephalus, and John Crawford, a paralytic, in A. Duncan, Sr., Clinical reports and commentaries, 1795.

281 Cases of Alex Lawson, in John Gregory, Clinical cases, 1771–1772; Bridget Wilson, in F. Home, Cases of patients, 1780–1781; and Robert Barron, in James Gregory, Clinical reports, 1795–1796. Also see cases of John Robb, in F. Home, Clinical cases, 1786–1787; John Black, in James Gregory, Cases of patients, 1781–1782; and finally James Robertson and A. Bolatis, both sailors in D. Rutherford, Clinical cases, 1799.

282 W. Cullen, Clinical lectures, 1772–1773, p. 32.

283 RIE. *Report of a Committee*, p. 90. In this document the Edinburgh infirmary is listed with a mortality rate of 6.4% whereas the Glasgow Infirmary has 8.% Guy's Hospital in London 9.4%, and the London Hospital 13.3%.

284 W. Cullen, Clinical lectures, 1772–1773, p. 567.

285 John Gregory, *Lectures on the Duties and Qualifications of a Physician*, new ed., London: Strahan & Cadell, 1772, p. 209.

286 Case of James Smyth, in A. Duncan, Sr., Clinical reports and commentaries, 1795.

287 Cases of Joan McDonald, in James Gregory, Clinical notes and lectures, 1779–1780; and Susan Philips, in T. C. Hope, Clinical casebook, 1796–1797.

288 See, for example, the cases of James Louden, in J. Hope, Cases of patients, 1781; and George Blair and Margaret Burton, in W. Cullen, Clinical cases and reports, 1773–1774.

289 Anonymous, *Practice of the British and French Hospitals*.

CHAPTER 5 *Clinical instruction*

1 J. Johnson, *A Guide for Gentlemen Studying Medicine at the University of Edinburgh*, London: Robinson, 1792, p. 45.

2 John Aikin, *Thoughts on Hospitals*, London: J. Johnson, 1771, p. 73; M. Iberti, *Observations Generales sur les Hôpitaux*, Paris, 1788, pp. 12–16. Iberti's work was reviewed in *Medical and Philosophical Commentaries* (by a Society of Physicians in Edinburgh), reprinted, Philadelphia: T. Dobson, 1793–1797, vol. 7 (1794), pp. 263–275.

3 Francis Home, *Clinical experiments, Histories, and Dissections*, 2nd corrected ed., London: Murray; Edinburgh: W. Creech, 1782, p. v.

4 William Cullen, *Clinical Lectures Delivered in the Years 1765 and 1766*, London: Lee & Hurst, 1797, p. 1.

5 Johnson, *Guide*, pp. 45–46.

6 Charles Newman, "Medical education in 1800," in his *Evolution of Medical Education in the Nineteenth Century*, London: Oxford University Press, 1957, pp. 25–33. For recent articles consult A. C. Chitnis, "Medical education in Edinburgh, 1790–1826, and some Victorian social consequences," *Med. Hist.* 17 (1973): 173–185; and W. B. Howie, "Medical education in 18th century hospitals," unpublished paper read before the Scottish Society of the History of Medicine, June 1970.

7 For a general view of medical education see Theodor Puschmann, *History of Medical Education*, trans. and ed. by E. H. Hare, London: H. K. Lewis, 1891, reprinted, New York: Hafner, 1966. The Renaissance experiences in clinical instruction are recounted in C. D. O'Malley, "Medical education during the Renaissance," in *The History of Medical Education*, ed. by O'Malley, Berkeley, CA: University of California Press, 1970, pp. 89–102; and L. Munster, "Die Anfänge eines klinischen Unterrichts an der Universität Padua im 16. Jahrhundert," *Med. Monatsschrift* 23 (1969): 171–174.

8   See G. A. Lindeboom, "Medical education in the Netherlands, 1575–1750," in O'Malley, *Medical Education*, pp. 201–216.

9   G. A. Lindeboom, "Boerhaave as a clinician," in his *Herman Boerhaave: The Man and His Work*, London: Methuen, 1968, chap. 13, pp. 283–292. For a brief overview also consult G. Rath, *Die Entwicklung des klinischen Unterrichts*, Göttinger Universitätsreden no. 47, Göttingen: Vanderhoeck & Ruprecht, 1965.

10 R. Scott, "The battle for students: medical teaching in Edinburgh in the first half of the eighteenth century," in *Edinburgh's Infirmary: A Symposium Arranged under the Auspices of the Scottish Society of the History of Medicine on 27th October, 1979*, Edinburgh: Lammerburn Press, 1979, p. 3.

11 For details see L. M. Zimmerman, "Surgeons and the rise of clinical teaching in England," *Bull. Hist. Med.* 37 (1963): 167–177.

12 See Toby Gelfand, *Professionalizing Modern Medicine: Paris Surgeons and Medical Science and Institutions in the Eighteenth Century*, Westport, CT: Greenwood Press, 1980.

13 A. Logan Turner, *Story of a Great Hospital: The Royal Infirmary of Edinburgh, 1729–1929*, Edinburgh: Oliver & Boyd, 1937, pp. 130–131. The information is based on the early minutes of the hospital.

14 See RIE, MB, vol. 3, meeting of Dec. 6, 1756, p. 267.

15 The minutes of the meetings held by the managers reflect this interest in the revenues obtained from the sale of the tickets. Predictably, the price of the "perpetual" ticket was raised in the 1780s to £10 10s. per student. Turner, *Story*, p. 131.

16 James Gregory, *Additional Memorial to the Managers of the Royal Infirmary*, Edinburgh: Murray & Cochrane, 1803, p. 464.

17 These data were obtained from a study of the Treasurer's Accounts, 1769–1795, 1796–1804, surviving in the MSS Collection, Medical Archives, University of Edinburgh.

18 See RIE, MB, vol. 2, meeting of Feb. 1, 1748, p. 169. There is confusion about the first course, one source indicating that it was taught in the winter of 1746–1747 (*Scots Magazine*) and one claiming the winter of 1747–1748 (letter of a student).

19 Taken from unpublished manuscript of Dr. Rutherford's clinical lectures delivered in 1758, in possession of and quoted by Turner, *Story*, p. 133. For details of Rutherford's teaching consult C. J. Lawrence. "Early Edinburgh medicine: theory and practice," in *The Early Years of the Edinburgh Medical School*, ed. by R. G. W. Anderson and A. D. C. Simpson, Edinburgh: Royal Scottish Museum, 1976, pp. 81–94.

20 Home, *Clinical Experiments*, pp. vi–vii.

21 RIE, MB, vol. 3, meeting of Jan. 1, 1750, p. 38.

22 Gregory, *Additional Memorial*, pp. 430–431.

23 RIE, MB, vol. 3, meeting of Dec. 29, 1755, p. 225.

24 Gregory, *Additional Memorial*, p. 431. See also James Gregory, Clinical lectures on cases (for the year 1785–1786) taken at the clinical ward of the Royal Infirmary, Edinburgh, and treated by James Gregory, M.D., Edinburgh, 1785–1786, MSS Collection, Wellcome Institute for the History of Medicine, London, p. 236.

25 RIE, MB, vol. 3, meeting of Dec. 6, 1756, p. 267.

26 *Ibid.*, vol. 6, meeting of July 5, 1790, p. 56. Since vol. 5 of the MB has been missing since 1800, we cannot follow the gradual expansion of the clinical ward for the period 1776–1788.

27 William Cullen, Clinical lectures, Edinburgh, 1772–1773, MSS Collection, RCP, Edinburgh.

28 See John Thomson, *An Account of the Life, Lectures, and Writings of William Cullen, M.D.*, 2 vols., Edinburgh: W. Blackwood & Sons, 1859, vol. 1, pp. 107–108.

29 James Gregory, *Memorial to the Managers of the Royal Infirmary*, Edinburgh: Murray & Cochrane, 1800, p. 35.

30 Edinburgh College Minutes, 1733–1790, session of the Senatus Academicus, Feb. 1, 1767, MSS, University of Edinburgh, pp. 173–177.

31 These figures were obtained by counting every student officially registered each year in the matriculation records kept in the MSS Collection, University of Edinburgh.

32 Edinburgh College Minutes, 1733–1790, session of the Senatus Academicus, Dec. 8, 1783, pp. 321–324. See Appendix C.
33 RIE, MB, vol. 6, session of Apr. 4, 1791, p. 84. Between 1763 and 1791 student attendance at the infirmary more than tripled, according to William Creech (from 100 to 323 students). See his *Letters Addressed to Sir John Sinclair . . .* Edinburgh, 1793, reprinted, New York: AMS Press, 1982, p. 23.
34 Separate Medical Matriculation records begin with vol. 1 (1783–1790), but no totals are available until 1794 (vol. 2, 1791–1795), MSS Collection, University of Edinburgh. These figures are slightly higher than those obtained from the official matriculation records, presumably because they count some of the students entered in pencil in the latter. The following list, published in the *Annals of Medicine for the Year 1799* 4 (1800): 537, gives the official number of medical students enrolled at the University of Edinburgh in the last decade of the eighteenth century:

1790–1791	510
1791–1792	547
1792–1793	581
1793–1794	527
1794–1795	525
1795–1796	508
1796–1797	577
1797–1798	591
1798–1799	592
1799–1800	634

35 RIE, MB, vol. 3, meetings of Jan. 2 and 3, 1758, p. 300.
36 *Ibid.*, vol. 3, meeting of Dec. 21, 1759, pp. 342–344; *ibid.*, vol. 4, meeting of Jan. 3, 1763, p. 52.
37 See Robert Dutch, ed., "A note on Peter Mark Roget," in *The Original Roget's Thesaurus of English Words and Phrases*, New York: St. Martin's Press, 1979, p. xxi.
38 Gregory, *Additional Memorial*, p. 347.
39 Andrew Duncan, Sr., to J. C. Smyth, May 15, 1802, in *Annals of Medicine* 8 (1803–1804): 462.
40 [John Stedman], *The History and Statutes of the Royal Infirmary of Edinburgh*, Edinburgh: Balfour & Smellie, 1778, pp. 74–75.
41 William Nolan, *An Essay on Humanity, or a View of Abuses in Hospitals*, London: J. Murray, 1786, pp. 36–37.
42 *Ibid.*, p. 38.
43 John Bell, *Answer for the Junior Members of the Royal College of Surgeons of Edinburgh*, Edinburgh: P. Hill, 1800, p. 38.
44 A handwritten notebook that contains a transcription of the documents relating to this dispute has been preserved in the archives of the Royal Medical Society of Edinburgh. The quotation is from the infirmary's missing MB, June 15, 1785, and appears on pp. 1–2 of this document.
45 *Ibid.,*. pp. 2–8.
46 *Ibid.*, p. 12.
47 The pamphlet was titled *A Narrative of Some Late Injurious Proceedings of the Managers of the Royal Infirmary Against the Students of Medicine in the University of Edinburgh*, Edinburgh: 1785. James Gray, in his *History of the Royal Medical Society, 1737–1937*, ed. by D. Guthrie, Edinburgh: University Press, 1952, mentions the existence of this publication (pp. 78–79), but no copies could be found in Edinburgh or anywhere else.
48 "To the learned and respectable Faculty of Medicine in the University of Edinburgh," transcribed in the notebook of the Royal Medical Society, p. 52.
49 "Answer from the professors to the address of the students of medicine," transcribed in the notebook of the Royal Medical Society, p. 61.
50 *Ibid.*, pp. 76–77.
51 *Ibid.*, pp. 89–91.
52 Students were also ordered to keep their hats off in the operating room, "that it may

not obstruct the view of others, and as a mark of respect to the operator." These regulations, dated 1792 and then again 1804, are contained in a pamphlet entitled *History of the Edinburgh Royal Infirmary* in the MSS Collection, University of Edinburgh; the rules for 1792 can also be found in RIE, MB, vol. 6, Oct. 1, 1792, pp. 157–158.

53 Gregory, *Memorial*, p. 60.
54 Letter from the managers of the RIE to the Royal Medical Society, Aug. 18, 1785, in the notebook of the Royal Medical Society, p. 40.
55 *Ibid.*, p. 68.
56 Gregory, *Additional Memorial*, p. 507.
57 Bell, *Answer*, p. 44.
58 Gregory, *Additional Memorial*, p. 427.
59 *Ibid.*, pp. 382–383.
60 *Ibid.*, p. 430.
61 *Ibid.*, p. 479.
62 *Ibid.*, p. 480.
63 *Ibid.*, p. 446.
64 Home, *Clinical Experiments*, p. ix. For more details about medical research in British hospitals of the period see U. Tröhler, "Britische Spitäler und Polikliniken als Heil- und Forschungsstatten, 1720–1820," *Gesnerus* 39 (1982): 115–131.
65 Gregory, *Additional Memorial*, pp. 380–381.
66 *Ibid.*, p. 497. Just as in private practice, patients would thus "not be distressed unnecessarily by knowing what medicines they are getting." Given the limited knowledge of medicine possessed by the sick poor and their widespread apprehensions about the experience of being hospitalized, the opposite argument could also be made.
67 Gregory, *Additional Memorial*, p. 472.
68 These statistics were gathered from a student casebook concerning Gregory's cases, MSS Collection, University of Edinburgh, and the official tabulations obtained from the infirmary Minute Books and patients' registers.
69 W. Cullen, Clinical lectures, 1772–1773, p. 29.
70 Francis Home, Clinical lectures delivered in the year 1769, taken by John Goodsir, Edinburgh, 1769, MSS Collection, RCP, Edinburgh, p. 1. The inaugural lecture was delivered May 15, 1769.
71 Bell, *Answer*, p. 46.
72 Discrepancies detected between admission dates appearing in the General Register of Patients and student casebooks often suggest that patients were transferred to the teaching ward one to three days after their initial admission to the hospital.
73 RIE, *Report of a Committee on the State of the Hospital*, Edinburgh, 1818, p. 68.
74 Gregory, *Additional Memorial*, pp. 476–477.
75 W. Cullen, Clinical lectures, 1772–1773, p. 49.
76 *Ibid.* See other portions of this manuscript.
77 James Gregory, Clinical notes and lectures, Edinburgh, 1779–1780, MSS Collection, RCP, Edinburgh.
78 Andrew Duncan, Sr., Clinical reports and commentaries, Feb.–Apr. 1795, presented by Alexander Blackhall Morison, Edinburgh, 1795, MSS Collection, RCP, Edinburgh. Unfortunately, the student who followed the lectures and clinical cases considered by Duncan left no information about their sequence of presentation, simply arranging them in his notes in accordance with Cullen's nosology. The title of his casebook and the brevity of the commentaries reproduced make it difficult to reach definite conclusions. The impression, however, is that during his tenure Duncan may have attempted to discuss every patient admitted to the teaching ward in an effort to expand the number and variety of cases judged useful for analysis.
79 Anonymous, "Ueber den neuesten Zustand der medicinischen Gelehrsamkeit in Frankreich und England: Auszug aus dem Briefe eines Reisenden an den Herausgeber," *Medicinisches Journal* 6 (1790): part 2, pp. 8–12.
80 W. Cullen, Clinical lectures, 1772–1773, p. 14.

81 *Ibid.*, p. 47.
82 *Ibid.*, p. 294.
83 *Ibid.*, p. 49.
84 Bell, *Answer*, p. 47.
85 Gregory, *Additional Memorial*, p. 478. One such patient, a young male labeled "melancholic," was admitted to Gregory's teaching ward in 1781 complaining of vertigo and stupor and with a history of head injuries during childhood. Nine days later, because there were no apparent physical problems to report and because of a background of previous depressive episodes, the man was transferred to the regular ward. See James Gregory, Cases of patients under the care of James Gregory, M.D., Edinburgh, 1781–1782, MSS Collection, RCP, Edinburgh.
86 James Parkinson, *The Hospital Pupil, or an Essay Intended to Facilitate the Study of Medicine and Surgery*, London: Symonds, 1800, p. 86. See also Home, *Clinical Experiments*, p. vii.
87 Home, *Clinical Experiments*, p. vii.
88 Bell, *Answer*, p. 7.
89 F. Home, Clinical lectures, 1769, p. 2. For a list of the items investigated during the teaching rounds and the organization of the lectures, see Andrew Duncan, Sr., "General view of the business of the Collegium Casuale or Case-Lectures," in his *Heads of Lectures on the Theory and Practice of Medicine*, 4th ed., corrected and enlarged, Edinburgh: C. Elliott, 1789, pp. 295–300.
90 Robert J. Thornton, *Dr. Cullen's Practice of Physic*, London: Lox & Son, 1816, p. 49.
91 F. Home, Clinical lectures, 1769, p. 8.
92 W. Cullen, Clinical lectures, 1772–1773, pp. 5–6.
93 Cullen, "On nosology," introductory lecture reprinted in *The Works of William Cullen, M.D.*, ed. by John Thomson, 2 vols., Edinburgh: Blackwood, 1828, vol. 1, p. 447. Cullen also remarked: "It is often convenient for a man to write a book and for this purpose he often feigns cases altogether, and the few he has observed he has dressed out in his closet with all the art he can." W. Cullen, Clinical lectures, 1772–1773, p. 6.
94 W. Cullen, Clinical lectures, 1772–1773, p. 7.
95 *Ibid.*, p. 7.
96 Home, *Clinical Experiments*, p. 58.
97 W. Cullen, Clinical lectures, 1772–1773, pp. 289–290.
98 *Ibid.*, p. 286.
99 *Ibid.*, pp. 650–651.
100 Gregory, *Additional Memorial*, p. 191.
101 W. Cullen, Clinical lectures, 1772–1773, p. 651.
102 *Ibid.*, p. 629.
103 *Ibid.*, p. 389.
104 William Cullen, Clinical lectures, delivered for John Gregory, Feb.–Apr. 1772, Edinburgh, 1772, MSS Collection, RCP, Edinburgh, p. 209.
105 W. Cullen, Clinical lectures, 1772–1773, p. 339.
106 William Cullen, original manuscript of clinical lecture delivered Apr. 21, 1772, MSS Collection, University of Glasgow. The statement is also quoted in Thomson, *Account*, vol. 1, p. 108.
107 F. Best Fynney, "The history of hydatids discharged with the wine," *Mem. Med. Soc.* (London) 2 (1794): 519.
108 [Stedman], *History and Statutes*, p. 63.
109 Gregory, *Additional Memorial*, pp. 159–160.
110 W. Cullen, Clinical lectures, 1772–1773, p. 578.
111 Gregory, *Additional Memorial*, pp. 270–271.
112 W. Cullen, Clinical lectures, 1772–1773, pp. 67–68; case of William Wilson, in James Gregory, Clinical cases, men's book, Edinburgh, 1785, MSS Collection, RCP, London.
113 RIE, MB, vol. 3, meeting of Feb. 5, 1750, p. 39.
114 Gregory, *Additional Memorial*, pp. 159–160.

115   RIE, MB, vol. 3, meeting of Dec. 21, 1759, pp. 342–344.
116   *Ibid.*, vol. 4, meeting of July 3, 1769, p. 203.
117   *Ibid.*, vol. 6, meeting of Oct. 1, 1792, p. 153.
118   *Ibid.*, vol. 6, meeting of Apr. 7, 1794, p. 197.
119   *Ibid.*, vol. 6, meeting of May 5, 1794, pp. 199–200.
120   James Russell, Surgical cases, 8 vols., Edinburgh, 1784–1792, MSS Collection, RCP, Edinburgh; William Brown, Casebooks, 5 vols., Edinburgh, 1790–1810, MSS Collection, RCS, Edinburgh. Brown's casebooks contain discussions of selected patients, many of them seen at the infirmary.
121   Brown, Casebooks, vol. 1, pp. 23–27, vol. 2, pp. 65–67.
122   The case of Gilbert Anderson, age 43, is contained in John Hope, Cases of patients in the Royal Infirmary under the care of John Hope, M.D., Edinburgh, 1781, MSS Collection, University of Edinburgh.
123   Case of David Rutherford, in John Gregory, Clinical cases of the Royal Infirmary of Edinburgh, Edinburgh, 1771–1772, MSS Collection, Medical Archives, University of Edinburgh.
124   Case of James Murrain, *ibid.*
125   W. Cullen, Clinical lectures, 1772–1773, pp. 397–409.
126   Case of William Simpson, in James Gregory, Clinical notes and lectures, 1779–1780.
127   Cases of Barbara Hope (chronic catarrh), James Gibb (anasarca), and Jane Berkeley (hydrothorax), in A. Duncan, Sr., Clinical reports and commentaries, 1795.
128   *Ibid.*, discussing a patient of William Brown's who died Feb. 14, 1795.
129   In the case of a so-called malignant fever presented by Home, the dissection was described to the students as follows: "Some serum was found in the cavity of the breast. Several livid spots in the intestines, probably the effects of the putrid fever and cause of his looseness. The lungs appeared sound but in the pericardium was contained about eight ounces of water. Here then, there were two different diseases, a malignant fever, and hydrops pericardii at the bitter end." Home never raised the possibility that fever and pericardial effusion could have been related. See F. Home, Clinical lectures, 1769.
130   Gregory, *Additional Memorial*, p. 133.
131   The terms of an eighteenth-century apprenticeship in surgery were described in Henry G. Graham, *The Social Life of Scotland in the Eighteenth Century*, London: A. & C. Black, 1909, p. 474.
132   Benjamin Bell, *The Life, Character and Writings of Benjamin Bell*, Edinburgh: Edmonston & Douglas, 1868, p. 23.
133   This summary of the surgical apprenticeship is contained in Bell, *Answer*, pp. 10–12.
134   RIE, MB, vol. 4, meeting of Oct. 2, 1769, pp. 206–207.
135   See the reprint of this document in Claredon H. Creswell, *The Royal College of Surgeons of Edinburgh*, Edinburgh: Oliver & Boyd, 1926, p. 234.
136   The information was obtained from a pamphlet entitled *At Surgeon's Hall Continues to Be Given, during the Sitting of the Classes of Medicine, a Complete Course of Surgery upon the Plan Which Has Been Followed for Some Years Past, Improved by the Cases Which Daily Occur in Practice*, in possession of the National Library of Scotland. The document is dated Edinburgh, Nov. 1772, and the quotation appears on p. 2.
137   *Ibid.*
138   *Ibid.*
139   Bell, *Answer*, p. 7.
140   "The students of medicine in the University of Edinburgh inform the managers of the Royal Infirmary," dated June 25, 1785, in notebook of the Royal Medical Society, p. 14.
141   *Ibid.*, p. 13.
142   Johnson, *Guide*, p. 44.
143   William Maitland, *The History of Edinburgh*, Edinburgh, 1753, book 7, p. 457.
144   Daniel Defoe, *A Tour through the Island of Great Britain*, 8th ed., London: Strahan, 1778, vol. 4, p. 81.
145   Gregory, *Memorial*, p. 20.

146 *Ibid.*, p. 19.
147 *Ibid.*, p. 22.
148 For details and the citation of the pertinent documents see R. E. Wright-St. Clair, *Doctors Monro: A Medical Saga*, London: Wellcome History of Medicine Library, 1964, chap. 11, pp. 82–86.
149 The history of midwifery education at Edinburgh still needs to be written. The essential names and dates are given in John D. Comrie, *History of Scottish Medicine*, 2nd ed., 2 vols., London: Wellcome History of Medicine Museum, 1932, vol. 1, pp. 299–300, 303–306.
150 RIE, MB, vol. 3, meeting of July 7, 1755, p. 211.
151 *Ibid.*, vol. 3, meeting of Oct. 6, 1755, p. 218.
152 *Ibid.*, vol. 3, meeting of Nov. 4, 1760, p. 365.
153 *Ibid.*, vol. 4, meeting of May 3, 1762, p. 39.
154 *Ibid.*, vol. 4, meeting of Aug. 7, 1764, pp. 80–81.
155 W. Cullen, Clinical lectures, Feb.–Apr. 1772, p. 338: "I received her at the desire of Dr. Young who thought it more convenient for her to die with us than in the lying-in ward."
156 Johnson, *Guide*, p. 29.
157 From the minutes of the Royal Infirmary meetings, Aug. 18, 1785, as transcribed in the previously cited notebook of the Royal Medical Society, p. 47.
158 RIE, MB, vol. 6, meeting of June 7, 1790, p. 52.
159 Gregory, *Additional Memorial*, p. 476: "For many years the managers permitted in the hospital a lying-in ward, but having learned by much experience that this was an improper institution, they very wisely abolished it."
160 RIE, MB, vol. 6, meeting of Nov. 7, 1791, p. 114.
161 *Ibid.*, vol. 6, meeting of Aug. 5, 1793, p. 178.
162 The quotation is from Joseph Warner, a surgeon at Guy's Hospital who wrote an account of his experiences in 1792. See Hector C. Cameron, *Mr. Guy's Hospital, 1726–1948*, London: Longmans, Green, 1954, pp. 92–93. For more details see chap. 2, "The beginnings of medical education in London and at Guy's," pp. 79–95.
163 Joseph Frank, *Reise nach Paris, London, und einem grossen Theile des uebrigen Englands und Schottlands*, 2 vols., Vienna: Camesina, 1804. Remarks about the Edinburgh infirmary are in vol. 2, pp. 226–257.
164 *Ibid.*, vol. 2, p. 227.
165 For an overview see E. Lesky, "Johann Peter Frank als Organisator des medicinischen Unterrichts," *Sudhoffs Archiv*. 39 (1955): 1–29. For further detail see Ramunas A. Kondratas, "Joseph Frank (1771–1842) and the development of clinical medicine," Ph.D. diss., Harvard University, 1977, especially chap. 5, pp. 173–234.
166 Samuel A. A. D. Tissot, *Essai sur les moyens de perfectionner les études de médecine*, Lausanne: Mourer, 1785, p. 114. More information about Tissot's ideas can be obtained from Antoinette S. Emch-Deriaz, "Towards a social conception of health in the second half of the eighteenth century: Tissot (1728–1797) and the new preoccupation with health and wellbeing," Ph.D. diss., University of Rochester, 1983, especially part III, section 2, titled "The hospital: a new conception in the eighteenth century," pp. 269–307.
167 *Ibid.*, p. 151.
168 *Ibid.*, p. 76.
169 *Ibid.*, pp. 118–121.
170 Johann P. Frank, "Von der speciellen Pathologie und Therapie," in his *System einer vollstaendigen medicinischen Polizey*, 6 vols., Vienna: C. Schaumburg, 1817, vol. 6, part 2, p. 262.
171 See Johann P. Frank, *Plan d'école clinique, ou methode d'enseigner la pratique de la médecine dans un hôpital academique*, Vienna: C. F. Wappler, 1790, pp. 18–21.
172 *Ibid.*, pp. 28–29. See also Johann P. Frank, *Ankuendigung des klinischen Instituts zu Goettingen*, Goettingen: J. C. Dieterich, 1784, p. 13.
173 Frank, *System*, vol. 6, part 2, pp. 262–307. See also C. Probst, "Johann Peter Frank als Arzt am Krankenbett," *Sudhoffs Archiv*. 59 (1975): 20–53.
174 For an overview see T. Gelfand, "Demystification and surgical power in the French

Enlightenment," *Bull. Hist. Med.* 57 (1983): 203–217. Gelfand furnishes greater detail in *Professionalizing Modern Medicine*.

175 T. Gelfand, "Gestation of the clinic," *Med. Hist.* 25 (1981): 169–180; Gelfand, "A confrontation over clinical instruction at the Hotel Dieu of Paris during the French Revolution," *J. Hist. Med.* 28 (1973): 268–282; Gelfand, "A clinical ideal: Paris 1789," *Bull. Hist. Med.* 59 (1977): 397–411.

176 The point was made by O. Temkin, "The role of surgery in the rise of modern medical thought," *Bull. Hist. Med.* 25 (1951): 248–259.

177 See Philippe Pinel, *The Clinical Training of Doctors: An Essay of 1793,* ed. and trans. with an introductory essay by Dora B. Weiner, Baltimore: Johns Hopkins University Press, 1980, especially pp. 91–94. A detailed account of the French ideas concerning clinical teaching can be found in Othmar Keel, "Cabanis et la généalogie de la médicine clinique," Ph. D. diss., McGill University, 1977. A summary of Keel's views can be found in a paper titled "The politics of health and the institutionalization of clinical practices in Europe in the second half of the eighteenth century," in *William Hunter and Medicine in the Enlightenment,* ed. by W. Bynum and R. Porter, Cambridge: Cambridge University Press, 1985.

178 C. Webster, "The crisis of the hospitals during the Industrial Revolution," in *Human Implications of Scientific Advance,* ed. by E. G. Forbes (Proceedings of the XVth Internat. Congress of the History of Science, Edinburgh, Aug. 10–15, 1977), Edinburgh: Edinburgh University Press, 1978, pp. 214–223.

179 For more details consult Christopher J. Lawrence, "Medicine as culture: Edinburgh and the Scottish Enlightenment," Ph.D. diss., University College, London, 1984, especially chap. 8 on William Cullen, pp. 312–416.

EPILOGUE

1 For a brief and concise sketch of this development see John H. Knowles, "The hospital," in *Life, Death, and Medicine,* ed. by K. L. White, San Francisco: W. H. Freeman, 1973, pp. 91–100.

2 A typical example was the career of Benjamin Bell, one of the most prominent infirmary surgeons, who was successively appointed dresser, surgical clerk, and attending surgeon. See Benjamin Bell, *The Life, Character and Writings of Benjamin Bell,* Edinburgh: Edmonston & Douglas, 1868.

3 See G. B. Risse, " 'Typhus' fever in eighteenth-century hospitals: new approaches to medical treatment," *Bull. Hist. Med.* 59 (1985): 176–195.

4 The remarks were made as part of a tribute to Benjamin Bell, *Scots Magazine* 63 (1801): 591.

5 Joseph Wilde, *The Hospital: A Poem in Three Books,* Norwich, England: Stevenson, Matchett & Stevenson, 1810, pp. 26–29.

6 James Gregory, Clinical lectures on cases (for the year 1785–1786) taken at the clinical ward of the Royal Infirmary, Edinburgh, and treated by James Gregory, M.D., Edinburgh, 1785–1786, MSS Collection, Wellcome Institute for the History of Medicine, London.

7 For details see Lester S. King, *The Medical World of the Eighteenth Century,* Chicago: University of Chicago Press, 1958; and Guenter B. Risse, "The History of John Brown's Medical System in Germany during the years 1790–1806," Ph.D. diss., University of Chicago, 1971, especially chap. 1.

8 James Gregory, *Memorial to the Managers of the Royal Infirmary,* Edinburgh: Murray & Cochrane, 1800, p. 218.

9 For details see Inci A. Bowman, "William Cullen and the Primacy of the Nervous System," Ph.D. diss., Indiana University, 1975.

10 G. B. Risse, "The Brownian system of medicine: its theoretical and practical implications," *Clio Medica* 5 (1970): 45–51. For an example of Cullen's empirical approach to treatment, see G. B. Risse, " 'Doctor William Cullen, physician, Edinburgh': a consultation practice in the eighteenth century," *Bull. Hist. Med.* 48 (1974): 338–351.

11 D. L. Cowen, "The Edinburgh Pharmacopoeia," *Med. Hist.* 1 (1957): 123–139.
12 Lewis Thomas, "Medical lessons from history," in his *Medusa and the Snail*, New York: Viking Press, 1979, p. 159.
13 For details see A. Berman, "The heroic approach to 19th century therapeutics," *Bull. Amer. Soc. Hosp. Pharm.* 2 (1954): 321–327; and G. B. Risse, "Calomel and the American medical sects during the 19th century," *Mayo Clin. Proc.* 48 (1973): 57–64.
14 William Cullen, Clinical lectures, Edinburgh, 1772–1773, MSS Collection, RCP, Edinburgh, p. 388.
15 Thomas, *Medusa and Snail*, p. 159.
16 See S. Cherry, "The hospitals and population growth: the voluntary general hospitals, mortality and local populations in the English provinces in the eighteenth and nineteenth centuries," 2 parts, *Popul. Stud.* 34 (1980): 59–75, 251–265.
17 L. S. Greenbaum, "Measure of civilization: the hospital thought of Jacques Tenon on the eve of the French Revolution," *Bull. Hist. Med.* 49 (1975): 43–56.
18 L. S. Greenbaum, "Health care and hospital building in eighteenth-century France: reform proposals of Du Pont de Nemours and Condorcet," *Studies on Voltaire* 152 (1976): 895–930.
19 L. S. Greenbaum, "The commercial treaty of humanity: la tournée des hopitaux anglais par Jacques Tenon en 1787," *Rev. d'Histoire des Sciences* 24 (1971): 319–350.
20 John Aikin, *Thoughts on Hospitals*, London: J. Johnson, 1771, p. 41.
21 W. F. Bynum, "Hospital, disease and community: the London Fever Hospital, 1801–1850," in *Healing and History*, ed. by C. E. Rosenberg, New York: Science History Publications, 1979, pp. 97–115.
22 The mortality figures for Amsterdam and Paris were furnished by Thomas Clarke, as cited by John Millar, *Observations on the Management of the Prevailing Diseases in Great Britain*, London: John Millar, 1779, p. 174. Statistics for Manchester and Newcastle were obtained from the annual reports of these hospitals, reproduced in John H. Woodward, *To Do the Sick No Harm: A Study of the British Voluntary Hospital System to 1875*, London: Routledge & Kegan Paul, 1974, app. 5, pp. 160–162.
23 These statistics were usually published in the Dec. issue of the year in question or the following Jan. The last year reported was 1786.
24 Michel Foucault, *The Birth of the Clinic: An Archeology of Medical Perception*, trans. from French by A. M. Sheridan Smith, New York: Vintage Books, 1975. See especially chap. 1, "Spaces and classes," pp. 3–21, and chap. 4, "The old age of the clinic," pp. 54–63. All of Foucault's references to Edinburgh are based on Aikin's *Hospitals*.
25 T. Gelfand, "Gestation of the clinic," *Med. Hist.* 25 (1981): 169–180.
26 Thomas Fowler, *Medical Reports on the Effects of Bloodletting, Sudorifics, and Blistering in the Cure of the Acute and Chronic Rheumatism*, London: J. Johnson, 1795, preface, p. vi. The composition of detailed clinic records on the Continent, specifically in Vienna, Jena, Goettingen, Bamberg, and Wuerzburg, was noted in *Med. & Phys. J.* 1 (1799): 180–181.
27 A successful example of the linkage of clinical appearances with local pathology is the work of James C. Smyth (1741–1821), an Edinburgh graduate shown to have been a precursor of Bichat in the field of histopathology: Othmar Keel, *La Généalogie de l'Histopathologie*, Paris: Vrin, 1979.
28 T. Gelfand, "The Hôspice of the Paris College of Surgery (1774–1793): a unique and invaluable institution," *Bull. Hist. Med.* 47 (1973): 375–393.
29 M. Joerger, "The structure of the hospital system in France in the ancien régime," *Annales E.S.C.* 32 (Sept–Oct. 1977): 1025–1051, trans. in *Medicine and Society in France*, ed. by Robert Foster, Baltimore: Johns Hopkins University Press, 1980, pp. 104–133.
30 For prerevolutionary conditions in Parisian hospitals, see Greenbaum, "Measure of civilization." Efforts to institute reforms are summarized by Greenbaum in "Health care."
31 P. A. Richmond, "The Hôtel-Dieu of Paris on the eve of the Revolution," *J. Hist.*

Med. 16 (1961): 335–353. For further details concerning this hospital see L. S. Green-baum, "Nurses and doctors in conflict: piety and medicine in the Paris Hôtel-Dieu on the eve of the French Revolution," *Clio Medica* 13 (1979): 247–267. Mortality figures for other Parisian hospitals were collected in 1785 in relation to a project to transfer the Hôtel-Dieu to another site and replace it with smaller hospitals: "Ta-bleau de la mortalité des differentes hôpitaux," in M. Foucault et al., *Les Machines à Guerir,* Paris: L'Institut de L'Environment, 1976, pp. 152–156.

32 René T. H. Laennec, *A Treatise on the Diseases of the Chest,* trans. from French by John Forbes, London, 1821, facsimile ed., New York: Hafner, 1962, pp. xxxii–xxxiii.

33 See Ludwig Fleck, "On the question of the foundations of medical knowledge," trans. by T. J. Trenn, *J. Med. & Philos.* 6 (1981): 237–256. For a more extensive view of Fleck's ideas, see his *Genesis and Development of a Scientific Fact,* ed. by T. J. Trenn and R. K. Merton, Chicago: University of Chicago Press, 1979.

34 See T. D. Murphy, "The French medical profession's perception of its social func-tion between 1776 and 1830," *Med. Hist.* 23 (1979): 259–278. This plan of profes-sional advancement was pointed out in Corvisart's work: W. R. Albury, "Heart of darkness: J. N. Corvisart and the medicalization of life," *Historical Reflection* 9 (1982): 17–31.

35 For details about their clinical histories, check James Gregory, Clinical notes and lectures, Edinburgh, 1779–1780, MSS Collection, RCP, Edinburgh. The General Register for the year 1780 lists their names, diagnoses, and dates of admission and discharge.

36 W. Cullen, Clinical lectures, 1772–1773, pp. 542, 266; case of Janet Clark, in An-drew Duncan, Sr., Clinical reports and commentaries, Feb.–Apr. 1795, presented by Alexander Blackhall Morison, 1795, MSS Collection, RCP, Edinburgh.

37 RIE, *Report of a Committee on the State of the Hospital,* Edinburgh, 1818, p. 68.

38 Wilde, *The Hospital,* p. 68.

APPENDIX A *Sources*

1 William Maitland, *The History of Edinburgh,* Edinburgh, 1753, book 7, p. 460.

2 Francis Clifton, *Tabular Observations, Recommended as the Plainest and Surest Way of Practicing and Improving Physick,* London: J Brindley, 1731, p. 17.

3 A. Logan Turner, *Story of a Great Hospital: The Royal Infirmary of Edinburgh, 1729–1929,* Edinburgh: Oliver & Boyd, 1937, p. 133.

4 Daniel Rutherford, Clinical cases, Edinburgh, 1799, MSS Collection, RCP, Edin-burgh.

5 See Appendix C.

6 RIE, MB, vol. 3, meeting of Dec. 29, 1755, p. 225.

7 *Ibid.,* vol. 6, meeting of Oct. 1, 1792, p. 157.

8 James Gregory, *Additional Memorial to the Managers of the Royal Infirmary,* Edinburgh: Murray & Cochrane, 1803, p. 431; see also William Nisbet, *The Clinical Guide, or a Concise View of the Leading Facts on the History, Nature, and Cure of Disease; to Which is Subjoined a Practical Pharmacopoeia,* Edinburgh: J. Watson, 1793, p. 180. By the end of the century casebooks achieved considerable popularity and were even sold by book dealers. Judging from surviving volumes, these notes were carefully bound in leather and placed in physicians' libraries side by side with the printed word.

9 Also consulted but not included in the statistical studies were the following case-books: Clinical cases and reports by Dr. Monro senior, Drs. Cullen and Whyte, Edinburgh, 1763–1765, MSS Collection, RCP, London; James Gregory, Clinical cases and reports, 2 vols., Edinburgh, 1777, MSS Collection, Royal Society of Med-icine, London; Francis Home, Cases in the clinical ward under the care of Dr. Home, Edinburgh, 1780, MSS Collection, Wellcome Institute for the History of Medicine, London; James Gregory, Clinical cases, men's book and women's book, Edinburgh, 1785, MSS Collection, RCP, London; James Gregory, Gregory's cases, women, probably by an anonymous student, Edinburgh, 1789, MSS Collection, Wellcome

Institute for the History of Medicine, London; and James Gregory, Clinical lectures for the History of Medicine, London; and James Gregory, Clinical lectures and cases, 1789–1796, MSS B51, National Library of Medicine, Bethesda, MD.

10 John Gregory, Clinical cases of the Royal Infirmary of Edinburgh, Edinburgh, 1771–1772, MSS Collection, Medical Archives, University of Edinburgh.

11 William Cullen, Clinical cases and reports taken at the Royal Infirmary of Edinburgh from Dr. Cullen, taken by Richard W. Hall, Edinburgh, 1772–1773, MSS Collection, National Library of Medicine, Bethesda, MD.

12 William Cullen, Clinical cases and reports taken at the Royal Infirmary of Edinburgh from Dr. Cullen, taken by Richard W. Hall, Edinburgh, 1773–1774, MSS Collection, National Library of Medicine, Bethesda, MD. The student who copied these cases subsequently became professor of obstetrics at the University of Maryland.

13 James Gregory, Clinical notes and lectures, Edinburgh, 1779–1780, MSS Collection, RCP, Edinburgh.

14 Francis Home, Cases of patients under the care of Francis Home, Edinburgh, 1780–1781, MSS Collection, RCP, Edinburgh.

15 John Hope, Cases of patients in the Royal Infirmary under the care of John Hope, M.D., Edinburgh, 1781, MSS Collection, University of Edinburgh.

16 James Gregory, Cases of patients under the care of James Gregory, M.D., Edinburgh, 1781–1782, MSS Collection, RCP, Edinburgh.

17 James Gregory, Clinical cases of Dr. Gregory in the Royal Infirmary of Edinburgh, taken by Nathan Thomas, Edinburgh, 1785–1786, MSS Collection, University of Edinburgh.

18 Francis Home, Clinical cases from the Royal Infirmary and reports with notes as delivered by Francis Home, by Robert Dunlop, Edinburgh, 1786–1787, MSS Collection, Edinburgh Room, Edinburgh City Library.

19 Andrew Duncan, Sr., Clinical reports and commentaries, Feb.–Apr. 1795, presented by Alexander Blackhall Morison, Edinburgh, 1795, MSS Collection, RCP, Edinburgh.

20 James Gregory, Clinical reports, Nov. 1, 1795– Feb. 1, 1796, Edinburgh, 1795–1796, MSS Collection, University of Edinburgh.

21 Thomas C. Hope, Clinical casebook, Edinburgh, 1796–1797, MSS Collection, RCP, Edinburgh.

22 D. Rutherford, Clinical cases, 1799. Rutherford, a student of William Cullen and Joseph Black, was also quite interested in chemistry.

23 See William Brown, Casebooks, 5 vols., Edinburgh, 1790–1810, MSS Collection, RCS, Edinburgh; and James Russell, Surgical cases, 8 vols., Edinburgh, 1784–1792, MSS Collection, RCP, Edinburgh.

24 This document is erroneously listed as a Ward Journal, 1773–1776, in the MSS Collection, Medical Archives, University of Edinburgh.

25 The Cullen papers at the University of Glasgow contain a few original clinical lectures, including one dated Apr. 21, 1772, that provides an excellent opportunity to check the accuracy of student notes. In the example, Cullen's remarks were faithfully reproduced and most details accurately recorded.

26 William Cullen, Clinical lectures, Edinburgh, 1772–1773, MSS Collection, RCP, Edinburgh. See Appendix C.

27 John Gregory, Clinical lectures, presented by John Abercrombie, 2 vols., Edinburgh, 1771–1772, MSS Collection, RCP, Edinburgh.

28 William Cullen, Clinical lectures, delivered for John Gregory, Feb.–Apr. 1772, Edinburgh, 1772, MSS Collection, RCP, Edinburgh.

29 Francis Home, Clinical lectures delivered in the year 1769, taken by John Goodsir, Edinburgh, 1769, MSS Collection, RCP, Edinburgh.

30 James Gregory, Clinical notes and lectures, 1779–1780.

31 A. Duncan, Sr., Clinical reports and commentaries, 1795. See Appendix C.

32 James Gregory, Lectures on medicine, probably taken by John Goodsir of Anstruther, Edinburgh, 1796–1797, MSS Collection, RCP, Edinburgh.

33 Daniel Rutherford, Clinical lectures by Dr. Daniel Rutherford, M.D., Edinburgh, 1799, MSS Collection, RCP, Edinburgh.

34 Also consulted for this study were the following lecture notes: James Gregory, Clinical lectures and cases, 1789–1786; James Gregory, Clinical lectures by John Henderson, Edinburgh, 1782, MSS Collection, Medical Society of London, now transferred to the Wellcome Institute for the History of Medicine, London; James Gregory, Clinical lectures on cases (for the year 1785–1786) taken at the clinical wards of the Royal Infirmary, Edinburgh, and treated by James Gregory, M.D., of Medicine, London; and Thomas C. Hope, Clinical lectures, Edinburgh, 1797, MSS Collection, Royal Society of Medicine, London.

APPENDIX B *Selected clinical cases*

1 For an expanded explanation of Duncan's treatments see Andrew Duncan, *Observations on the Operation and Use of Mercury in the Venereal Disease*, Edinburgh: Kincaid & Creech, 1772, pp. 107–143.

2 *Ibid.*, p. 150: "To keep the patient upon the verge of a salivation is all that is necessary."

3 See John Rotheram, ed., *The New Edinburgh Dispensatory*, 3rd American from 4th Edinburgh ed. (1794), Boston: Thomas & Andrews, 1796, pp. 410–411; and Andrew Duncan, Sr., ed., *The Edinburgh New Dispensatory*, 2nd ed., Edinburgh: C. Elliot, 1789, pp. 448–449.

4 Rotheram, *New Dispensatory*, pp. 228–229.

5 William Cullen, *A Treatise of the Materia Medica*, 2 vols., Edinburgh: J. Cruikshank & R. Campbell, 1789, vol. 2, pp. 325–332.

6 See Duncan, *Edinburgh Dispensatory*, p. 302.

7 For details about potio cretacea see Rotheram, *New Dispensatory*, pp. 498–499.

8 See discussion of Peggy Maitland in Daniel Rutherford, Clinical cases, Edinburgh, 1799, MSS Collection, RCP, Edinburgh.

9 *Ibid.;* see discussion dated July 19, 1799.

10 Rotheram, *New Dispensatory*, p. 137.

11 Cullen, *Materia Medica*, vol. 2, pp. 251–252.

12 See "The dispensatory for the use of the poor in the Royal Hospital at Edinburgh," in *The Pharmacopoeia of the Royal College of Physicians at Edinburgh*, ed. by William Lewis, London: J. Nourse, 1748, p. 356.

13 *Ibid.*

14 Rotheram, *New Dispensatory*, pp. 95–96.

15 *Ibid.*, p. 147.

16 *Ibid.*, pp. 441–442; Cullen, *Materia Medica*, vol. 2, pp. 256–257.

17 Lewis, *Pharmacopoeia*, pp. 347–348.

18 Duncan, *Edinburgh Dispensatory*, p. 573.

19 *Ibid.*, p. 266

APPENDIX D *Drug usage at the infirmary*

1 Andrew Duncan, Sr., Clinical reports and commentaries, Feb.–Apr. 1795, presented by Alexander Blackhall Morison, Edinburgh, 1795, MSS Collection, RCP, Edinburgh.

2 J. W. Estes, *Hall Jackson and the Purple Foxglove: Medical Practice and Research in Revolutionary America, 1760–1820*, Hanover, NH: University Press of New England, 1979, pp. 141–163.

3 William Withering, *An Account of the Foxglove and Some of Its Medical Uses*, Birmingham: M. Swinney, 1785, p. 8.

4 Estes, *Hall Jackson*, pp. 152, 206, 208.

5 For more far-reaching assessments of this important concept, see C. E. Rosenberg, "The therapeutic revolution: medicine, meaning, and social change in nineteenth-

century America," *Perspect. Biol. Med.* 20 (1977): 485–506; and Rosenberg, "Medical text and social context: explaining William Buchan's Domestic Medicine," *Bull. Hist. Med.* (1983): 22–42.

6   Case of Robert Grant, admitted for paralysis hemiplegica on Mar. 24, 1795, in A. Duncan, Sr., Clinical reports and commentaries, 1795.

7   J. W. Estes, "Therapeutic practice in colonial New England," in *Medicine in Colonial Massachusetts, 1620–1820,* ed. by Philip Cash, Eric H. Christianson, and J. Worth Estes, Boston: Colonial Society of Massachusetts, 1980, pp. 289–383; Estes, "Naval medicine in the age of sail: the voyage of the New York, 1802–1803," *Bull. Hist. Med.* 56 (1982): 238–253.

8   J. W. Estes, "Making therapeutic decisions with protopharmacologic evidence," *Trans. & Stud. Coll. Phys.* (Philadelphia), 5th ser., 1 (1979): 116–137.

9   *Ibid.;* see also Estes, *Hall Jackson,* pp. 111, 124–125.

Index